# CLINICAL LABORATORY MEDICINE

## Application of Laboratory Data

### RICHARD RAVEL, M.D.

Clinical Instructor in Pathology, University of Miami Medical School
Director of Laboratories, St. Francis Hospital, Miami Beach, Florida

SECOND EDITION

## YEAR BOOK MEDICAL PUBLISHERS, INC.

35 EAST WACKER DRIVE · CHICAGO

Reprinted, November 1969

Reprinted, September 1970

Reprinted, February 1972

Second Edition, 1973

Library of Congress Catalog Card Number:   72-95729

0-8151-7095-5

# Preface to Second Edition

It is always flattering to write a new edition. I hope the previous one was useful and that the present edition will be even better. New tests have been introduced, and some existing ones have been given added significance by new techniques or additional experience. As in the previous edition, there is a definite degree of selection in those tests which are included. However, this time there is a chapter entitled "Special Category Tests" containing various procedures which are worth mentioning for some special reason but which seem better left out of the regular text for the sake of continuity and brevity.

Among notable changes, the chapter on thyroid disease has been mostly rewritten, and significant alterations have been made in many other areas. New tests such as fetoprotein, homovanillic acid, lecithin/sphingomyelin ratio, Australia antigen, "corrected" thyroxine-by-isotope, plasma testosterone, and protamine sulfate have been added. Subjects such as lipoprotein phenotyping, rubella serologic methods, and disseminated intravascular coagulation tests have been significantly expanded. Also greatly expanded is a section in the Appendix on drugs which interfere with laboratory tests. These are only a fraction of the additions and alterations.

Richard Ravel

# Preface to First Edition

The clinical laboratory has a major role in modern medicine. A bewildering array of laboratory procedures is available, each of which has its special usefulness and its intrinsic problems, its advantages and its drawbacks. Advances in biochemistry and radio-isotopes, to name only two conspicuous examples, are continually adding new tests or modifying older methods toward new usefulness. It seems strange, therefore, that medical education has too often failed to grant laboratory medicine the same prominence and concern that are allotted to other subjects. If ever a comprehensive, systematic and critical teaching system were needed, it is for this complex and heterogeneous topic. It would seem that if one were to consider ordering any laboratory procedure, several things should be known about that test, including:

1. In what situations is the test diagnostic, and in what situations does the test provide useful information without being diagnostic?

2. What commonly available tests give similar information, and when should one be used in preference to the others?

3. What are the disadvantages of the test and possibilities of error or false results?

The fact that this type of information is not adequately disseminated is quickly brought home to a clinical pathologist, who supervises the clinical laboratory and at the same time acts as liaison to clinicians on laboratory problems. It becomes quickly evident in two ways—the continually rising number of laboratory procedure requests and even a casual inspection of patients' hospital charts. Unnecessary tests represent severe financial and personal inconvenience to the patient; inappropriate tests or tests done under improper conditions mean wasted or misleading information, and often a loss of precious time.

In laboratory medicine, textbooks are available, as in all areas
of general medicine considered detailed enough to warrant a specialty
status. These fall into two groups: those mainly for the technician
and those designed for clinicians. Technician-oriented books necessarily stress the technical aspects of individual tests, with emphasis
on cookbook methodology. Textbooks for the clinician vary considerably in approach. Some excellent works concentrate almost exclusively on one subject or subspecialty, such as hematology. Many
others combine technician methodology with discussion to varying degrees of the clinical aspects of tests. The latter aspect often suf-
fers due to inevitable limitations imposed by mere length. Some
texts which emphasize the clinical approach may be criticized on the
grounds that they neglect either adequate attention to possible limitations and sources of error in each particular laboratory procedure,
or fail to delineate the background or the technical aspects of the
tests enough to provide a clear picture as to just what information
the test actually can provide.

This volume attempts to meet these criticisms. Its aim is to
provide enough technical and clinical information about each laboratory procedure included so as to allow adequate understanding, selection, and interpretation of these procedures. Many of the laboratory
tests require varying amounts of individual discussion. Others are
noted in the context of the diseases in which they may be useful. In
addition, most of the common diseases in which laboratory tests
render significant assistance are briefly outlined, and the role of the
laboratory in each is explained. Also included are a considerable
number of diseases or conditions which are uncommon or even rare,
but which may be considered important from various points of view—
either as well-known entities, diagnostic problems, or cases which
may benefit from early diagnosis and therapy.

There is a great temptation for a work of this type to become
encyclopedic. Brevity and succinctness are preserved, therefore,
at some cost, hopefully with more gain than loss. Probably the most
striking examples are the chapters on infectious diseases and parasitology. In most cases, description of clinical syndromes and
specific organisms has been eliminated or markedly reduced, because this book is not intended to be a treatise on internal medicine.
Emphasis is on material which seems more directly concerned with
selection and interpretation of laboratory tests. Nevertheless, a few
diseases (such as leptospirosis) are important from the standpoint of
laboratory diagnosis because their signs and symptoms mimic other
conditions, so the clinical findings are included in some detail. On
the other hand, syphilis serology has a chapter to itself due to confusion which surrounds the multiplicity of available tests. Likewise,
certain subjects are discussed at unusual length. These are topics
which, in my experience, seem to be common problem areas. The
aim is to provide a reasonably thorough, yet compact, survey of
laboratory medicine. This book is meant to provide some area of

assistance to anyone who is engaged in clinical medicine, and to provide, in a sense, a reasonably comprehensive course in clinical pathology.

It is anticipated that the style and format of this book may be criticized; either because the uninitiated reader might gain an impression that laboratory medicine can be reduced to a relatively few rules or protocols, or that one approach to diagnosis is presented as though all others were invalid. Such inferences are not intended.

It should be obvious that no person could write a book covering clinical pathology entirely from his own experience. On the other hand, adequate citation of references would be a tremendous undertaking in itself. A compromise is therefore offered. At the ends of the chapters there are lists of suggested readings, composed of selected references which include textbooks with general or specific coverage, papers on certain specific subjects, and occasionally an article selected because of an unusually inclusive bibliography. Due to space considerations, those references with more than two authors have been listed in the first author's name only. This book is only a beginning; the reader is urged to consult these papers and others on individual subjects in order to broaden the information presented here, and to evaluate contrasting points of view.

An Appendix is provided, in order to include certain information which is useful but which seemed better presented separately from the regular text. Much of this is in tabular form.

I wish to express my deep appreciation to the following members of the University of Miami Medical School faculty, and to several others, who critically reviewed portions of the manuscript and made many valuable suggestions:

J. Walter Beck, Ph.D., Associate Professor of Pathology, Department of Parasitology.

George W. Douglas, Jr., M.D., Chief, Microbiology Section, Communicable Disease Center, U.S. Public Health Service.

N. Joel Ehrenkranz, M.D., Professor of Medicine, Division of Infectious Diseases.

Mary J. Harbour, M.D., Instructor, Department of Radiology.

Martin H. Kalser, M.D., Ph.D., Professor of Medicine, Division of Gastroenterology.

Robert B. Katims, M.D., Assistant Professor of Medicine, Department of Endocrinology.

Howard E. Lessner, M.D., Associate Professor of Medicine, Division of Hematology.

Joel B. Mann, M.D., Assistant Professor of Medicine, Division of Renal Disease and Endocrinology.

Leslie C. Norins, M.D., Chief, Venereal Disease Research Laboratory, Communicable Disease Center, U.S. Public Health Service.

William L. Nyhan, M.D., Ph.D., Professor of Pediatrics.

John A. Stewart, M.D., Assistant Chief, Virology Section, Com-
    municable Disease Center, U.S. Public Health Service.
Thomas B. Turner, M.D., Director, John Elliot Blood Bank, Miami,
    Fla.

                                                    Richard Ravel

# Table of Contents

# CHAPTER 1

# Basic Hematologic Tests and Classification of Anemia

Hematology is the study of the blood, the cellular elements of the blood, and the metabolic processes by which the blood components are formed. The major emphasis in hematology is given to the three cellular elements of the blood—red cells, white cells, and platelets—the plasma proteins, electrolytes, fluid, and other constituents being covered elsewhere in this book. Each of the three cellular elements will be discussed separately for reasons of convenience.

There are several tests which form the backbone of laboratory diagnosis in hematology.

## 1. Hemoglobin (Hb)

This is the oxygen-carrying compound contained in red cells. Hemoglobin can be measured chemically, and the amount of hemoglobin per 100 ml. of blood can be used as an index of the oxygen-carrying capacity of the blood. Total blood Hb depends mostly on the number of RBC (the Hb carriers) but also (to a much lesser extent) on the amount of Hb in each RBC. A low hemoglobin level thus indicates anemia. Depending on the method used and the care with which the laboratory checks its spectrophotometers, hemoglobin values are accurate to 2-3%. Older methods (Sahli) used a chemical technique in which the final compound was compared visually against a colored glass standard; at best, this gives 2-3 times the average error of methods using a good spectrophotometer. Normal values are 12-17 Gm. per 100 ml. (grams per 100 ml. is often abbreviated Gm. %) for males and 11-15 Gm. per 100 ml. for females (p. 439).

11

## 2. RBC Count

The number of RBC per cubic millimeter gives an indirect estimate of the hemoglobin content of the blood. Blood cell counting chamber (hemocytometer) methods give average errors of 4-8%, or even more—depending on the experience of the technician. New machine counting techniques (Coulter Counter) reduce this error to about 2-4%. However, most smaller laboratories do not yet have these machines. Normal values are 4.5-6.0 million/cu. mm. for males and 4.0-5.5 million/cu. mm. for females.

## 3. Hematocrit (HCT)

After centrifugation, the height of the red cell column is measured and compared with the height of the original whole blood. The percentage of red cell mass to original blood volume is the hematocrit. Anticoagulated whole blood is centrifuged in a special tube. Since whole blood is made up essentially of RBC and plasma, after centrifugation the percentage of packed red cells gives an indirect estimate of the number of RBC per 100 ml. of whole blood (and thus, in turn, is an indirect estimate of the amount of hemoglobin). Hematocrit thus depends mostly on the number of RBC, but there is some effect (to a much lesser extent) from the average size of the RBC. Normal values are 40-54% for males and 37-47% for females. The hematocrit is usually about three times the hemoglobin value (assuming no marked hypochromia). The average error in hematocrit procedures is about 1-2%. Microhematocrits are generally as accurate as the older standard Wintrobe (macrohematocrit) technique.

## 4. Indices (Wintrobe Indices)

Wintrobe introduced a very useful method to demonstrate certain characteristics of red cells.

a) Mean Corpuscular Volume (MCV): This concept utilizes the effect that the average size of the RBC has on the hematocrit. If the average RBC size is increased, the same number of RBC will have a slightly larger cell mass and thus a slightly increased hematocrit reading, whereas the opposite happens if the average RBC size is smaller than normal. The MCV is therefore calculated from the hematocrit and RBC count as follows:

$$\frac{HCT \times 10}{*RBC\ Count} = MCV \quad \text{(HCT in \%; RBC in millions/cu. mm.*;}$$
$$\text{MCV in cubic microns } [cu.\mu])$$

Normal values are $87 \pm 5$ cu.$\mu$ (manual) and $90 \pm 10$ cu.$\mu$ (Coulter Counter).

b) Mean Corpuscular Hemoglobin (MCH): This concept gives an estimate of the amount of hemoglobin in the average red cell; this

*Use the number of millions rather than the actual count; e. g., 4,560,000 = 4.56 millions.

is done by comparing the blood hemoglobin level to the RBC count as follows:

$$\frac{Hb \times 10}{*RBC\ Count} = MCH$$   (Hb in Gm./100 ml.; RBC in millions/cu. mm.*; MCH in micro-micrograms [$\mu\mu$g.])

Normal values are $29 \pm 2\mu\mu$ (manual) and $30 \pm 4\mu\mu$ (Coulter Counter).

c)  Mean Corpuscular Hemoglobin Concentration (MCHC): This concept estimates the average concentration of hemoglobin in the average RBC.  It differs from MCH in that the average RBC concentration of hemoglobin depends on red cell size as well as on the actual amount of hemoglobin contained in the RBC.  MCHC is calculated as follows:

$$\frac{Hb \times 100}{HCT} = MCHC$$   (Hb in Gm./100 ml.; HCT in %; MCHC in %)

Normal values are $34 \pm 2\%$ (manual) and $34 \pm 3\%$ (Coulter Counter).

There are several factors which should be mentioned.  First, as an index of red cell hemoglobin, the MCHC is often more reliable than the MCH, since the MCHC does not incorporate the relatively inaccurate RBC count procedures.  It is true that macrocytic or microcytic (larger or smaller than normal) RBC will alter the MCHC independently of the hemoglobin values.  However, in those diseases where there is significant over-all macrocytosis or microcytosis, the red cell counts of the blood are changed (decreased) in addition to the changes in average red cell size.  Since hematocrit depends on the number of RBC even more than on the average RBC size, the decrease in RBC number more than compensates for the relatively small effects that RBC size have on the hematocrit.  Therefore, in most clinical situations, alterations in average RBC size alone do not affect the MCHC significantly.  Secondly, the various indices are affected only by average cell measurements, either of size or quantity of hemoglobin.  This is especially noticeable in the indices dependent on average RBC size (MCV and, to some extent, MCHC).  There may be considerable variation in size between individual red cells (anisocytosis), but the indices do not show this, since they take into account only the average size.  Third, examination of a well-made peripheral blood smear will give most of the same information as the indices.  Indices are not a substitute for examination of the peripheral blood smear, but may be helpful in confirming equivocal cases.  The indices are only as accurate as the various counts and procedures (plus calculation) that went into their preparation.

5.  Examination of Wright-Stained Peripheral Blood Smear

This procedure gives a vast amount of information.  It allows visual estimation of the amount of hemoglobin in RBC and the over-

*See footnote, p. 12.

all size of RBC. In addition, alterations in size, shape, and structure of individual red cells or white cells are visible which may have
diagnostic significance in certain diseases. Pathologic early forms
of the blood cells are also visible. Finally, a good estimate of the
platelet count can be made in most cases from the peripheral smear
alone.

The peripheral smear is the most useful laboratory procedure
in hematology. There obviously are many limitations; for example,
a peripheral smear cannot demonstrate the presence of anemia per
se, which must be detected by means of either the Hb, HCT, or
RBC count. Also, many etiologies of anemia show peripheral blood
changes which are nonspecific. In some cases where the peripheral
smear is highly suggestive, it may not be so in early stages of the
disease. Even if characteristic cell changes are present, there may
be different underlying causes for the same particular morphologic
type of anemia, different causes which call for different treatment.
Finally, there are some conditions which produce anemia without
any demonstrable morphologic changes in the peripheral smear.
The same comments about RBC may, in general, also be applied to
the white cells of the peripheral smear. However, it is often possible to predict greatly increased WBC number by comparison with
the normal over-all visual ratio of WBC to RBC. A differential
count of the various WBC forms is done from the peripheral smear.

6. Reticulocyte Count

Reticulocytes occupy an intermediate position between nucleated RBC in the bone marrow and mature (non-nucleated fully hemo-
globinated) RBC. After the normoblast (metarubricyte) nucleus is
extruded from the cell, some remnants of nuclear material remain
for a short time. It is possible to stain this material using vital
staining techniques and dyes such as methylene blue or cresyl blue.
The material then is seen microscopically in the form of dark blue
dots arranged in loose aggregates or reticulum. The reticulocyte
count is an index of the production of mature red cells by the blood-
forming organs, mostly the bone marrow. Increased reticulocyte
counts mean an increased number of RBC being put out into the
peripheral blood in response to some stimulus. In exceptionally
great reticulocyte responses, there may even be nucleated RBC
pushed out into the peripheral blood due to massive red cell production activity of the bone marrow. Except in a very few diseases
such as erythroblastosis, the number of peripheral blood nucleated
RBC is usually small in the few situations when they do appear.
Reticulocytes are not yet completely mature RBC, so that when
reticulocytes appear in the peripheral blood they may be slightly
larger than normal RBC. This may give a slightly macrocytic MCV
and show macrocytes on peripheral smear. Also, reticulocytes
may sometimes have a slightly bluish (basophilic) tinge with Wright's
stain (although this often does not occur); this phenomenon is called

polychromatophilia, and results from the fact that the reticulocyte is not yet a mature RBC, and therefore does not have a full complement of (reddish-staining) hemoglobin.

### 7. WBC Count

This may be done using either a hemocytometer or machine (such as the Coulter Counter). The error produced by hemocytometer counts is about 4-8%, but may be higher with inexperienced personnel. Coulter counts have approximately 2-4% error. The machine has the disadvantage that WBC counts over 100,000/cu. mm. become increasingly inaccurate unless a dilution is used. Also, some of the abnormal lymphocytes of lymphocytic leukemia are unusually fragile and may be destroyed when the specimen is prepared for a machine count, thus giving a falsely somewhat lower value. With either hemocytometer or machine, nucleated RBC are counted as WBC, so a correction has to be made on the basis of the percentage of nucleated RBC (to 100 WBC) found on the peripheral smear.

### 8. Platelet Count

This is done using a hemocytometer counting chamber. The usual procedure using a standard microscope has approximately a 10-20% error. A somewhat similar method that makes use of a phase contrast microscope has a reported error of about 8%. Normal values are 150,000-300,000/cu. mm. for direct counts.

### 9. Bone Marrow Aspiration

Bone marrow aspiration is of help in several situations: (1) to demonstrate the diagnosis of megaloblastic anemia; (2) to establish the diagnosis of leukemia or multiple myeloma; (3) to show whether deficiency of one or more of the peripheral blood cellular elements is due to a deficiency in the bone marrow precursors (bone marrow hypoplasia); (4) to document a deficiency in body iron stores in certain cases of suspected iron-deficiency anemia; (5) in certain selected cases, to demonstrate metastatic neoplasm or some types of infectious disease (culture or histologic sections may be preferred to routine Wright-stained smears).

These nine procedures are the basic tests of hematology. Intelligent selection and interpretation of these procedures usually can go far toward solving the vast majority of hematologic problems. Other tests may be ordered to confirm or rule out a diagnosis suggested by the results of preliminary study. These other tests will be discussed in association with the diseases in which they are useful.

However, once again, certain points should be made. Laboratory tests in hematology are no different from any other laboratory tests. Two or more tests should not be ordered which give essentially the same information in any particular situation. For example, it is rarely necessary to order Hb, HCT, and RBC count all together unless indices are needed. As a matter of fact, either the Hb or the HCT is usually sufficient alone, although, initially, the two are often ordered together as a check on each other (being the least accurate, the RBC count is rarely helpful). The WBC count and differential are usually both done initially. If both are normal, there usually is no need to repeat the differential count if the (total) WBC count remains normal and there are no morphologic abnormalities of the RBC and WBC.

Another point to be stressed is the proper collection of specimens. The timing of collection is sometimes extremely important. Transfusion therapy may cause a megaloblastic bone marrow to lose its diagnostic megaloblastic features, sometimes in as little as 12 hours. On the other hand, transfusion will not affect a bone marrow which has no iron. Capillary blood (finger puncture) is best for making peripheral blood smears, because oxalate anticoagulant causes marked artifacts in WBC morphology and even will slightly alter the RBC. EDTA anticoagulant will cause a false decrease in hematocrit (Hb is not affected) if the amount of blood collected is less than half the proper volume (for the amount of EDTA in the tube). When capillary (fingerstick) blood is used to make HCT, Hb, or cell counts, too much squeezing of the finger or other poor technique may result in dilution of the blood by tissue juice and give falsely low values. On the other hand, dehydration may result in hemoconcentration and produce falsely high values. This may mask an anemia actually present, or when the patient is properly hydrated, a repeat determination may give the false impression of a sudden drop in values, such as might otherwise come from an acute bleeding episode. If very severe, hemoconcentration may simulate polycythemia.

## ANEMIA—CLASSIFICATION

Although anemia may be defined as a decrease in hemoglobin concentration, it may result from a pathologic decrease in the red cell count. Since mature RBC are fully saturated with hemoglobin, such a decrease means that total blood hemoglobin will also be affected. Anemia is a symptom of some underlying disease, and is not a diagnosis. There always is a cause, and most of the causes may be discovered by a relatively few simple procedures. The greatest help in finding the underlying disease responsible comes from knowing the common causes of anemia, getting a good history, doing a thorough physical examination, and ordering a logical sequence of laboratory tests based on what the situation and other findings suggest.

Classification of anemia is helpful because it provides a handy reference for differential diagnosis. There are several possible classifications; each is helpful in some respects.

Anemia may be classified according to pathogenesis. Using this concept, three mechanisms may be responsible:

1. Deficiency of Vital Hematopoietic Raw Material—"Factor Deficiency Anemia." The most common causes of deficiency anemia are iron deficiency and deficiency of vitamin $B_{12}$ and/or folic acid.

2. Failure of the Blood-Forming Organs to Produce or to Deliver Mature RBC to the Peripheral Blood—"Production-Defect Anemia." This may be due to: (a) replacement of marrow by fibrosis or by neoplasm (primary or metastatic); (b) hypoplasia of the bone marrow, most commonly produced by certain chemicals; or (c) toxic suppression of marrow production or delivery without actual marrow hypoplasia, found to variable extent in some patients with certain systemic diseases. The most common of these are severe infection, chronic renal disease, widespread malignancy (without extensive marrow replacement), rheumatoid-collagen diseases, and hypothyroidism (these conditions may sometimes be associated with an element of hemolytic anemia).

3. RBC Loss from the Peripheral Blood—"Depletion Anemia." This is commonly due to: (a) hemorrhage, acute or chronic (causing escape of red cells from the vascular system); (b) hemolytic anemia (RBC destroyed or RBC survival shortened within the vascular system); or (c) hypersplenism (splenic sequestration).

A second classification is based on a morphologic approach. Using the appearance of the red cells on a peripheral blood smear and/or Wintrobe indices, anemias may be characterized as microcytic, normocytic, or macrocytic. They may be further subdivided according to the average amount of RBC hemoglobin, resulting in hypochromia or normochromia (macrocytic RBC may appear hyperchromic on peripheral smear, but this is an artifact due to an enlarged and therefore thicker cell which, being thicker, does not transmit light through the central portion as it would normally).

I. Microcytic
   A. Hypochromic
      (1) Chronic iron deficiency (most frequent cause)
      (2) Thalassemia
      (3) Occasionally in certain chronic systemic diseases
   B. Normochromic
      Very uncommon; may be simulated by spherocytosis; present to mild degree in some cases of infection
II. Normocytic
   A. Hypochromic
      (1) Some cases of anemia due to systemic diseases
      (2) Many cases of lead poisoning
   B. Normochromic
      (1) Acute blood loss
      (2) Hemolytic anemia
      (3) Bone marrow replacement or hypoplasia

    (4)  Hypersplenism
    (5)  Many cases of anemia due to systemic diseases
    (6)  Some cases of lead poisoning

III.  Macrocytic
    A.  Hypochromic
       Some cases of macrocytic anemia with superimposed iron
       deficiency
    B.  Normochromic
       (1)  Pernicious anemia
       (2)  Malabsorption (vitamin $B_{12}$ and/or folic acid)
       (3)  Folic acid deficiency
       (4)  Reticulocytosis
       (5)  Some cases of chronic liver disease and hypothyroidism
       (6)  Some cases of aplastic anemia

The more common causes of anemia will be discussed in greater detail in the following chapters.  Only the more common hematologic diseases will be covered.  No attempt will be made to list every known entity or every disease which either produces or is associated with anemia.  For a more complete coverage, several excellent textbooks on hematology are available.

## REFERENCES

Bishop, C. , and Surgenor, D. M. (eds.):  The Red Blood Cell (New
    York: Academic Press, Inc. , 1964).
Diggs, L. W. , et al.:  The Morphology of Blood Cells (North Chicago,
    Ill.:  Abbott Laboratories, 1954).
Dutcher, T. F.:  Erythrocyte indices and corpuscular constants re-
    visited, Lab. Med. 2:32, 1971.
Harris, J. W. , and Kellermeyer, R. W.:  The Red Cell (2d ed. ;
    Cambridge, Mass.:  Harvard University Press, 1970).
Hillman, R. S. , and Finch, C. A.:  The misused reticulocyte,
    Brit. J. Haemat. 17:313, 1969.
Jacobson, L. O. , and Doyle, M. (eds.):  Erythropoiesis (New York:
    Grune & Stratton, Inc. , 1962).
Miale, J. B.:  Laboratory Medicine—Hematology (4th ed.; St. Louis:
    The C. V. Mosby Company, 1972).
Perrotta, A. L. , et al.:  The polychromatophilic erythrocyte, Am.
    J. Clin. Path. 57:471, 1972.
Sandoz Atlas of Haematology (2d ed. ; Basel, Switzerland:  Sandoz
    Ltd. , 1952).
Smith, C. H.:  Blood Diseases of Infancy and Childhood (2d ed. ; St.
    Louis:  The C. V. Mosby Company, 1966).
Sunderman, F. W. , and Boerner, F. (eds.):  Normal Values in
    Clinical Medicine (Philadelphia: W. B. Saunders Company, 1949).

Wheby, M. S. :  Using a clinical laboratory in the diagnosis of anemia, M. Clin. North America 50:1689, 1966.

Whitfield, C. L. : The patient with anemia: Diagnosis, The New Physician 16:184, 1967.

Williams, W. J. , et al. :  Hematology (New York:  McGraw-Hill Book Co. Inc. , 1972).

Wintrobe, M. M. :  Clinical Hematology (6th ed. ; Philadelphia:  Lea & Febiger, 1967).

# CHAPTER 2

# Factor Deficiency Anemia

## I. IRON

Iron is utilized from the diet in the ferrous form, absorbed mostly in the upper and middle small intestine, and coupled to a protein known as transferrin after a series of complicated physiologic reactions. The bone marrow RBC precursors utilize part of the iron; some of the excess is stored by bone marrow reticulum cells in the form of hemosiderin. This creates a storehouse of available iron in cases of deficiency. Deficiency may be created in two ways: a chronic deficiency in dietary or available iron, or a loss of blood hemoglobin of such magnitude that normal amounts of dietary iron are not sufficient for replacement.

Acute blood loss can usually be handled without difficulty, if the bleeding episode is not too prolonged and if tissue iron stores are adequate. The anemia which develops from acute bleeding is normocytic and normochromic, and is not the type characteristic of chronic iron deficiency. Changes in hematocrit are discussed elsewhere (p. 111). Chronic bleeding, however, is often sufficient to exhaust body iron stores from continued attempts by the bone marrow to restore the blood hemoglobin level. If this occurs, a hypochromic-microcytic type of anemia eventually develops. Chronic bleeding may be in the form of slow tiny daily loss, intermittent losses of small to moderate size not evident clinically, or repeated more widely spaced larger bleeding episodes. Chronic iron deficiency may develop with normal diet, but naturally is hastened if the diet is itself borderline or deficient in iron.

In adults, anemia due to pure dietary iron deficiency is extremely uncommon. Most of these cases are due to such malabsorption diseases as sprue, which, strictly speaking, is not a dietary problem. A more common etiology is from iron deficiency of pregnancy, brought on by a combination of iron utilization by the fetus superimposed on previous iron deficiency due to excessive menstrual bleeding or multiple pregnancies.

By far the most common cause of chronic iron deficiency in adolescents or adults is excessive blood loss. In males, this is usually from the gastrointestinal tract. In females, it may be either GI or vaginal bleeding. Therefore in females, a careful inquiry about the frequency, duration, and quantity of menstrual bleeding is essential. An estimate of quantity may be made from the number of menstrual pads used. In males and females below age 40, peptic ulcer is probably the most frequent GI etiology. After age 40, GI carcinoma should always be ruled out. Hemorrhoids are sometimes the cause of chronic iron deficiency anemia; but, since hemorrhoids are very common, it should never be assumed, without further investigation, that the anemia is due only to hemorrhoids.

If excessive vaginal bleeding is suspected, a careful vaginal examination with a Papanicolaou (Pap) smear should be done. If necessary, a gynecologist should be consulted. For possible GI bleeding, a stool for occult blood should be ordered on at least three separate days. However, one or more negative stool guaiacs do not rule out GI cancer or peptic ulcer, since these lesions may bleed intermittently. If a patient is over age 40 and stool guaiacs are negative, it would probably be the best thing to do a sigmoidoscopy and a barium enema. If the barium enema is negative and no other cause for the iron-deficiency anemia can be demonstrated, it would be wise to repeat the barium enema in 3-4 months, in case a lesion was missed. The lower GI tract studies are particularly stressed as important for detection of carcinoma because gastric carcinoma has a very poor cure rate by the time it becomes demonstrable, whereas colon carcinoma has an excellent cure rate if discovered in the early stages. The detection of peptic ulcer and the differential diagnosis of gastrointestinal lesions by selection of appropriate laboratory tests is discussed in more detail in Chapter 26 (Gastrointestinal Function). In addition to peptic ulcer, gastric hiatus hernia is sometimes associated with iron deficiency anemia.

In infancy, there is a different situation. The infant grows rapidly and must make hemoglobin to keep up with his expanding blood volume. The demands of rapid growth may lead to iron depletion at age 6 months to 2 years because the majority of the infant's iron comes from the hemoglobin he possessed at birth. Premature infants are therefore more likely to develop iron deficiency because their hemoglobin volume at birth was less. Since milk contains relatively small amounts of iron, infants on prolonged milk diets are more likely to develop iron deficiency.

Under the experimental situation of a normal adult on a normal diet made iron-deficient by repeated phlebotomy, it takes about 3 months before significant anemia (hemoglobin more than 2 Gm. per 100 ml. below normal) appears. The first laboratory indication

of iron deficiency is a bone marrow showing absent marrow iron.
The next test to become abnormal is the serum iron level. When
anemia becomes manifest, it is moderately hypochromic but only
slightly microcytic; marked hypochromia and microcytosis are relatively late manifestations of iron lack. When treated, these tests
return to normal in the reverse order. It takes several months before bone marrow iron appears again, despite adequate therapy.

    The reticulocyte count is normal in uncomplicated chronic
iron-deficiency anemia. Superimposed acute blood loss or other
factors such as adequate iron in the hospital diet may cause reticulocytosis. For a short time following recent (acute) hemorrhage, the
Wintrobe MCV may be normal or even increased due to the reticulocytosis. The reticulocyte response to iron therapy (3-7%) is somewhat less than that seen with treatment of megaloblastic anemia.

    Serum iron (SI) levels are decreased in iron-deficiency ane-
mia. Normal values vary according to the method used, but less
than 50 $\mu$g./100 ml. is usually considered low. The plasma total
iron-binding capacity (TIBC) is increased. Since both the serum
iron and the plasma iron-binding capacity have fairly wide normal
ranges, a simultaneous plasma iron and TIBC is more helpful than
the SI alone, when the serum iron level is not markedly decreased.
Normally, the TIBC is about one third saturated. It will be much
less saturated in chronic iron-deficiency anemia (p. 442).

    The peripheral blood smear in severe cases shows marked
hypochromia and microcytosis and, in addition, considerable anisocytosis and poikilocytosis. This means that not all the RBC are
microcytes. The microcytes of iron deficiency have to be differentiated from spherocytes; this is usually not difficult, since in
chronic iron deficiency even the microcytes have hypochromia.
Bone marrow aspiration shows mild erythroid hyperplasia and absent marrow iron.

## II.   VITAMIN B$_{12}$

    Vitamin B$_{12}$ is absorbed in the ileum with the aid of "intrinsic
factor" produced by the gastric glands of the stomach. Vitamin B$_{12}$
deficiency may be due to three causes: (1) dietary lack, which is
rarely sufficient by itself to cause anemia, (2) deficiency of intrinsic
factor, leading to pernicious anemia, and (3) malabsorption syndromes involving the ileum mucosa or B$_{12}$ handling by the ileum.
There may be associated folic acid deficiency.

    Deficiency of either vitamin B$_{12}$ or folic acid eventually leads
to development of megaloblastic anemia. The red cell precursors
in the marrow become slightly enlarged and develop a peculiar
sieve-like appearance of the nuclear chromatin called megaloblastic
change. This affects all stages of the red cell precursors. The
bone marrow typically shows considerable erythroid hyperplasia as
well as megaloblastic change. Not only are the red cells affected

but also WBC and platelets.  In far-advanced megaloblastic anemia there is a peripheral blood leukopenia and thrombocytopenia in addition to anemia; in early cases there may be anemia only.  The bone marrow shows abnormally large metamyelocytes and band neutrophils.  A macrocytosis is usually present in the peripheral blood, along with considerable anisocytosis and poikilocytosis.  Hypersegmented polymorphonuclear neutrophils are characteristically found in the peripheral blood, although their number may be few or the degree of hypersegmentation may be difficult to separate from normal variation.

The diagnosis of megaloblastic anemia is made from bone marrow aspiration.  This should be done as soon as possible and definitely before transfusion, since the characteristic megaloblastic changes can quickly disappear even though the anemia is not affected by such a small amount of $B_{12}$ or folic acid.  The diagnosis of pernicious anemia is made by gastric aspiration and the Schilling test with and without intrinsic factor, as described in Chapter 25 (p. 299). The classic Schilling test response in pernicious anemia is low absorption ("positive test") without intrinsic factor and normal absorption with added intrinsic factor, while primary small bowel disease produces impaired $B_{12}$ absorption with and without intrinsic factor. However, some cases of pernicious anemia are reported to display Schilling test response typical of primary small bowel malabsorption; after treatment with parenteral $B_{12}$, the Schilling test results then became typical of pernicious anemia.  A bone marrow should be the first procedure done in cases of macrocytic anemia because not all cases of megaloblastic anemia have positive Schilling test results (without intrinsic factor).

Treatment with intrinsic factor plus $B_{12}$ evokes a reticulocyte response of 5-15%.  The same thing will occur after a Schilling test, due to the nonisotopic $B_{12}$ given parenterally.


## III.   FOLIC ACID

The main causes of folic acid deficiency are:  (1) dietary deficiency (most common cause), (2) primary small intestine malabsorption syndrome, (3) pregnancy, and (4) anticonvulsant drugs.

Folic acid deficiency causes a megaloblastic anemia which may be indistinguishable from pernicious anemia in every laboratory respect (except the behavior of the Schilling test with and without intrinsic factor).  It may also be indistinguishable clinically, except that neurologic symptoms do not occur from folic acid deficiency.  Folic acid therapy will improve most of the hematologic abnormalities of pernicious anemia, even though the pernicious anemia defect is vitamin $B_{12}$ and not folic acid, but folic acid therapy alone can make pernicious anemia neurologic damage worse.  Therefore, it is necessary to differentiate $B_{12}$ and folic acid problems.

Malabsorption syndromes associated with folic acid deficiency are most often due to primary small bowel disease. These are discussed in Chapter 25. A small but significant percentage of pregnant women develop folic acid deficiency, although by far the most common cause of deficiency anemia in pregnancy is iron deficiency. Folic acid deficiency in pregnancy may be due to dietary defect plus fetal demands; sometimes no good explanation is possible. One clue may be a report that oral contraceptive pills can be associated with folic acid and vitamin B6 deficiency. Dietary defect occasionally causes megaloblastic anemia in nonpregnant adult females or in adult males. This is most common in chronic alcoholics with liver disease. Certain anticonvulsant drugs, especially Dilantin and Mysoline, can on occasion produce a macrocytic megaloblastic anemia which responds best to folic acid. A considerable number of patients taking these drugs have macrocytosis without anemia. The actual percentage of those developing anemia is extremely small. It should be noted that megaloblastic anemia due to pregnancy, diet, or anticonvulsant drugs shows normal Schilling test results.

The "Therapeutic Trial."—In deficiency diseases, treatment with the specific agent which is lacking will give a characteristic response in certain laboratory tests. This response may be used as a confirmation of the original diagnosis. Failure to obtain the expected response means either that doubt is cast on the original diagnosis, that treatment has been inadequate either in dosage, absorption, utilization, or the type of agent used, or that some other condition is present which is interfering with treatment or possibly is superimposed on the more obvious deficiency problem. The two usual deficiency diseases are chronic iron deficiency and vitamin B12 or folic acid deficiency. When a test agent such as iron is given in therapeutic dose, a reticulocyte response should be manifest in 3-7 days, with values at least twice normal (or significantly elevated over baseline values if the baseline is already elevated). Usually, the reticulocyte count is normal or only slightly elevated in uncomplicated hematologic deficiency diseases. If the baseline reticulocyte values are already significantly elevated over normal range in a suspected deficiency disease, this suggests either previous treatment (or, in some cases, a response to hospital diet), wrong diagnosis, or some other superimposed factor (such as recent acute blood loss superimposed on chronic iron deficiency anemia). If the baseline values are already over twice normal, it may not be possible to document a response. Once the correct replacement substance is given in adequate dosage, hemoglobin values generally rise toward normal at a rate of approximately 1 gram per 100 ml. per week.

Two major cautions must be made regarding the "Therapeutic Trial": (1) it never takes the place of a careful systematic search for the etiology of a suspected deficiency state and (2) the patient may respond to one agent and at the same time have another factor deficiency or more serious underlying disease.

A "Therapeutic Trial" usually is initiated using therapeutic doses of the test agent. This standard procedure will not differentiate vitamin $B_{12}$ from folic acid deficiency, since therapeutic doses of either will invoke a reticulocyte response in deficiency due to the other. If a therapeutic trial is desired in these circumstances, a small physiologic dose should be used—such as 1 microgram of vitamin $B_{12}$ per day for 10 days, or 100 micrograms of folic acid per day for 10 days. At least 10 days should elapse between completion of one trial agent and beginning of another. Also, the patient should be on a diet which is deficient in folic acid or $B_{12}$, and baseline reticulocyte studies should be performed for a week on this diet before initiation of the actual trial. Generally, in vitamin $B_{12}$ deficiency, the Schilling test (without intrinsic factor) gives the same information, and can be repeated with the addition of intrinsic factor to pinpoint the etiology. In folic acid deficiency, a therapeutic trial may be helpful in establishing the diagnosis. The main drawback of the "Therapeutic Trial" in diagnosis is the time involved.

Other methods for diagnosis of $B_{12}$ and folic acid deficiency include serum assay of these substances. Serum folic acid determination is still done by a bacterial assay technique, so it is available only in larger hospitals or reference laboratories. Serum should be frozen immediately and sent to the laboratory in dry ice. Antibiotic therapy will interfere with any microbiological assay method, so that therapy must cease for a full week before such tests are carried out. Vitamin $B_{12}$ determination can now be done by radioimmunoassay and should be more readily available. Blood can be drawn with crossmatch specimens before transfusion, the serum frozen, and these tests (as well as others) done later if needed.

## REFERENCES

Alparin, J. B., et al.: Studies of folic acid requirements in megaloblastic anemia of pregnancy, Arch. Int. Med. 117:681, 1966.

Beutler, E., et al.: A comparison of the plasma iron, iron-binding capacity, sternal marrow iron and other methods in the clinical evaluation of iron stores, Ann. Int. Med. 48:60, 1958.

Briggs, M., and Staniford, M.: Oral contraceptives and blood-iron, Lancet 2:742, 1969.

Brown, E. B.: Clinical aspects of iron metabolism, Seminars Hemat. 3:314, 1966.

Carmel, R., and Herbert, V.: Correctable intestinal defect of vitamin $B_{12}$ absorption in pernicious anemia, Ann. Int. Med. 67:1201, 1967.

Chanarin, I.: The Megaloblastic Anaemias (Oxford, England: Blackwell Scientific Publications, 1969).

Conrad, M. E., and Crosby, W. H.: The natural history of iron
  deficiency induced by phlebotomy, Blood 20:173, 1962.
Corcino, J. J., et al.: Absorption and malabsorption of vitamin $B_{12}$,
  Am. J. Med. 48:562, 1970.
Crosby, W. H.: Mucosal block: An evaluation of concepts relating
  to control of iron absorption, Seminars Hemat. 3:299, 1966.
DeLeeuw, N. K. M., et al.: Iron deficiency and hydremia in normal
  pregnancy, Medicine 45:291, 1966.
Drapanas, T., et al.: Role of the ileum in the absorption of vitamin
  $B_{12}$ and intrinsic factor (NF), J.A.M.A. 184:337, 1963.
Editorial: Pyridoxine-responsive anemia, J.A.M.A. 180:684, 1962.
Editorial: Achlorhydria and anaemia, Lancet 2:27, 1960.
Eichner, E. R., and Hillman, R. S.: The evolution of anemia in
  alcoholic patients, Am. J. Med. 50:218, 1971.
Emerson, P. M., and Wilkinson, J. H.: Lactate dehydrogenase in
  the diagnosis and assessment of response to treatment of megalo-
  blastic anemia, Brit. J. Haemat. 12:678, 1966.
Erlandson, M. E.: Iron metabolism and iron deficiency anemia,
  Pediat. Clin. North America 9:673, 1962.
Fudenberg, H., and Estren, S.: Non-addisonian megaloblastic ane-
  mia, Am. J. Med. 25:198, 1958.
Harris, J. W., and Kellermeyer, R. W.: The Red Cell (2d ed.;
  Cambridge, Mass.: Harvard University Press, 1970).
Hawkins, C. F., and Meynell, M. J.: Macrocytosis and macro-
  cytic anemia caused by anticonvulsant drugs, Quart. J. Med.
  27:45, 1958.
Layrisse, M., et al.: Megaloblastic anemia of pregnancy: Charac-
  teristics of pure megaloblastic anemia and megaloblastic anemia
  associated with iron deficiency, Blood 15:724, 1960.
Lindenbaum, J.: Folic acid deficiency in sickle cell anemia, New
  England J. Med. 269:875, 1963.
Luhby, A. L., and Cooperman, J. M.: Folic Acid Deficiency in
  Man and Its Interrelationship with Vitamin $B_{12}$ Metabolism, in
  Levine, R., and Luft, R. (eds.): Advances in Metabolic Dis-
  orders (New York: Academic Press, Inc., 1964), Vol. I, p. 263.
Pollycove, M.: Iron metabolism and kinetics, Seminars Hemat.
  3:235, 1966.
Pritchard, J. A.: Hemoglobin regeneration in severe iron-deficien-
  cy anemia, J.A.M.A. 195:717, 1966.
Spector, I., and Hutter, A. M., Jr.: Folic acid deficiency in neo-
  plastic disease, Am. J. M. Sc. 252:419, 1966.
Spurling, C. L., et al.: Juvenile pernicious anemia, New England
  J. Med. 271:995, 1964.
Waxman, S., et al.: Drugs, toxins and dietary amino acids affecting
  vitamin $B_{12}$ or folic acid absorption or utilization, Am. J. Med.
  48:599, 1970.

Weir, D. R., et al.: Serum proteins and blood vitamins in anemia
of the chronically ill—Possible role of protein undernutrition, J.
Chron. Dis. 22:407, 1969.
Wenk, R. E.: Significance of Iron Measurements, Postgrad. Med.
45:59, 1969.
Zimmerman, H. J., et al.: Serum enzymes in disease. II. Lactic
dehydrogenase and glutamic oxaloacetic transaminase in anemia,
A. M. A. Arch. Int. Med. 102:115, 1958.

# CHAPTER 3

# Production-Defect Anemia

Anemia due to inadequate erythropoiesis without factor deficiency may be classified in several ways. One system is based on the mechanism involved; either marrow failure to incorporate adequate supplies of hematopoietic raw materials (such as iron) into red cell precursors, failure to release mature red cells from the marrow, or destruction of red cell precursors in the marrow. From a clinical point of view, it is easier to divide production-defect anemias into two categories—those due to a hypoplastic bone marrow, and those with normally cellular marrow which are associated with certain systemic diseases.

## I. HYPOPLASTIC MARROW

Conditions which produce a hypoplastic marrow affect the bone marrow directly, either by actual replacement or by toxic depression of red cell precursors. Bone marrow examination is the main diagnostic or confirmatory test.

1. Replacement of Marrow by Fibrosis: This condition is commonly termed myelofibrosis, is usually idiopathic, and leads to a clinical syndrome called myeloid metaplasia. The peripheral blood picture is similar in many ways to that of chronic myelogenous leukemia. Many include this condition in the group of "myeloproliferative syndromes," and a more complete discussion is given in Chapter 6.

2. Replacement of Marrow by Neoplasm: The types of tumors most commonly metastatic to bone marrow, the laboratory abnormalities produced and the main hematologic findings are covered in Chapter 32. The anemia of neoplasia is usually normocytic and normochromic. Iron-deficiency anemia secondary to hemorrhage may be present if the tumor has invaded or originated from the gastro-

intestinal tract. Besides extensive marrow replacement ("mye-lophthisic anemia"), neoplasia may produce anemia with minimal bone involvement or even without any marrow metastases; in these patients, there seems to be some sort of toxic influence on the mar-row production and release mechanism. In occasional cases of widespread neoplasm, a hemolytic component (shortened RBC life span) has been demonstrated.

Multiple myeloma is a neoplasm which is difficult to separate from the group of leukemias on one hand and the category of malig-nant lymphomas on the other. Myeloma initially or eventually in-volves the bone marrow and produces anemia of moderate degree which is normocytic and normochromic. The diagnosis of multiple myeloma is covered in Chapters 21 and 32. Despite proliferation of plasma cells in the bone marrow, appearance of more than an oc-casional plasma cell in the peripheral blood is very uncommon. Peripheral blood RBC often display the phenomenon of rouleau for-mation, a piling up of red cells like a stack of coins. This is not specific for myeloma, and is most often associated with hyper-globulinemia.

3. Aplastic Anemia: Patients with this disease develop se-vere anemia, often progressive and fatal, and bone marrow aspira-tion reveals hypoplasia or aplasia of red cell precursors. WBC and/or platelets may also be involved. In 50% or more of the pa-tients, the reason for bone marrow changes is unknown. In the re-mainder, the most common known etiologies are destruction by toxins and idiosyncratic reactions. Of course, the two terms are related, but one group of cases is caused by exposure to chemicals or toxins which affect everyone, whereas another group develops marrow aplasia as an idiosyncratic reaction to a drug or chemical which does not have this effect on most other people. The exact cause of aplastic anemia cannot be found in at least 50% of cases.

The most common known causes in the general toxin group are chemicals such as benzene; also excessive x-ray and radioactive compound exposure. This group causes pancytopenia (anemia, leukopenia, and thrombocytopenia) and is most often fatal, although occasionally persons do recover. Leukemia is an occasional late development if the patient survives long enough.

A great variety of drugs and chemicals have been reported to cause idiosyncratic reactions. The effects range from pancytopenia to any combination of single or multiple blood element defect. Bone marrow aspiration usually shows a deficiency in the particular cell precursor involved, although, especially with megakaryocytes, this is not always true. These patients most often recover if they can be supported long enough, although a considerable number die from superimposed infection.

The drugs most often implicated are:

Pancytopenia—Chloramphenicol (Chloromycetin), Mesantoin, gold preparations, nitrogen mustard compounds, Myleran and other antileukemic drugs.

Leukopenia—Chlorpromazine (Thorazine), promazine (Sparine),
          Butazolidin, thiouracil, antileukemic drugs.
Thrombocytopenia—Quinidine, Furadantin, ristocetin (Spontin).

The anemia produced in those people who do have anemia is of the normocytic-normochromic type. Reticulocyte counts are usually low (although they sometimes might be slightly elevated if the patient is in a recovery phase). About one third of aplastic anemia patients have a macrocytic peripheral blood smear.

As noted, bone marrow aspiration is usually essential for diagnosis, and can be used to follow any response to therapy. However, there are problems not always taken into account. A false impression of marrow hypocellularity may be produced by hemodilution of the marrow specimen, by aspiration at a place which has unusually large amounts of fatty tissue, and by poor slide preparation technique. Occasional completely "dry" puncture is not uncommon in normal persons, due to considerable variability in the bone marrow distribution. Therefore, the diagnosis should never be made on the basis of a single failure to obtain marrow. Also, a bone marrow section—or at least a clot section (processed like an ordinary histologic specimen)—is more reliable than a smear for estimating cellularity. This is especially true for megakaryocytes. On the other hand, a smear is definitely more valuable for demonstrating abnormal morphology. Both can usually be done at the same time.

## II. SYSTEMIC DISEASE

1. Renal Disease: Anemia of moderate degree is frequently found in association with uremia. Some investigators claim it is almost always present when the BUN is persistently over twice normal, and often appears before this level. Patients with prolonged but potentially reversible azotemia (such as acute renal failure) often develop anemia until the kidneys recover. Transient types of azotemia usually do not produce anemia unless azotemia is prolonged or unless due to the underlying cause itself. The anemia of actual renal insufficiency develops regardless of the cause of the uremia.

The peripheral blood RBC are usually normocytic and normochromic; there is often mild-to-moderate anisocytosis. There sometimes may be mild hypochromia, and occasionally some degree of microcytosis. In some cases "burr" cells are found; these are triangular shrunken RBC with irregular pointed projections from the surface.

Bone marrow usually shows normal cellularity, although some cases have mild RBC hypoplasia. Marrow iron is adequate. Serum iron is usually normal, but about 20-30% of patients have low serum iron even though they do not have iron deficiency. Reticulocyte counts are usually normal; occasionally, they may be slightly elevated.

The pathophysiology involved is not well understood. The primary known abnormality is a lack of incorporation of iron into RBC within the bone marrow. There is depression both of hemoglobin synthesis and of formation and release of mature RBC into the peripheral blood. In 10-15% of patients there is also decreased RBC survival in the peripheral blood, although the hemolytic aspect is usually not severe. In the late stages of uremia there may be a bleeding tendency due to coagulation defects, most commonly thrombocytopenia. Platelet function may be abnormal even with normal numbers of platelets. The effect of hemorrhage, if it occurs, is separate and additional to the anemia of chronic renal disease.

2. <u>Anemia of Neoplasia</u>: This was mentioned earlier (p. 28), and is discussed also in Chapter 32. This anemia is usually normocytic-normochromic with normal reticulocyte counts, unless there is hemorrhage or chronic blood loss. A hemolytic component is present in a considerable minority of patients, but hemolysis is generally mild and is not detectable except with radioisotope red cell survival procedures. Occasionally, hemolysis may be severe, especially with chronic lymphocytic leukemia and malignant lymphomas. Thrombocytopenia may be found in certain types of leukemia and in myelophthisic anemias. Fibrinolysins may appear in occasional cases of widespread malignancy, most often prostate carcinoma.

3. <u>Anemia of Infection</u>: Mild-to-moderate anemia is frequently seen in association with subacute or chronic infection. The mechanism of this anemia is not well understood, but there seems to be a decreased rate of erythropoiesis, coupled in some patients with slightly shortened RBC survival and failure to utilize iron normally. The anemia of infection does not usually develop unless the infection lasts a month or more, although occasionally anemia may develop rapidly in severe acute infection such as septicemia. Also, chronic infection generally is of at least moderate severity. Such situations include bronchiectasis, salpingitis, abscess of visceral organs or body cavities, or severe pyelonephritis. Anemia is a common finding in subacute bacterial endocarditis and in the granulomatous diseases such as tuberculosis or sarcoidosis. The anemia is usually normocytic and normochromic, but sometimes is hypochromic. Reticulocyte counts are usually normal, although occasionally they may be slightly increased. Bone marrow aspiration shows either normal marrow or hyperplasia of the granulocytes. Serum iron is usually low or low normal, and plasma total iron-binding capacity is reduced (in iron-deficiency anemia the TIBC is elevated).

4. <u>Rheumatoid-Collagen Disease Group</u>: This frequently is associated with mild-to-moderate normocytic-normochromic anemia. Again, reticulocytes are usually normal and the bone marrow is unremarkable. Apparently there is decreased erythropoiesis with

a slightly shortened RBC survival, but there is disagreement about the factor of RBC survival.

5. Chronic Liver Disease: The type and frequency of anemia in liver disease vary with the type and severity of hepatic dysfunction, but has been reported in up to 75% of patients. It is most frequently seen in far-advanced cirrhosis. Extensive metastatic carcinoma of the liver may produce the same effect, although it is difficult to say whether the liver involvement or the neoplasm itself is the real cause. About one third to one half of those with anemia have a macrocytosis; about one third are normocytic. Some have a hypochromia due to gastrointestinal blood loss. Target cells in varying numbers are a fairly frequent finding on peripheral blood smear.

Macrocytic anemia in liver disease is most often found in severe chronic liver damage; such anemia is not usually caused by acute liver disease, even when severe, or by chronic disease of only slight or mild extent. A small but significant percentage of hepatic macrocytic anemias are megaloblastic, usually secondary to folic acid dietary deficiency, although most are not megaloblastic and will not be corrected by folic acid treatment. A macrocytic peripheral blood smear may be present even when there is a normal Hb or HCT, and sometimes even with a normal MCV.

Gastrointestinal bleeding occurs in a considerable number of cirrhotic patients; often it is very slight and very intermittent. Esophageal varices are present in some; other lesions may be demonstrated in other patients, but in a considerable proportion of cases the source of the bleeding cannot be located.

Anemia and other cytopenias, especially thrombocytopenia, may be occasionally produced by the effects of liver disease on the spleen. Hypersplenism occurs in some of the patients with portal vein hypertension and its resulting splenic congestion (see p. 49). In severe chronic (or massive acute) liver disease, coagulation problems may occur due to insufficient hepatic synthesis of several blood coagulation factors.

Some liver-diseased patients have shortened RBC survival demonstrated only by using radioactive isotope studies, without evidence of gastrointestinal bleeding. There is no clinical or laboratory evidence of hemolysis otherwise. Zieve's syndrome is a rare combination of hyperlipemia, cirrhosis, and hemolytic anemia. This hemolytic anemia has reticulocytosis and the other classic findings of hemolysis.

Unless blood loss is a factor, and excluding those cases of megaloblastic anemia, the bone marrow is unremarkable in liver disease, and reticulocytes are usually close to normal. Not all cases of anemia in liver disease can be explained.

6. Hypothyroidism: Anemia is found in 30-60% of cases. About one third of the anemic patients have a macrocytic type, most of the remainder being either normocytic-normochromic or normocytic-hypochromic.

The normocytic-hypochromic type responds to a combination of iron and thyroid hormone preparation. The iron deficiency component is frequently produced by excessive menstrual bleeding; in patients without demonstrable blood loss there is speculation that decreased intestinal iron absorption may occur, since thyroid hormone is known to increase intestinal carbohydrate absorption. Most of the macrocytic cases respond only to thyroid hormone. Occasional macrocytic cases respond to $B_{12}$ and are presumably secondary to decreased intestinal absorption; most do not. The bone marrow is not megaloblastic (except in the few $B_{12}$ deficiency cases), and is sometimes slightly hypocellular. Reticulocytes are usually normal. Isotope studies reportedly show normal survival time in most cases. Lack of thyroid hormone seems to have a direct effect on erythropoiesis, since thyroid extract therapy cures both the myxedema and the anemia (unless there is superimposed iron deficiency).

To conclude this discussion, it should be noted that the normocytic-normochromic anemia of systemic diseases has often been called "simple chronic anemia"—although the pathophysiology is apparently far from simple. The disease categories listed are only the most common. In many cases, the diagnosis is one of exclusion; the patient has anemia for which no definite etiology can be found, so whatever systemic disease he has is blamed for the anemia. In these patients, it is important to rule out treatable serious diseases; this especially is true for hypochromic anemias (where blood loss might be occurring) and macrocytic anemias (which may be due to $B_{12}$ or folic acid deficiency). A normocytic-normochromic picture may be due to an occult underlying disease such as malignant lymphoma or multiple myeloma.

## REFERENCES

AMA Council on Drugs: Drug-induced blood dyscrasias, J. A. M. A. 188:531, 1964.

Burns, S. L.: Anemia in rheumatoid arthritis, M. Clin. North America 52:527, 1968.

Cartwright, G. E.: The anemia of chronic disorders, Seminars Hemat. 3:351, 1966.

Cartwright, G. E., and Wintrobe, M. M.: The Anemia of Infection: A Review, in Dock, W., and Snapper, I. (eds.): Advances in Internal Medicine (Chicago: Year Book Medical Publishers, Inc., 1952), Vol. V, p. 165.

Clement, D. H.: Aplastic anemia, Pediat. Clin. North America 9:703, 1962.

Corr, W. P., et al.: Hematologic changes in tuberculosis, Am. J. M. Sc. 248:709, 1964.

Dawson, R. B., Jr.: Drug-induced blood dyscrasias—prevention and diagnosis, M. Times 96:671, 1968.

Ellis, L. D., and Westerman, M. P.: Autoimmune-hemolytic anemia and cancer, J. A. M. A. 193:962, 1965.

Friedman, I. A., and Schwartz, S. O.: The Relation Between the Liver and the Hematopoietic System, in Popper, H., and Schaffner, F. (eds.): Progress in Liver Diseases (New York: Grune & Stratton, Inc., 1961), Vol. 1, p. 134.

Harris, J. W., and Kellermeyer, R. W.: The Red Cell (2d ed.; Cambridge, Mass.: Harvard University Press, 1970).

Hattersley, P. G.: Macrocytosis of the erythrocytes: A preliminary report, J. A. M. A. 189:997, 1964.

Havard, C. W. H.: An investigation of refractory anemias, Quart. J. Med. 31:21, 1962.

Hines, J. D., and Grasso, J. A.: The sideroblastic anemias, Seminars Hemat. 7:86, 1970.

Huguley, C. M.: Hematological reactions, J. A. M. A. 196:122, 1966.

Leikin, S. L.: Hematologic aspects of renal disease, Pediat. Clin. North America 11:667, 1964.

Leithold, S. L., et al.: Hypothyroidism with anemia demonstrating abnormal vitamin $B_{12}$ absorption, Am. J. Med. 24:535, 1958.

Maldonado, J. E., et al.: The thymus gland and its relationship to the hematopoietic and immunologic systems: A review, Mayo Clin. Proc. 39:60, 1964.

Marks, P. A., et al.: Hemolytic anemia associated with liver disease, M. Clin. North America 47:711, 1963.

Movitt, E. R., et al.: Idiopathic true bone marrow failure, Am. J. Med. 34:500, 1963.

Pisciotta, A. V.: Drug-induced leukopenia and aplastic anemia, Clin. Pharmacol. & Therap. 12:13, 1971.

Scott, J. L., et al.: Acquired aplastic anemia, Medicine 38:119, 1959.

Waldon, H. A.: Anemia of lead poisoning: A review, Brit. J. Indust. Med. 23:83, 1966.

Weiss, A. J.: Hematologic complications of renal disease, M. Clin. North America 47:1001, 1963.

Zieve, L.: Jaundice, hyperlipemia, and hemolytic anemia: A heretofore unrecognized syndrome associated with alcoholic fatty liver and cirrhosis, Ann. Int. Med. 48:471, 1958.

# CHAPTER 4

# Depletion Anemia

Two types of depletion anemia are possible: abnormal loss of red cells from the circulation and abnormal destruction of red cells within the circulation. Red cell loss due to hemorrhage has been covered elsewhere (blood volume, p. 110; iron-deficiency anemia, p. 20 ). Intravascular RBC destruction is called hemolytic anemia. In general, there are two major types of hemolytic anemia. In one category, destruction is relatively slow, and, although RBC survival is shortened, the only laboratory test which demonstrates this fact is radioisotope study using tagged RBC. In the other category, hemolysis or shortened RBC life span is sufficient to cause abnormality in one or more standard laboratory tests.

Two etiologic groups comprise most of the hemolytic anemias: those primarily due to intracorpuscular RBC defects and those primarily due to extracorpuscular agents acting on the RBC. This provides a rational basis for classification.

I. Due Primarily to Intracorpuscular Defects

    A. Hemoglobinopathies
    B. Glucose-6-phosphate dehydrogenase (G-6-PD) defect
    C. Hereditary (congenital) spherocytosis
    D. Paroxysmal nocturnal hemoglobinuria

II. Due Primarily to Extracorpuscular Agents

    A. Isoimmune antibodies
    B. Autoimmune antibodies
    C. Toxins (lead, bacterial toxins)
    D. Parasites (malaria)
    E. Systemic diseases
    F. Hypersplenism

Certain laboratory tests are extremely helpful in suggesting or demonstrating the presence of hemolytic anemia. Which tests are abnormal, and to what degree, depends of course on the severity of the hemolytic process and possibly also on its duration.

1. Reticulocyte Count: This is significantly elevated in nearly all active hemolytic anemias, and the degree of reticulocytosis corresponds to some extent with the degree of anemia. The highest counts appear after acute hemolytic episodes. The reticulocyte count is a valuable screening test for active hemolytic anemia, and reticulocyte counts of over 5% should suggest this diagnosis. Other conditions which give a similar reticulocyte response are acute bleeding and deficiency anemias after initial treatment (note that sometimes the treatment may be dietary only). It usually takes 2-3 days after acute hemolysis to obtain the characteristic reticulocyte response.

2. Serum Haptoglobin: Haptoglobins are alpha-2 globulins which bind any free hemoglobin liberated by intravascular RBC destruction. Haptoglobin quantity can be measured in several ways, most commonly by electrophoresis. Decreased serum or plasma haptoglobins usually mean that hemolysis has occurred, and that some of the haptoglobins have been made unavailable because of binding to free hemoglobin. Haptoglobins also are decreased in situations with considerable extravascular RBC destruction, such as congenital spherocytosis or Rh incompatibility reactions. Haptoglobins are fairly sensitive indicators of hemolytic anemia; however, congenital absence of haptoglobin occurs in about 3% of Negroes and rarely in whites.

3. Plasma Methemalbumin: After the binding capacity of haptoglobin is exhausted, free hemoglobin combines with albumin to form a compound known as methemalbumin. This can be demonstrated with a spectroscope. The presence of methemalbumin means that intravascular hemolysis has occurred to a considerable extent. It also suggests that the episode was either continuing or relatively recent, because otherwise the haptoglobins would be replenished and once again take over the hemoglobin removal duty from albumin.

4. Free Hemoglobin in Plasma or Urine: This occurs when all the plasma protein-binding capacity for free hemoglobin is exhausted, including albumin. There normally is a small amount of free hemoglobin in the plasma, probably because some artifactual hemolysis is unavoidable in drawing blood and processing the specimen. This is less when plasma is used instead of serum. If increased amounts of free hemoglobin are found in plasma, and artifactual hemolysis due to poor blood-drawing technique (very frequent, unfortunately) can be ruled out, then a relatively severe degree of intravascular hemolysis is probable. If the degree of hemolysis is marked, this is often accompanied by free hemoglobin in the urine (hemoglobinuria).

5. Direct Coombs Test: This test is helpful when a hemolytic process is suspected or demonstrated. It detects a wide variety of both isoantibodies and autoantibodies which have attached to the patient's red cells. This is discussed in Chapter 9. The indirect Coombs test is often wrongly ordered in such situations. The indirect Coombs test forms a part of certain special techniques for antibody identification and is usually not helpful in most clinical situations when ordered by itself. If an antibody is demonstrated by the direct Coombs test, an antibody identification test should be requested and the laboratory will decide what techniques to use, depending on the situation.

6. Serum Unconjugated ("Indirect-Acting") Bilirubin: This is often elevated in hemolysis which is of at least moderate degree. Slight or mild degrees of hemolysis will often show no elevation. The direct-acting (conjugated) fraction is usually not elevated significantly in jaundice due to purely hemolytic cause. Serum bilirubin is not as helpful in diagnosis of hemolytic anemias as most of the other tests except in blood bank problems, and often shows equivocal results.

7. RBC Survival Studies: Red blood cell survival can be estimated in vivo by tagging some of the patient's red cells with a radioactive isotope such as $^{51}Cr$, drawing daily blood samples for isotope counting, and determining in this way how long it takes for the tagged cells to disappear from the circulation. Survival studies are most useful to demonstrate low-grade hemolytic anemias, situations in which bone marrow production is able to keep pace with red cell destruction, but is not able to keep the red cell count at normal levels. Low-grade hemolysis often presents as anemia whose etiology cannot be demonstrated by the usual methods. There are, however, certain drawbacks to this procedure. If anemia is actually due to chronic occult extravascular blood loss, tagged red cells will disappear from the circulation by this route and simulate decreased intravascular survival. A minor difficulty is the fact that survival data are only approximate, because certain technical aspects of isotope red cell tagging limit the accuracy of measurement.

I A.   The Hemoglobinopathies

At birth, approximately 80% of the infant's hemoglobin is fetal-type hemoglobin (Hb F), which has a greater affinity for oxygen than the adult type. By age 6 months, all except 1-2% is replaced by adult hemoglobin (Hb A). Persistence of large amounts of fetal hemoglobin is abnormal. There are a considerable number of abnormal hemoglobins, which differ structurally and biochemically to varying degrees from normal adult hemoglobin. The clinical syndromes produced in persons having certain of these abnormal types are called the hemoglobinopathies. The most important of these syndromes are thalassemia, sickle cell anemia, and hemoglobin C disease. All the abnormal hemoglobins are genetically transmitted, just as normal adult hemoglobin is.  Therefore, since each person has two genes for each trait (such as hemoglobin type), one gene on one chromosome received from the mother and one gene on one chromosome received from the father, a person can be either homozygous (two genes with the trait) or heterozygous (only one of the two genes with the trait).  When present in double dose (homozygous, or both genes), the syndrome produced by the abnormal hemoglobin is usually much more severe than if the gene were present only in a single dose (heterozygous, only one of the two genes carrying the abnormal trait).  This also allows genes for two different abnormal hemoglobins to be present in the same person.

1.  Sickle Cell Hemoglobin: Several disease states may be due to the abnormal hemoglobin gene called sickle hemoglobin (Hb S).  When the gene is present in double dose (SS), the disease produced is called sickle cell anemia.  When the gene is present in single dose only (S plus another hemoglobin), it is called sickle trait.  Sickle cell hemoglobin is found mostly (although not exclusively) in Negroes.  The incidence of sickle trait in Negroes is about 10% and of sickle cell anemia about 1%.

a) Sickle cell anemia: Sickle cell (SS) anemia symptoms are not usually manifest until age 6 months or later.  On the other hand, survival over age 40 is not frequent.  Anemia is of moderate or severe degree, and the patient often has slight jaundice (manifested by scleral icterus).  The patients seem to adapt surprisingly well to their anemic state, and apart from easy fatigability, or perhaps weakness, have few symptoms until a so-called crisis develops.  The crisis of sickle cell disease is often due to small infarcts in various organs, but in some cases the reason is unknown.  Abdominal pain or bone pain are the two most common symptoms, and the pain may be extremely severe.  There usually is an accompanying leukocytosis, which, if associated with abdominal pain, may suggest acute intra-abdominal surgical disease.  The crisis ordinarily lasts 5-7 days.  In most cases, there is no change in hemoglobin levels during the crisis.

Other commonly found abnormalities in sickle cell disease are chronic leg ulcers (usually over the ankles), hematuria, and a loss of urine-concentrating ability.  Characteristic bone abnormalities are frequently seen on x-ray films, especially of the skull.  Gallstones are increased in frequency.  There may be various neurologic signs and symptoms.  The spleen may be palpable in a few early cases, but eventually it becomes smaller than normal, due to repeated infarcts.  The liver is palpable in occasional cases.

As mentioned, the anemia is moderate to severe.  There is moderate anisocytosis.  Target cells are characteristically present, but are fewer than 30% of the RBC.  Sickled cells are found in the peripheral blood smear in many, although not all, of the patients.  Sometimes they are very few and take a careful search.  There are

usually nucleated RBC of the orthochromic or polychromatophilic
normoblast stages, most often ranging from 1 to 10 per 100 WBC.
Polychromatophilic RBC are usually present. Howell-Jolly bodies
appear in a fair number of patients. The WBC count may be normal
or there may be a mild leukocytosis, which sometimes may become
moderate in degree. There is often a "shift to the left" (when in
crisis, this becomes more pronounced) and sometimes even a few
myelocytes are found. Platelets may be normal or even moderately
increased.

The laboratory features of active hemolytic anemia are present, including moderate or even marked reticulocytosis.

Diagnosis rests on first demonstrating the characteristic
sickling phenomenon, and then doing paper hemoglobin electrophoresis to find out if the abnormality is SS disease or some combination
of another hemoglobin with the S gene. Bone marrow shows marked
erythroid hyperplasia, but a bone marrow is not helpful and is therefore not indicated for diagnosis of suspected sickle cell disease.

Sickle hemoglobin is less soluble than normal adult hemoglobin when oxygen tension is lowered, and the sickle hemoglobin forms
crystalline aggregates under these circumstances which distort the
RBC shape into a sickle shape. A sickle preparation ("sickle cell
prep") may be done in two ways. A drop of blood from a finger
puncture is placed on a slide, coverslipped, and the edges sealed
with petrolatum jelly. The characteristic sickled forms are seen
after 6 hours (or earlier), but may not appear until nearly 24 hours.
A more widely used procedure is to add a reducing substance, 2%
sodium metabisulfite, to the blood before coverslipping. This speeds
the reaction markedly, with the preparation becoming readable in 15-
60 minutes. The sickle preparation may be negative early in life,
presumably because most of the hemoglobin is still fetal hemoglobin
(Hb F). Other sickle hemoglobin tests are available (p. 38).

Hemoglobin electrophoresis on filter paper allows good separation of Hb S from Hb A and C. In SS disease, 75-95% is sickle
hemoglobin and the remainder is fetal (F) hemoglobin.

The sickle cell preparation is almost always positive in homozygous (SS) disease, except in young infants, if the test is properly
done. On peripheral smear, certain other abnormal RBC shapes
may be confused with sickle cells. The most common of these are
ovalocytes, schistocytes, and burr cells. Ovalocytes are somewhat
rod-shaped RBC which, on occasion, may be found normally in small
numbers, but which may also appear due to another genetically inherited abnormality, hereditary ovalocytosis. Compared to sickle
cells, the ovalocytes are not usually curved and are fairly well
rounded at each end, lacking the sharply pointed ends of the classic
sickle cell. Schistocytes may be found in certain severe hemolytic
anemias, usually of a toxic or an antigen-antibody type. They are
red cells being destroyed, and have an irregular, stubby, crescent-
shaped form, not the longer more slender and regular sickle cell

shape.  Burr cells are small, roughly elongated, triangular cells
with short spinous processes protruding from various places.  They
are found most often in uremia.  Again, they do not have the long,
slender, smooth form of the typical sickle cell.

b)  Sickle cell trait:  This is the (heterozygous) combination of
one gene for sickle (S) hemoglobin with one gene for normal adult (A)
hemoglobin.  There is no anemia, and no clinical evidence of any
disease except for two situations:  some persons with S trait develop
splenic infarction when flying at high altitudes in nonpressurized
airplanes, and some persons develop hematuria for unknown reasons.  On paper electrophoresis, 20-45% of the hemoglobin is sickle
type, with the remainder being normal adult (A) type.  The metabisulfite sickle preparation is usually positive; although a few patients
have been reported negative, some believe that every person with
sickle hemoglobin will have a positive sickle preparation if properly
done.

c)  Sickle-cell hemoglobin C (SC) disease:  This combines one
gene for sickle (S) hemoglobin with one for hemoglobin C.  About 20%
of patients do not have anemia and are asymptomatic.  In the others,
a disease is produced which may be much like that of SS disease, but
is usually milder.  Compared to sickle cell (SS) disease, the anemia
is usually only of mild or moderate degree, although sometimes it
may be severe.  Crises are less frequent; abdominal pain has been
reported in 30%.  Bone pain is almost as common as in SS disease,
but is usually much milder.  Idiopathic hematuria is found in a substantial minority of cases.  Chronic leg ulcers occur but are not
frequent.  Skull x-ray abnormalities are not frequent, but may be
present.

There are some differences from SS disease.  In SC disease,
aseptic necrosis in the head of the femur is common; this can occur
in SS disease but is not frequent.  Splenomegaly is common in SC
disease, with a palpable spleen in 65-80% of the patients.  Finally,
target cells are more frequent on the average than in SS disease
(due to the Hb C gene), although the number present varies considerably from patient to patient and cannot be used as a differentiating point unless over 30% of the RBC are involved.  Nucleated
RBC are not common in the peripheral blood.  Sickle cells may or
may not be present in the peripheral smear; if present, they are
usually few in number.  WBC counts are usually normal except in
crises or with superimposed infection.

Sickle preparations are usually positive.  Hemoglobin electrophoresis establishes a definitive diagnosis.

2.  Hemoglobin C:  a) Hemoglobin C disease:  This is the double
dose homozygous state (CC) for the Hb C gene.  The C gene is said to
be present in about 2% of Negroes, so that homozygous (CC) Hb C
disease is not common.  The C gene may be homozygous (CC), in
combination with normal hemoglobin (AC), or in combination with
any of the other abnormal hemoglobins (such as SC disease).  Epi-

sodes of abdominal and bone pain may occur, but usually are not severe. Splenomegaly is generally present. The most striking feature of the peripheral blood smear is the large number of target
cells, always over 30% and often close to 90%.

Diagnosis is by means of hemoglobin electrophoresis.

b) Hemoglobin C trait: This is the combination of the C gene
and the normal hemoglobin (A) gene. There is no anemia, nor any
symptoms. The only abnormality is the presence of variable numbers of target cells in the peripheral blood smear.

3. Thalassemia: Strictly speaking, there is no thalassemia
hemoglobin. Thalassemia is a complex group of genetically inherited abnormalities in hemoglobin synthesis. There are three main
clinical types: thalassemia major, which has over 50% fetal (F)
hemoglobin, thalassemia minor, which has normal amounts of fetal
hemoglobin but usually has increased amounts of a variant of normal
hemoglobin called Hb $A_2$, and combinations of the thalassemia gene
with other abnormal hemoglobins. The thalassemia gene is found
most commonly in persons who originated from Greece or southern
Italy, and is also rather frequent in other countries which border
the Mediterranean.

Actually, the situation is much more complicated than this de-
scription implies. The globin portion of normal hemoglobin (hemoglobin $A_1$) is composed of two pairs of polypeptide (amino acid)
chains, one pair called alpha and the other beta. All hemoglobins
have two alpha chains, but certain hemoglobins have amino acid
chains different from beta comprising the second chain pair. Thus,
hemoglobin $A_2$ has two delta chains, and hemoglobin F has two gamma chains. All three of these hemoglobins ($A_1$, $A_2$, and F) are normally present in adult RBC, but $A_2$ and F normally are only in trace
amounts. One polypeptide chain from each pair is inherited from
each parent, so that one alpha chain and one beta chain are derived
from the mother, and the other alpha and beta chain from the father.
The thalassemia gene may involve either the alpha or the beta chain.
In the great majority of cases, the beta is affected; genetically speaking, it would be more correct to call such a situation a beta thalassemia. If the condition is heterozygous, only one of the two beta
chains is affected; this supposedly leaves only one beta chain (instead of two) available for Hb $A_1$ synthesis, thus resulting in a partial decrease of normal hemoglobin ($A_1$) synthesis, and a relative
increase in $A_2$ hemoglobin. This produces the clinical picture of
thalassemia minor. In a homozygous beta thalassemia, both of the
beta chains are affected; this apparently results in marked suppression of normal hemoglobin $A_1$ synthesis and leads to a compensatory
increase in gamma chains; the combination of increased gamma
chains with the nonaffected alpha chains produces marked elevation
of hemoglobin F. This gives the clinical syndrome of thalassemia
major. It is also possible for the thalassemia gene to affect the
alpha chains; in heterozygous alpha thalassemia, hemoglobin $A_1$

production is mildly curtailed, but no hemoglobin $A_2$ or F increase occurs, because they also need alpha chains. If the alpha thalassemia is homozygous, apparently hemoglobin production, in most cases, is curtailed enough to be lethal in utero or in neonatal life.

a) Thalassemia major (Cooley's anemia): This disease produces a severe anemia, which is accompanied by a considerable number of normoblasts in the peripheral blood. The nucleated RBC are most often about a third or half the number of WBC, but may even exceed them. There are often Howell-Jolly bodies and considerable numbers of polychromatophilic RBC. The mature red cells are usually very hypochromic, with considerable anisocytosis and poikilocytosis, and there are moderate numbers of target cells. The mean corpuscular volume (MCV) is microcytic. WBC counts are often mildly increased, and there may be mild granulocytic immaturity, sometimes even with myelocytes present. Platelets are normal. Skull x-ray films show abnormal patterns similar to those in sickle cell anemia, but even more pronounced. Death most often occurs in childhood or adolescence.

Diagnosis is suggested by a severe anemia with very hypochromic RBC, moderate numbers of target cells, many nucleated RBC, and a family history of Mediterranean origin. The sickle preparation is negative. Definitive diagnosis depends on the fact that in thalassemia major, fetal hemoglobin (Hb F) is elevated (10-90% of the total hemoglobin, usually over 50%). Hb F has approximately the same migration rate as Hb $A_1$ on paper electrophoresis, so the two cannot easily be separated by this technique. However, Hb F is much more resistant to denaturation by alkali than is Hb $A_1$. This fact is utilized in the alkali denaturation test. The hemoglobin solution is added to a certain concentration of NaOH and, after filtration, the amount of hemoglobin in the filtrate (the undenatured Hb) is measured and compared to the original total quantity of hemoglobin.

b) Thalassemia minor: This variation of thalassemia produces a mild (or sometimes moderate) anemia which is most often asymptomatic. It is characterized by mildly or moderately hypochromic and microcytic RBC with moderate poikilocytosis and a varying (usually not great) number of target cells. Nucleated RBC are not found in the peripheral smear. Splenomegaly may be present.

The main laboratory abnormality in thalassemia minor is an increased amount of $A_2$ hemoglobin (this is true for heterozygous beta thalassemia; $A_2$ is not elevated in the less common heterozygous alpha thalassemia). As noted previously, $A_2$ is a variant of adult Hb $A_1$, and is normally present in quantities up to 2.5 or 3.0%. In (beta) thalassemia minor, $A_2$ is elevated, ranging from 3.5 to 10%. Fetal (F) Hb is normal. $A_2$ Hb cannot be demonstrated on paper electrophoresis; cellulose acetate or the more complicated and time-consuming starch block electrophoresis is required for diagnosis. These methods, especially starch techniques, are not available in many laboratories.

Thalassemia minor must sometimes be differentiated from iron-deficiency anemia because of the hypochromic microcytic status of the red cells. The serum or plasma iron is high-normal or elevated and the plasma total iron-binding capacity is considerably decreased (i.e., the TIBC is much more saturated than normal). Bone marrow iron is increased.

c) Sickle-thalassemia: This produces a condition analogous to S-C disease—clinically similar in many respects to SS anemia but considerably milder. Sickle cell preparations are positive. There is often a considerable number of target cells. In these patients, 60-80% of the hemoglobin is Hb S, with 0-2% being Hb F and the remainder, if any, composed of Hb A. This means that paper electrophoresis may give either an SS or an SA pattern. When the hemoglobin is SA (rather than the SF combination that may be found in some cases of homozygous sickle cell disease) type, and there is over 50% sickle hemoglobin, this suggests S-thalassemia. Also, sickle trait does not usually have the clinical picture of S-thalassemia. When the pattern is SS, the diagnosis is difficult. Clues are a syndrome much milder than one would expect with SS disease, and the presence of more target cells and hypochromia than one would expect. Family studies are often necessary, looking for thalassemia minor in one of the parents.

To conclude the hemoglobinopathies, certain observations should be made. First, a sickle preparation should be done on all Negro patients who have anemia, hematuria, abdominal pain, or arthralgias. This should be followed up with paper electrophoresis if the sickle preparation is positive or peripheral blood smears show significant numbers of target cells. However, if the patient had these studies done previously, there is no need to repeat them. Secondly, these patients may have other diseases superimposed on their hemoglobinopathies. For example, unexplained hematuria in a person with sickle hemoglobin may be due to carcinoma and should not be blamed on the hemoglobinopathy without investigation. Likewise, when there is hypochromia and microcytosis, one should rule out chronic iron deficiency (e.g., chronic bleeding). This is especially true when the patient has sickle trait only, since this does not usually produce anemia. The leukocytosis found as part of SS disease (and to a lesser degree in S-C and S-thalassemia) may mask the leukocytosis of infection. As mentioned, finding significant numbers of target cells suggests one of the hemoglobinopathies. However, target cells are often found in chronic liver disease; they may be seen in any severe anemia in relatively small numbers, and may sometimes be produced artifactually at the thin edge of a blood smear.

I B.   Glucose-6-Phosphate Dehydrogenase (G-6-PD) Defect

This is a sex-linked genetic defect carried on the female (X) chromosome. To obtain full expression of its bad effects, the gene must not be opposed by a normal X chromosome. Therefore, the defect is most severe in males (XY) and in the much smaller number of females who have both X chromosomes having the abnormal gene. Those females with only one abnormal gene ("carrier" females) have varying expressions of bad effect, ranging from completely asymptomatic to only moderate effects even under stimulation which is greater than that needed to bring out the defect clinically in affected males or homozygous females.

The G-6-PD defect is found mainly in Negroes and to a lesser extent in persons whose ancestors came from Mediterranean countries such as Italy or Greece. The defect centers in the key role of G-6-PD in the pentose phosphate glucose metabolic cycle of RBC. When RBC get older, they normally have less ability to utilize the pentose phosphate (oxidative) cycle, which is an important pathway for utilization of glucose, although secondary to the Embden-Meyerhof (nonoxidative) glycolysis cycle. When the defective G-6-PD status is superimposed on the older erythrocyte, utilization of the pentose phosphate shunt is lost. This cycle is apparently necessary to protect the integrity of the RBC against certain chemicals. Currently it is thought that these chemicals act as oxidants and that TPNH from the pentose cycle is the reducing agent needed to counteract their effects. At any rate, exposure to certain chemicals in sufficient dosage results in destruction of erythrocytes with a sufficiently severe G-6-PD defect. In Negroes, only older RBC are affected; in Mediterranean people, the defect is more severe and most RBC are sensitive.

As noted, before drug exposure the susceptible patients do not have anemia. After a hemolytic drug is given, acute hemolysis is usually seen on the second day, but sometimes not until the third or fourth day. All the classic laboratory signs of nonspecific acute hemolysis are present. The degree of anemia produced in Negroes is only moderate, because only the older cell population is destroyed. If the drug is discontinued, hemolysis stops in 48-72 hours. If the drug is continued, anemia continues at a plateau level, with only a small degree of active hemolysis taking place as the RBC advance to the susceptible cell age.

Many drugs have been reported to cause this reaction in G-6-PD defective persons. The most common ones are the following: antimalarials, sulfas, nitrofurantoin (Furadantin) family, aspirin and similar analgesics, such as phenacetin. Hemolysis induced by various infections has been frequently reported.

There are several tests available to demonstrate G-6-PD deficiency. The most commonly used is Brewer's test. This depends on the fact that when oxyhemoglobin is turned to methemoglobin chemically, the addition of methylene blue will reduce the methemoglobin back to oxyhemoglobin. G-6-PD deficient RBC are not able to accomplish the methemoglobin reduction process in the same

amount of time as in a normal person. The amount of methemoglobin is measured after the standard test time limit.

Once again, the same caution applies to G-6-PD that was necessary with the hemoglobinopathies. Hemolytic anemia in those
groups known to have a high incidence of this defect should always
raise the suspicion of its presence. However, even if the patient
has the defect, this does not exclude the possibility that the actual
cause of hemolysis was something else.

I C.  Hereditary (Congenital) Spherocytosis

This is another genetically transmitted red cell defect. Most
of the patients involved are English or northern Europeans. A dominant gene is involved, whose incidence apparently is not frequent,
but also not rare. The defect is manifest as spherocytosis of varying numbers of the red cells, in some patients relatively few, in
other patients many.

Most patients are asymptomatic unless a crisis develops. The
development of symptoms most often begins in childhood. There
may be no anemia at all, or any variation from mild to moderate.
The crisis of congenital spherocytosis is intermittent and varies in
frequency. It is due to sudden hypoplasia of the bone marrow of unknown cause which usually lasts 6-10 days. During the crisis, anemia may become severe. Between crises, patients may be completely asymptomatic or may have very mild jaundice (scleral icterus). If anemia is present, there may be a slight or mild reticulocytosis and slightly to mildly elevated serum indirect bilirubin.
There is a considerably increased incidence of gallstones.

The spherocytes are not destroyed in the blood stream, but
are sequestered, removed, and destroyed in the spleen. Splenomegaly usually is present. Therefore, splenectomy satisfactorily
cures the patient's symptoms because marrow RBC production can
then keep up with the presence of spherocytes, which have a shorter
life span than normal RBC.

The most useful diagnostic test in congenital spherocytosis is
the osmotic fragility test. RBC are placed in bottles containing decreasing concentrations of NaCl. When the concentration becomes
too dilute, normal RBC begin to hemolyze. Spherocytes are more
susceptible to hemolysis in hypotonic saline than normal RBC, so
that spherocytes begin hemolyzing at concentrations above the normal range. This will be true when there are significant degrees of
spherocytosis from any cause, not just congenital spherocytosis.
Incidentally, target cells are resistant to hemolysis in hypotonic
saline and begin to hemolyze at concentrations below those of normal RBC.

I D.  Paroxysmal Nocturnal Hemoglobinuria

This is a rare but famous etiology for hemolytic anemia. The disease consists of a chronic hemolytic anemia with crisis episodes of hemoglobinuria which most often occur at night. It usually affects young or middle-aged adults. The anemia is usually of moderate degree except during crisis, when it may be severe. A crisis is reflected by all the usual laboratory parameters of severe hemolysis, including elevated plasma hemoglobin. No spherocytosis or demonstrable antibodies are present. The disease gets its name because hemoglobinuric episodes change urine collected during or just after sleep a red or brown color due to large amounts of hemoglobin, whereas urine formed during the day is clear. Various stimuli are known to precipitate attacks in some cases; these include infections, surgery, and blood transfusion.

In addition to severe anemia, leukopenia is extremely common and thrombocytopenia is fairly common. This is in contrast to most other hemolytic anemias, where hemolysis usually provokes leukocytosis.

A good screening test is a urine hemosiderin examination. However, a positive urine hemosiderin may be obtained in many cases of chronic hemolytic anemia of various types, and also may be produced by frequent blood transfusions, especially if given over periods of weeks or months. A much more specific test is the acid hemolysis (Ham) test. The RBC of paroxysmal nocturnal hemoglobinuria (PNH) are more susceptible to hemolysis in acid pH. Therefore, serum is acidified to a certain point which does not affect normal RBC but will hemolyze the RBC of PNH.

A more recently reported test, claimed to be as good or better than the Ham procedure, is called the sugar-water test.

## II A. Hemolytic Anemia Due to Isoagglutinins (Isoantibodies)

As explained in Chapter 10 these are hemolytic reactions caused by antibodies within the various blood group systems. The classification, symptomatology, and diagnostic procedures necessary for detection of such reactions and identification of the etiology are discussed in that chapter.

## II B. Hemolytic Anemia Due to Autoagglutinins (Autoantibodies)

These are antibodies produced by an individual against certain of his own body cells. In this discussion, those produced against his own red blood cells are the ones in question. This disease has been called "autoimmune hemolytic anemia" or "acquired hemolytic anemia."

Autoantibodies of the autoimmune hemolytic anemias form two general categories: those which react best in vitro above room temperature (37º C, warm autoantibodies) and those which react best in vitro at cold temperatures (cold autoantibodies or cold agglutinins). For each type there are two general etiologies, idiopathic and secondary to some known disease.

Warm autoantibodies are the most frequent type, and the idiopathic variety is twice as frequent as that secondary to known disease. Clinically, in the warm type, the anemia appears at any age and may be either chronic or acute. When chronic, it is more often relatively low grade. When acute, it is often severe and fatal. The laboratory signs are those of any hemolytic anemia and depend on the degree of anemia. Thus, there are varying degrees of reticulocyte elevation. The direct Coombs test (p.91) is usually, although not always, positive. Most of the patients have spherocytes in the peripheral blood, especially if the anemia is acute. There is often splenomegaly.

Cold agglutinins are much less frequent. They are seen mostly in adults and more often in the elderly. The idiopathic and secondary forms have a nearly equal incidence. Clinically, the disease is often worse in cold weather. Raynaud's phenomenon is common. Splenomegaly is not common. Laboratory abnormalities are not as marked as in the warm autoantibody type, except for a usually positive direct Coombs test. The anemia tends to be less severe. The reticulocyte count is usually increased, but often only slightly. Spherocytes are more often absent than present. WBC and platelets are usually normal unless altered by underlying disease. However, exceptions to the above statements may occur, with severe hemolytic anemia present in all its manifestations. As noted in the discussion of primary atypical pneumonia (p. 194), cold agglutinins may occur in many normal persons, but only in titers up to 1:64. In symptomatic anemia due to cold agglutinins (cold autoantibodies), the cold agglutinin titer is almost always over 1:1000.

The causes of acquired hemolytic anemia of the secondary type, either warm or cold variety, can be divided into three main groups. The most frequent occurrence is with chronic lymphocytic leukemia, to a lesser extent in lymphocytic lymphoma, and occasionally with Hodgkin's disease. The second group in order of frequency is the collagen diseases, notably lupus. The third is a miscellaneous category, including systemic diseases in which the development of overtly hemolytic anemia is relatively rare, but which does happen from time to time. These diseases include viral infections, severe liver disease, ovarian tumors, and carcinomatosis. It should be emphasized that in all the groups of diseases mentioned above, anemia is a common or even frequent finding, but that the anemia is usually not due to hemolytic anemia—at least not of the overt or symptomatic type. Anemias of systemic disease were discussed earlier (p. 30).

## II C. Hemolytic Anemia Due to Toxins

1. Chemical: Lead poisoning is the most frequent in this group. Ingestion of paint containing lead used to be frequent in children and still happens occasionally. Working with auto storage

batteries and gasoline fumes is the most common cause in adults. It takes several weeks of chronic exposure to develop symptoms, unless a large dose is ingested. The anemia produced is most often mild to moderate, and the usual reason for seeing the patient is development of other systemic symptoms such as convulsions from lead encephalopathy, abdominal pain, or paresthesias of hands and feet. The anemia is more often hypochromic, but may be normochromic; it is usually normocytic. Basophilic stippling of red cells is often very pronounced, and forms a classic diagnostic clue to this condition. Basophilic stippling may occur in any severe anemia, especially the hemolytic anemias, but when present in unusual quantity should suggest lead poisoning unless the cause is already obvious. The stippled cells are reticulocytes, which, for some unknown reason, appear in this form in these patients. However, in some patients, basophilic stippling is minimal or absent. In lead poisoning there is usually increased urinary excretion of coproporphyrin type III, and this fact provides a very useful screening test (however, in a few cases there may be normal results).

Other chemicals were mentioned in the discussion on glucose-6-phosphate dehydrogenase deficiency anemia (p. 44). Benzene toxicity was discussed in the hypoplastic bone marrow anemias (p. 29). Other chemicals which often produce a hemolytic anemia if taken in sufficient dose include naphthalene, toluene, phenacetin, and distilled water given intravenously. Severe extensive burns often produce acute hemolysis to varying degree.

2. Bacterial: Clostridium welchii septicemia often produces a severe hemolytic anemia with spherocytes. Hemolytic anemia is rarely seen with tuberculosis. The anemia of infection is usually not overtly hemolytic, although there may be a minor hemolytic component (not demonstrable by the usual laboratory tests).

II D. Hemolytic Anemia Due to Parasites

Malaria is by far the most frequent. It has to be considered in persons who have visited endemic areas and who have suggestive symptoms or no other etiology for their anemia. The diagnosis is made from peripheral blood, best obtained morning and afternoon for 3 days. Organisms within parasitized RBC may be few, and often will be missed unless the laboratory is notified that malaria is suspected. A thick-drop special preparation is the method of choice for diagnosis. With heavy infection, the parasites may be identified in an ordinary (thin) peripheral blood smear. A hemolytic anemia is produced with the usual reticulocytosis and other laboratory abnormalities of hemolysis. Most patients have splenomegaly. Bartonella infection occurs in South America, most often in Peru. This is actually a bacterium rather than a parasite, but in many textbooks is usually retained in the parasite category. The organisms infect RBC and cause hemolytic anemia similar clinically to malaria.

## II E. Hemolytic Anemia Due to Systemic Diseases

This is most often seen with certain types of reticuloendothelial malignancy (chronic lymphocytic leukemia and lymphocytic
lymphoma), but may occur in collagen diseases and rarely in systemic illnesses or severe acute infections (p. 31 ). In most diseases where it occurs the actual incidence is very low or rare.
Even in the higher-incidence groups such as certain reticuloendothelial malignancies and, to a lesser extent, the collagen diseases,
it is not very common. Further discussion is located in the section
on hemolytic anemias due to autoimmune antibodies (p. 93).

## II F. Hypersplenism

This is a poorly understood entity whose main feature is an
enlarged spleen associated with a deficiency in one or more blood
cell elements. The most common is thrombocytopenia, but there
may be a pancytopenia or any combination of anemia, leukopenia,
and thrombocytopenia. Hypersplenism may be primary or, more
commonly, secondary to any disease which causes splenic enlargement. However, it should be noted that splenic enlargement in many
cases does not produce hypersplenism effects. Portal hypertension
with secondary splenic congestion is the most common etiology; the
usual cause of this is cirrhosis. If anemia is produced in hypersplenism, it is normocytic and normochromic without reticulocytosis. Bone marrow examination in hypersplenism shows either mild
hyperplasia of the deficient peripheral blood element precursors, or
normal marrow.

Several mechanisms have been proposed to explain the various
effects of hypersplenism. To date, the weight of evidence favors
sequestration in the spleen. In some cases, the spleen may destroy
blood cells already damaged by immunologic or congenital agents;
in some cases, the action of the spleen cannot be completely explained.

## INVESTIGATION OF A PATIENT WITH ANEMIA

To conclude the presentation of anemia, the thing most needed
is a rational and systematic approach to diagnosis. Anemia is a
symptom, not a disease. Most of the causes can be localized by
utilizing available information plus a relatively few laboratory tests.
When anemia is discovered (usually by the appearance of a low hemoglobin or hematocrit value), the first thing is to determine whether
anemia really exists or is due to hemodilution. If the patient is not
getting intravenous fluids, the next step is to get a WBC count, differential, red cell indices, reticulocyte count and a description of
RBC morphology from the peripheral smear. Naturally, it is better to personally look at the peripheral smear in addition, because
many technicians do not routinely pay much attention to the RBC of

a peripheral smear (this is the main reason for getting indices).  A
careful history and physical examination must be performed.  To
some extent, the findings on the peripheral smear and indices help
suggest areas to particularly emphasize (p. 441).

1.  If the RBC are hypochromic and microcytic, chronic blood
loss must always be ruled out carefully.

2.  If the RBC show macrocytosis, the possibility of megaloblastic anemia must always be investigated.

3.  If the RBC are not markedly hypochromic and microcytic,
if macrocytosis due to megaloblastic anemia is ruled out, and if the
reticulocyte count is significantly elevated, two main possibilities
should be considered: acute blood loss and hemolytic anemia.  The
reticulocyte count is usually 5% or over in these cases.  However,
the possibility of a deficiency anemia responding to therapy should
not be forgotten, and also the possibility that macrocytosis may be
due to a reticulocytosis.

4.  In a basically normocytic-normochromic anemia where no
significant reticulocytosis is present, and either leukopenia or
thrombocytopenia (or both) is present, hypersplenism, bone marrow
depression, or a few systemic diseases such as lupus are the main
possibilities.

5.  Appearance of certain RBC abnormalities in the peripheral
blood suggests certain diseases.  Considerable numbers of target
cells suggest one of the hemoglobinopathies or chronic liver disease.
Marked basophilic stippling points toward lead poisoning.  Sickle
cells mean sickle cell anemia.  Nucleated RBC indicate either bone
marrow replacement or unusually marked bone marrow erythropoiesis, most commonly seen in hemolytic anemias.  Significant
rouleau formation suggests abnormal globulins or hyperglobulinemia.  Spherocytes usually indicate an antigen-antibody type of hemolytic anemia, but may mean congenital spherocytosis or a few
other kinds of hemolytic anemia.

Once the basic underlying process is identified, the etiology
can usually be isolated by selective laboratory tests plus the help of
physical examination and careful history.

In general, it is best to perform diagnostic studies before
giving blood transfusions, although in many cases the diagnosis can
be made despite transfusion.  Usually, appropriate blood specimens
for the appropriate tests can be obtained before transfusion of blood
is actually begun, since blood for type and crossmatching must first
be drawn anyway.  A peripheral blood smear is often helpful to indicate what tests will be needed.

## REFERENCES

Amorosi, E. L.: Hypersplenism, Seminars Hemat. 2:249, 1965.

Crosby, W. H.: Hypersplenism, in DeGraff, A. C., and Creger, W. P. (eds.): Annual Review of Medicine (Palo Alto, Calif.: Annual Reviews, Inc., 1962), Vol. 13, p. 127.

Crosby, W. H.: Diagnosing hemolytic anemias in the laboratory, Postgrad. Med. 43:93, 1968.

Dacie, J. V.: The Haemolytic Anemias (2d ed.; New York: Grune & Stratton, Inc., 1962).

Fairbanks, V. F., and Fernandez, M. N.: The identification of metabolic errors associated with hemolytic anemia, J. A. M. A. 208:316, 1969.

Gaither, J. C.: Paroxysmal nocturnal hemoglobinuria, New England J. Med. 265: 421, 1961.

Giblett, E.: Haptoglobin: A review, Vox sang. 6:513, 1961.

Githens, J. H., and Hathaway, W. E.: Autoimmune hemolytic anemia and the syndrome of hemolytic anemia, thrombocytopenia, and nephropathy, Pediat. Clin. North America 9:619, 1962.

Goldwein, M. I.: Autoimmune hemolytic anemia: A review, Am. J. Clin. Path. 56:293, 1971.

Grossbard, L., and Marks, P. A.: Enzymes in Hematologic Disease, in Cooley, E. L. (ed.): Diagnostic Enzymology (Philadelphia: Lea & Febiger, 1970), p. 73.

Harris, J. W., and Kellermeyer, R. W.: The Red Cell (2d ed.; Cambridge, Mass.: Harvard University Press, 1970).

Jonxis, J. H. P.: The Hemoglobinopathies, in Levine, S. Z. (ed.): Advances in Pediatrics (Chicago: Year Book Medical Publishers, Inc., 1966), Vol. XIV, p. 91.

Kruger, H. C., and Burgert, E. O.: Hereditary spherocytosis in 100 children, Mayo Clin. Proc. 41:821, 1966.

McCurdy, P. R.: Abnormal hemoglobins and pregnancy, Am. J. Obst. & Gynec. 90:891, 1964.

McElfresh, A. E.: Congenital microspherocytosis, Pediat. Clin. North America 9:665, 1962.

Motolsky, A. G., and Stamatoyannopoulos, G.: Clinical implications of glucose-6-phosphate dehydrogenase deficiency, Ann. Int. Med. 65:1329, 1966.

Osgood, E. F.: Antiglobulin-positive hemolytic anemias, Arch. Int. Med. 107:313, 1961.

Pearson, H. A.: Newer concepts in the genetics of the thalassemias, Pediat. Clin. North America 9:635, 1962.

River, G. L., et al.: S-C hemoglobin: A clinical study, Blood 18:385, 1961.

Sanford, H. N.: The hemolytic anemias of infancy and childhood, Pediat. Clin. North America 9:443, 1962.

Woods, W. E., and O'Neill, B.: Sucrose haemolysis: A simple screening test for paroxysmal nocturnal haemoglobinuria, M. J. Australia 56:21, 1969.

# CHAPTER 5

# White Blood Cells and Leukocytosis

White blood cells (leukocytes) form the first line of defense by the body against invading microorganisms. Neutrophils and mono-cytes respond by phagocytosis; lymphocytes and plasma cells apparently produce antibodies. Besides nonspecific response to infection by either bacteria or virus, alterations in the normal leukocyte blood picture may provide a diagnostic clue in certain specific diseases, both benign and malignant. Non-neoplastic leukocyte alterations may be quantitative, qualitative, or both, the qualitative aspects demonstrating an increased degree of immaturity, morphologic alteration in cellular structure, or increased quantity of certain less commonly found types of WBC.

Normal white cell maturation sequence begins with the blast form, presumably itself derived from fixed tissue reticulum cells. In the myelocytic (granulocytic) series (Table 1) the blast is characterized by a large nucleus with delicate interlacing chromatin, one or more nucleoli, and a relatively scanty basophilic cytoplasm without granules. Next in sequence is the progranulocyte (promyelocyte), which is essentially similar to the blast except for the appearance of cytoplasmic granules. This gives rise to the myelocyte. The myelocyte nuclear chromatin is more condensed, no nucleolus is present, and the nucleus itself is round cr oval, sometimes with a slight flattening along one side. The cytoplasm is mildly basophilic and has granules to varying degrees, although sometimes granules are absent. There often is a small localized pale or clear area next to the flattened portion (if present) of the nucleus, the so-called myeloid spot. Next, the nucleus begins to indent; when it does, the cell is called a metamyelocyte (juvenile). As the metamyelocyte continues to mature, the nucleus becomes more and more indented, the nuclear chromatin becomes more and

52

## TABLE 1.—TERMINOLOGY OF BLOOD CELLS

| Series | Classic Terminology | Synonyms |
|---|---|---|
| Granulocytic | Myeloblast | |
| | Promyelocyte | Progranulocyte |
| | Myelocyte | |
| | Metamyelocyte | "Juvenile" |
| | Band granulocyte | "Stab" |
| | Segmented granulocyte | Polymorphonuclear |
| Erythroid | Pronormoblast | Rubriblast |
| | Basophilic normoblast | Prorubricyte |
| | Polychromatophilic normoblast | Rubricyte |
| | Orthochromic normoblast | Metarubricyte |
| | Reticulocyte | |
| | Erythrocyte | |
| Lymphocytic | Lymphoblast | |
| | Prolymphocyte | |
| | Lymphocyte | |
| Plasmocytic | Plasmablast | |
| | Proplasmocyte | |
| | Plasmocyte | Plasma cell |
| Monocytic | Monoblast | |
| | Promonocyte | |
| | Monocyte | |

more condensed and clumpy, and the cytoplasm becomes less and less basophilic. The entire cell size becomes somewhat smaller, with the nucleus taking up less and less space. Finally, the band (stab) neutrophil stage is reached. There is some disagreement over just what constitutes a band as opposed to a metamyelocyte on the one hand and a mature polymorphonuclear on the other. Basically, a band is distinguished from a late metamyelocyte when the nucleus has indented over half its diameter, and the nucleus has formed a curved rod structure which is roughly the same thickness through-out. The final stage is the polymorphonuclear neutrophil. The nucleus has segmented into two or more lobes, at least one of which is connected only by a thread-like filament to the next. The nuclear chromatin is dense and clumpy. The cytoplasm is a very slightly eosinophilic color, or at least there is no basophilia. There usu-ally are small irregular granules, which often are indistinct. The separation point of the polymorphonuclear from the band is the pres-ence of the filament connection between lobes. Beginning lobe for-mation occurs in late band forms. When the constriction becomes at least reasonably thin, it may be called a polymorphonuclear ("poly"). Naturally, there are transition forms between any of the maturation stages just enumerated (Fig. 1).

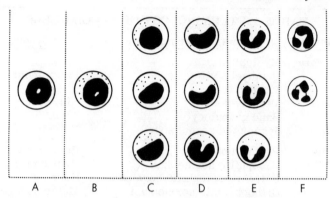

Fig. 1.—Maturation sequence of granulocytic (myelocytic) series.  A, blast; B, promyelocyte; C, myelocyte (top, early stage;
bottom, late stage); D, metamyelocyte (top, early stage; bottom,
late stage); E, band (top, early stage; bottom, late stage); F, segmented granulocyte (top, early stage).

Monocytes are often confused with metamyelocytes or bands.
The monocyte tends to be a larger cell.  Its nuclear chromatin is a
little less dense than the myeloid cell and instead of being clumpy it
is a little more strand-like.  The nucleus typically has several
pseudopods, which sometimes are obscured by being superimposed
on the remainder of the nucleus and have to be looked for carefully.
Sometimes, however, a band monocyte nuclear shape is present.
The nuclear membrane (outline) is less well defined than that of the
metamyelocyte or band.  The cytoplasm of the monocyte tends to be
greater and often has a light gray color, different from either the
basophilia of the early myeloid cells or the adult neutrophil color.
However, the monocyte sometimes has a cytoplasm whose color is
close to that of a neutrophil.  The granules of a monocyte, when
present, usually are very tiny or pinpoint in size, a little smaller
than those of a neutrophil.  In some cases, the best differentiation
is to find undisputed bands and compare their nucleus and cytoplasm with that of the cell in question.

The normal range for peripheral blood WBC is 4,500-11,000/
cu. mm.  Most persons fall into the range of 5,000-10,000/ cu. mm.,
but there is significant overlap between normal and abnormal in the
wider range, especially between 10,000 and 11,000/cu. mm.

| | |
|---|---|
| Total neutrophils | 50-70% |
| Segmented neutrophils (polys) | 50-70% |
| Bands (stabs) | 3- 5% |
| Metamyelocytes (juveniles) | 0- 1% |
| Lymphocytes | 20-40% |
| Monocytes | 0- 7% |
| Eosinophils | 0- 5% |
| Basophils | 0- 1% |

A. Neutrophilic Leukocytosis

　　1. Infection and Inflammation: This is the most frequent cause. Besides an increase in total neutrophil count, there often is some degree of immaturity ("shift to the left"—the maturation sequence of Schilling used to be diagramed with the more mature forms going toward the right and the immature forms progressing toward the left). Usually a shift to the left centers in the early segmented and band neutrophil stages. Leukocytosis is most often seen with bacterial infection; viral infections, in general, tend to have normal counts or even leukopenia. The granulomatous infections (tuberculosis, sarcoid) most often have normal WBC counts, but tuberculosis may have a leukocytosis. Typhoid fever is a bacterial infection which usually does not have a leukocytosis; on the other hand, chickenpox is one viral disease which does. Overwhelming infection, particularly in debilitated persons or the elderly, may fail to show leukocytosis.

　　2. Tissue Destruction: This may be due to burns, abscess, trauma, hemorrhage, infarction, carcinomatosis, or surgery, and is often accompanied by varying degrees of leukocytosis. The leukocytosis varies in severity and frequency according to the etiology and the amount of tissue destruction.

　　3. Metabolic Toxic States: The most frequent of these include uremia, diabetic acidosis, acute gout attacks, and convulsions. A similar situation prevails to some extent during the last phase of pregnancy.

　　4. Certain Drugs and Chemicals: Adrenal cortical steroid therapy has been reported to frequently produce significant leukocytosis. Poisoning by various chemicals, especially lead, is another cause (certain drugs may, on the other hand, sometimes cause leukopenia due to idiosyncratic bone marrow depression).

　　5. Following acute hemorrhage or during severe hemolytic anemia, acute or chronic.

B. Monocytosis

　　Monocytosis may occur in the absence of leukocytosis. It is most frequently found in typhoid fever, tuberculosis, subacute bacterial endocarditis, and during the recovery phase of some cases of acute infection. Malaria and leishmaniasis (kala-azar) are frequent causes outside the United States.

C. Eosinophilia

　　1. Parasites: Eosinophilia is most often associated with roundworms and infestation by the various flukes. In the United States, roundworms predominate, such as Ascaris, Strongyloides, and Trichinella (Trichina). The condition known as visceral larva migrans, caused by the nematode Toxocara canis (common in dogs)

is sometimes seen in man. In Trichinella infection an almost diagnostic triad is bilateral upper eyelid edema, severe muscle pain,
and eosinophilia (eosinophilia, however, may be absent in overwhelming infection).

2. Acute Allergic Attacks: Asthma, etc.

3. Certain Extensive Chronic Skin Diseases—especially pem-
phigus; also may appear in psoriasis and several others.

4. Miscellaneous Conditions: Eosinophilia is reported in 20%
of periarteritis nodosa cases and 25% of sarcoidosis. It also has
been reported in up to 20% of Hodgkin's disease, but is usually not
impressive. Many diseases, including metastatic carcinoma, have
been reported to produce eosinophilia, but these are either unusual
diseases or unusual findings in more common diseases, and the fact
is mentioned only as a reminder of this possibility.

## D.  Basophilia

The most frequent cause is chronic myelogenous leukemia.
Basophils may be increased in the other "myeloproliferative" diseases, and occasionally in certain nonmalignant conditions.

## E.  Lymphocytosis

Usually this accompanies a normal or decreased total white
count. Viral infection is the most common etiology. Sometimes a
neutropenia (such as occurs with agranulocytosis) will produce a
"relative" type of lymphocytosis (actually a pseudolymphocytosis),
since the total lymphocytes remain the same but the neutrophils are
greatly decreased. A real lymphocytosis with leukocytosis occurs
in pertussis, infectious lymphocytosis, and infectious mononucleosis.

## F.  Neonatal Leukocytosis

At birth, there is a leukocytosis of 18,000-22,000 for the first
1-3 days. This drops sharply at 3-4 days to levels between 8,000
and 16,000. At roughly 6 months, approximate adult levels are
reached, although the upper limit of normal is more flexible. Although the postnatal period is associated with neutrophilia, lymphocytes slightly predominate thereafter until about age 4-5 years,
when adult values for total WBC count and differential become established (p. 439).

## REFERENCES

Conrad, M. E.: Hematologic manifestations of parasitic infections,
    Seminars Hemat. 8:267, 1971.
Donohugh, D. L.: Eosinophils and eosinophilia, California Med.
    104:421, 1966.

Ferenzi, G. W.: The significance of neutropenia, M. Clin. North America, 46:245, 1962.

Hildebrand, F. L., et al.: Eosinophilia of unknown cause, Arch. Int. Med. 113:129, 1964.

John, T. J.: Leukocytosis during steroid therapy, Am. J. Dis. Child. 111:68, 1966.

Kuvin, S. F., and Brecher, G.: Differential neutrophil counts in pregnancy, New England J. Med. 266:877, 1962.

Lemon, B. K., and Kaump, D. H.: Infectious lymphocytosis: A report of an epidemic in children, J. Pediat. 36:61, 1950.

Maldonado, J. E.: Monocytosis: A current appraisal, Mayo Clin. Proc. 40:248, 1965.

Miller, F. F.: Eosinophilia in the allergic population, Ann. Allergy 23:177, 1965.

Twomey, J. J., and Leavell, B. S.: Leukemoid reactions to tuberculosis, Arch. Int. Med. 116:21, 1965.

Welsh, J. D., et al.: The incidence and significance of the leukemoid reaction in patients hospitalized with pertussis, South. M. J. 52:643, 1959.

Wood, T. A., and Frenkel, E. P.: The atypical lymphocyte, Am. J. Med. 42:923, 1967.

Zacharski, L. R., et al.: The lymphocyte, Mayo Clin. Proc. 42:431, 1967.

# CHAPTER 6

# Leukemia, Lymphomas, and Myeloproliferative Syndromes

A consideration of the origin and maturation sequence of white blood cells is helpful in understanding the classification and behavior of the leukemias and their close relatives, the malignant lymphomas. Most authorities agree that the basic cell of origin is the fixed tissue reticulum cell. Figure 2 shows the normal WBC development sequence. Corresponding malignancy is included in parentheses at each stage.

Note that malignancy may be centered at each major stage in the development sequence of the blood cells. In general, the earlier the stage at which malignancy is centered, the worse the patient's prognosis. Thus, a leukemia whose predominant cell is the myeloblast has a much worse prognosis than one whose predominant cell is the myelocyte.

Acute leukemia is a term originally defined as a leukemia which, if untreated, would be expected to allow an average life span of less than 6 months. The predominant cell is usually the blast (or closely related cells such as the promyelocyte). In most cases, there are over 25% blasts in the peripheral blood and this criterion is the usual basis for establishing the diagnosis of acute leukemia. The one major exception to this is monocytic leukemia, which behaves like acute leukemia even though the number of monoblasts may be very low.

Chronic leukemia is one which, if untreated, would on the average be expected to permit a life span of more than 1 year. The predominant cell forms are more mature; generally, the prognosis is best for those with the most mature forms. Thus, chronic lymphocytic leukemia has a better prognosis than chronic granulocytic (myelocytic) leukemia.

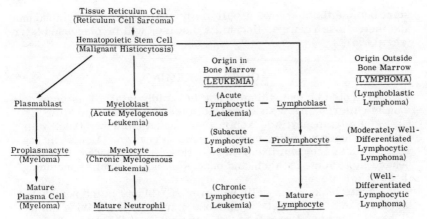

Fig. 2.—Relationship of leukemia and malignant lymphoma to normal WBC maturation sequence.

Subacute leukemia falls between the acute and chronic types.

Leukemia itself is a term which implies malignancy of one of the white cell types, ordinarily implying a situation in which the total number of white cells in the peripheral blood is increased (above the normal range).

Subleukemic leukemia is sometimes used to characterize a leukemia in which the total peripheral blood WBC count is within normal range, but a significant number of immature cells (usually blasts) are present. Aleukemic leukemia is used when the peripheral blood count is normal (or, more often, decreased) and no abnormal cells are found in the peripheral blood. The diagnosis of subleukemic or aleukemic leukemia is made by bone marrow examination. Over 20% blasts in the bone marrow usually means leukemia, and 10-20% is suspicious.

Stem cell leukemia or acute blastic leukemia are terms often applied when nearly all the white cells are blasts and no definite differentiating features are present. Myeloblasts and lymphoblasts are morphologically almost identical. In some cases, it is possible to distinguish between blast types, but for practical purposes it should not be considered reliable. In most cases, the differentiation is made on other information, such as the age of the patient and the types of cells accompanying the blasts. Auer rods are small rod-shaped structures which sometimes are present in the cytoplasm of blasts. When present, these are diagnostic of myeloid cells. They may also be found in the myelomonocytic form of monocytic leukemia.

The malignant lymphomas are basically similar to the lymphocytic leukemias; both derive from the lymphocyte series, but the leukemias originate in the bone marrow, whereas the lymphomas start outside the marrow, usually in lymph nodes.  The lymphomas and their close relative, Hodgkin's disease, will be discussed later (see p. 66).

## ACUTE LEUKEMIA

As noted before, this disease is rapidly fatal.  It is most common in children, but a second peak in frequency is found after age 60.  Acute lymphocytic leukemia is the usual childhood type, with acute myelogenous being most frequent thereafter.  Monocytic leukemia is less frequent than lymphocytic or myelogenous; it tends to behave in an acute fashion, and occurs mainly in adults, including those of middle age.

Acute leukemia usually has over 25% blasts in the peripheral blood and over 50% blasts in the bone marrow.  Sometimes the peripheral blood has fewer than 25%, especially if there is a leukopenia.  The total peripheral WBC count is most often mildly to moderately elevated (15,000-50,000), but a sizable minority of patients have counts in the normal range or leukopenia.  Anemia is present and is generally of moderate to severe degree.  If not present initially, it develops later.  Thrombocytopenia is also found in most cases.

Lymph nodes are often not palpable, although lymphadenopathy of mild degree may be present—especially late in the disease.  The spleen is either normal or only slightly enlarged in most cases.  Generally speaking, enlargement of visceral organs is related to the duration of leukemia, so that the chronic leukemias are usually the ones with marked organomegaly or adenopathy.  A fair number of acute leukemia cases develop ulcerative lesions in the oral mucous membranes or gums—occasionally elsewhere, as in the gastrointestinal tract.  Hemorrhagic phenomena are frequent, due to the thrombocytopenia.  Superimposed infection is common, and is probably the most frequent cause of death.

Several diseases can simulate the clinical and sometimes part of the laboratory picture of acute leukemia.

Infectious mononucleosis is frequently a problem because of the leukocytosis (or initial leukopenia) plus the atypical lymphocytes.  However, infectious mononucleosis almost never has anemia and only rarely has thrombocytopenia.  The bone marrow of infectious mononucleosis is normal, and is not infiltrated by significant numbers of the atypical lymphocytes.  The Paul-Bunnell test is negative in leukemia.

Aplastic anemia may simulate acute leukemia because of peripheral blood pancytopenia.  The bone marrow, however, is usually hypoplastic.  Agranulocytosis often has mouth lesions and has leukopenia, but there is no anemia or thrombocytopenia.

Certain viral diseases, such as mumps, measles, and whooping cough, are occasionally associated with considerably elevated

WBC counts. There may be occasional atypical lymphocytes. There is no anemia or thrombocytopenia. A disease called infectious lymphocytosis occurs in children, but is uncommon. WBC counts may be 40,000-90,000—all mature lymphocytes. This condition lasts only a few days. There are no abnormal cells, no anemia and thrombocytopenia, and there is a normal bone marrow.

Overwhelming infection may cause immature cells and even a few blasts to appear in the peripheral blood of infants and young children, and sometimes other toxic bone marrow stimulation does likewise. There is often anemia and sometimes thrombocytopenia. Bone marrow aspiration may be hypercellular and show marked myeloid hyperplasia, but does not usually have the number of blasts found in leukemia. The peripheral blood blasts are usually less than 5%. They decrease in number and disappear when the underlying disease is treated.

## MONOCYTIC LEUKEMIA

As noted, this entity has the clinical and laboratory aspects of acute leukemia. In monocytic leukemia, however, the number of actual blasts may be low in both the peripheral blood and bone marrow. Instead of blasts there are cells resembling monocytes.

Monocytic leukemia has been subdivided into two types: (1) the so-called pure type (monocytic leukemia of Schilling) and (2) the myelomonocytic type (monocytic leukemia of Naegeli).

Myelomonocytic leukemia is by far the most frequent variety. It actually is a form of myelogenous leukemia, in which the leukemic cells have features both of the more differentiated myeloid line and the more primitive histiocytic precursors of the myeloid cells. The nucleus is histiocytic; the cytoplasm tends to be myelocytic. There may be accompanying myeloid cells which are nonmonocytic less immature forms; if so, this helps make the diagnosis. Sometimes the cells are indistinguishable from those of "pure" monocytic leukemia (Schilling type), but eventually some of them develop myeloid features. If Auer rods are found, this establishes the myeloid derivation of the cells.

Diseases which are accompanied by a monocytosis are sometimes confused with monocytic leukemia. Bone marrow aspiration provides the differentiation. The most common of these diseases are tuberculosis, subacute bacterial endocarditis, and typhoid fever.

## CHRONIC LYMPHOCYTIC LEUKEMIA

This disease is usually found after the age of 50. It is more common in males. Average survival is 3-7 years, with an appreciable number of patients alive even at 8-10 years. WBC counts usually range from 50,000 to 200,000. Most of the white cells are lymphocytic; of these lymphocytes, most (often nearly all) are mature types. In some cases, there may be a considerable number of prolymphocytes and even some blasts, but this is not common. There is mild-to-moderate normocytic-normochromic anemia, usually without reticulocytosis. Platelets are often decreased, but this may not occur until late in the disease. The bone marrow shows over 20% lymphocytes—usually over 50%. There is splenomegaly, usually to at least moderate degree, and often moderate adenopathy. Occasionally, the splenomegaly and adenopathy are marked. There is a considerable tendency to infection, and this is often the cause of death. A Coombs-positive autoimmune hemolytic anemia is reported in about 5-10% of cases; a Coombs-negative hemolytic anemia, often without a reticulocytosis, eventually develops in 15-25% of cases.

## CHRONIC MYELOGENOUS (GRANULOCYTIC) LEUKEMIA

This entity is most common between the ages of 20 and 50 and is rare in childhood. There usually is an increased (total) peripheral white blood cell count. This most often is in the 50,000-200,000 range. There is usually a predominance of myeloid cells having intermediate degrees of maturity, such as the myelocyte and early metamyelocyte. As a matter of fact, the peripheral blood often looks like a bone marrow. Anemia is usually present, although initially it is often slight. Later, anemia becomes moderate. There may be mild reticulocytosis with polychromatophilia and there occasionally are a few nucleated RBC in the peripheral blood. Platelets are either normal or increased. Average patient survival is 2-4 years. Terminally, a picture of acute leukemia often develops, the so-called blast crisis, associated with severe anemia, thrombocytopenia, and myeloblastic type of peripheral blood and bone marrow.

Bone marrow aspiration in chronic myelogenous leukemia shows a markedly hypercellular marrow due to the granulocytes, with intermediate degrees of immaturity. In this respect, it resembles the peripheral blood picture.

On physical examination, there are varying degrees of adenopathy and organomegaly. The spleen is often greatly enlarged, and the liver may be moderately enlarged. Lymph nodes are often easily palpable, but generally only slightly to moderately.

One characteristic of chronic myelogenous leukemia is the finding of increased numbers of basophils in the peripheral blood. The reason for the basophilia is not known.

One interesting nonhematologic aspect of chronic myelogenous leukemia is the presence, in most but not all cases, of a specific chromosome abnormality in the leukemic cells. No other neoplasm thus far has such a consistent finding. The chromosome involved is number 21 in the 21-22 group (of the Denver classification); this contains a characteristic deformity and is called the Philadelphia chromosome. The significance of this genetic abnormality is not clear, since most cases of chronic myelogenous leukemia have no apparent inheritance. Also, acute myelogenous leukemia or the cells of the acute (blastic) terminal crisis of chronic myelogenous leukemia do not possess the Philadelphia chromosome.

When chronic myelogenous leukemia has the typical picture of a WBC count over 100,000 with myelocytic predominance, increased platelets, and a basophilia, the diagnosis is reasonably safe. The two conditions which otherwise may be hard to differentiate are myeloid metaplasia and leukemoid reaction. Leukemoid reaction is an abnormally marked granulocytic response to some bone marrow stimulus, most commonly infection. Leukemoid reaction is basically the same process as an ordinary leukocytosis, except in the degree of response. The expected peripheral blood WBC count elevation is even more marked than usual, and may reach the 50,000-100,000 range in some cases. Instead of the mild degree of immaturity expected which would center in the band neutrophil (stab neutrophil) stage, the immature tendency ("shift to the left") may be extended to earlier cells such as the myelocyte. The bone marrow may show considerable myeloid hyperplasia with unusual immaturity. However, the number of early forms in either the peripheral blood or bone marrow is not usually as great as the classic case of granulocytic leukemia. There is no basophilia, although the increased granulation often seen in neutrophils during severe infection ("toxic granulation") is sometimes mistaken for basophilia. The bone marrow in leukemoid reaction is moderately hyperplastic and may show mild immaturity, but again is not quite as immature as chronic myelogenous leukemia. Splenomegaly and lymphadenopathy may be present in a leukemoid reaction due to the underlying infection, but the spleen is usually not as large as the spleen found in classic chronic myelogenous leukemia.

A disease which is often very difficult to separate from chronic myelogenous leukemia (CML) is agnogenic (idiopathic) myeloid metaplasia (AMM). This is most common in the age group 50-60. The syndrome results from bone marrow failure and subsequent extramedullary hematopoiesis on a large scale by the spleen and sometimes in the liver and lymph nodes. Actually, the extramedullary hematopoiesis is compensatory and therefore not idiopathic (agnogenic), but the reason for the bone marrow failure is. The bone marrow is most commonly replaced by fibrous tissue (myelofibrosis), but sometimes the syndrome of AMM may occur with normally cellular or even hypercellular marrow, at least in the early stages. The average life span is 5-7 years. There is a normochromic anemia of mild-to-moderate degree. There usually is a moderate degree of reticulocytosis and polychromatophilia, more so than with CML. There tends to be a moderate degree of anisocytosis and poikilocytosis, somewhat more than with CML. Abnormal RBC shapes are fairly frequent in AMM, and teardrop forms are very characteristic, although sometimes similar shapes may be found in CML. Nucleated RBC are more frequent in AMM than in CML.

The WBC counts in AMM are most often in the 20,000-50,000 range and very seldom reach 100,000. WBC counts within normal range are not uncommon. Peripheral blood differential counts are similar to CML. There may be basophilia, although this is not as common as in CML. Splenomegaly is usually marked, just as in CML, even when the WBC count is relatively low. Platelets are normal or increased, and giant platelets are often found. Giant platelets may be found in CML but are not too common.

Bone marrow examination is the most valuable differentiating test between CML and AMM. CML has a hypercellular marrow with moderate immaturity. AMM most often has a hypocellular or fibrotic marrow. Often no marrow can be obtained, and sometimes a bone biopsy is necessary to make sure the difficulty was not due to poor technique rather than actual absence of marrow. Sometimes x-ray films will show bone sclerosis, but this is not always true.

Although it would seem by the preceding discussion that differentiation between CML and AMM should be easy, the differences outlined may be slight and may at times appear in either disease. In fact, CML and AMM have been classified together under the term "myeloproliferative syndrome."

A useful test to differentiate leukemoid reaction, CML, and AMM is the neutrophil alkaline phosphatase stain. A fresh peripheral blood smear is stained with a reagent which colors the alkaline phosphatase granules normally found in the cytoplasm of mature and moderately immature neutrophils. One hundred neutrophils are counted, and after each neutrophil is graded 0 to 4 plus, depending on the amount of alkaline phosphatase it possesses, the total count (score) for the 100 cells is added up. In most patients with leukemoid reaction, simple leukocytosis, and leukocytosis of pregnancy or estrogen therapy (birth control pills), and in 80-90% of polycythemia vera patients, the score is higher than normal range. In AMM, about two thirds of patients have elevated values; about 25% fall within normal limits; and about 10% are low. In CML, about 90% are below normal, but 5-10% reportedly have normal values. In acute leukemia, values may be low, normal, or high; the percentage in each category differs in cell types but not enough to provide adequate cell type diagnosis. Infectious mononucleosis in early stages is associated with low or normal values in 95% cases. Enough overlap and borderline cases occur to limit the usefulness of the test in establishing a definitive diagnosis; however, when values are obtained which are well out of normal range, the result can be very helpful in problem cases. However, an experienced technician is needed to make the test reliable, because the test reagents often give trouble, and the reading of the results is often not easy. Therefore, diagnosis should not be based on this test alone. In obvious cases, there is no need to do this test. Values may be normal or elevated in CML during remission, blast crisis, or superimposed bacterial infection.

One other source of confusion with CML is the so-called leu-koerythroblastic marrow response seen occasionally with certain diseases such as septicemia and widespread carcinomatous replace-ment of bone marrow. Anemia is present, and both immature white cells and also nucleated RBC may sometimes appear in the periph-eral blood. A bone marrow usually is diagnostic in widespread marrow neoplasia; blood cultures and neutrophil alkaline phospha-tase are helpful in septicemia.

## POLYCYTHEMIA

Polycythemia is an increase in the total blood red cells over normal range. This usually entails a concurrent increase in hemo-globin and hematocrit. Since various studies disagree somewhat on the values which should be considered the upper limits of normal, partially arbitrary criteria are used to define polycythemia. A he-moglobin of over 18 Gm./100 ml. for men and 16 Gm./100 ml. for women and a hematocrit of over 55% for men and 50% for women are generally considered polycythemic levels.

Polycythemia may be divided into three groups: primary (poly-cythemia vera), secondary, and relative.

Polycythemia vera has sometimes been included with chronic myelogenous leukemia and agnogenic myeloid metaplasia as myelo-proliferative diseases. Polycythemia vera is most frequent between the ages of 40 and 70. In classic cases, peripheral blood WBC and platelets are also increased along with the RBC; however, this is not always found. The peripheral blood WBC count is over 10,000/cu. mm. in 50-70% of the cases. About 20-30% have a leukocytosis over 15,000/cu. mm. of relatively mature forms; about 10% have a leuko-cytosis over 15,000/cu. mm. with a moderate degree of neutrophil immaturity (myelocytes and metamyelocytes present). Platelets are elevated in about 25% of cases. There may be small numbers of polychromatophilic RBC in the peripheral blood, but these are not usually prominent. Splenomegaly occurs in 60-90% of patients, and is more common in those with a leukocytosis. Hepatomegaly is less frequent, but still common (40-50%). Bone marrow aspiration usu-ally shows marrow hyperplasia, with classically an increase in all three blood element precursors—WBC, RBC, and megakaryocytes. A marrow section is much more valuable than marrow smears to demonstrate this. Serum uric acid is elevated in up to 30-40% of cases, due to the increased red cell turnover.

Clinically, there is an increased incidence of peptic ulcer and gout, and a definite tendency toward the development of venous thrombosis.

The classic triad of greatly increased red cell mass (Hb and HCT), leukocytosis with thrombocytosis, and splenomegaly, make the diagnosis obvious. However, often the hemoglobin and hemato-crit are only moderately elevated, and some or all of the other fea-tures may be lacking. The problem then is to differentiate between polycythemia vera and the other causes of polycythemia.

True polycythemia refers to an increase in the total red cell mass (quantity). Relative polycythemia is a term used to describe a normal total red cell mass which falsely appears increased, due to decrease in plasma volume. Dehydration is the most common etiology for relative polycythemia; in most cases, the hematocrit is high normal or only mildly increased, but occasionally it may be substantially elevated. In simple dehydration, other blood constituents such as the WBC, electrolytes, and urea nitrogen (BUN) also tend to be (falsely) elevated. The most definitive test is a blood volume study (p. 111), which will demonstrate that the red cell mass is normal. Stress polycythemia (Gaisböck's syndrome) also is a relative polycythemia due to diminished plasma volume. Most persons affected are middle-aged males; there is a strong tendency toward mild degrees of hypertension, arteriosclerosis, and obesity.

Secondary polycythemia is a true polycythemia, but, as the name implies, it has some specific underlying etiology for the increase in red cell mass. The most common cause is hypoxia. This usually is due to chronic lung disease or to congenital heart disease (although it is also seen in those who live at high altitudes). Cushing's syndrome is rather frequently associated with mild, sometimes moderate, polycythemia. A much less common etiology is certain tumors, most frequently renal carcinoma (hypernephroma) and hepatic carcinoma (hepatoma). There are several other causes, but these are rare. Marked obesity is one (Pickwickian syndrome).

Laboratory tests allow differentiation of these conditions from polycythemia vera.

1. Blood volume measurements (red cell mass plus total blood volume, p. 111) can rule out relative polycythemia. Relative polycythemia has a decreased total blood volume (or plasma volume) and a normal red cell mass.

2. Blood oxygen saturation studies can rule out hypoxic polycythemia. Arterial oxygen saturation is normal in polycythemia vera, and is decreased in hypoxic (secondary) polycythemia.

3. Bone marrow aspiration is often useful, as stated earlier. A marrow section (from clotted marrow left in the syringe and fixed in formalin, then processed like a tissue biopsy) is much better than marrow smears for this purpose. However, even bone marrow sections are not always diagnostic.

4. Serum uric acid levels may be useful in some cases. If the uric acid is elevated, this would be a point in favor of polycythemia vera, since secondary polycythemia has normal uric acid values. However, since uric acid is normal in many cases of polycythemia vera, a normal value is not helpful.

## MALIGNANT LYMPHOMAS

The malignant lymphomas are derived from lymphoid tissue, such as lymph nodes. Lymph nodes are composed of two parts, germinal centers and lymphoreticular tissue. The germinal centers contain lymphoblasts and reticulum cells; these produce the mature lymphocytes and reticulum cells which form the remainder of the lymphoid tissue. Therefore, three main types of cells exist in lymph nodes (and other lymphoid tissue): reticulum cells, lymphoblasts, and lymphocytes. Malignancy may arise from any of these three cell types, as noted before in the early discussion on leukemia. Depending on the cell origin, the malignant lymphomas are divided into three types—reticulum cell sarcoma, lymphocytic lymphoma, and Hodgkin's disease. Lymphocytic lymphoma (lymphosarcoma) may in turn be subdivided into poorly differentiated (lymphoblastic), moderately well differentiated, and well differentiated, depending of course on the predominant degree of differentiation of the lymphoid cells (Table 2). Besides the degree of differentiation, malignant lymphomas may exist in two architectural patterns—nodular and diffuse. In the nodular type, the lymphomatous tissue is distributed in focal aggregates or nodules. In the diffuse type, the lymphoma-tous cells diffusely and completely replace the entire lymph node or the nonlymphoid area invaded. Hodgkin's disease, which will be discussed later, also exists in a nodular or diffuse form, although the nodular variety is rare. In the malignant lymphomas as a whole, the diffuse pattern is more frequent than the nodular one.

TABLE 2.—HISTOLOGIC CLASSIFICATION OF
MALIGNANT LYMPHOMAS

| Cell Type | Histologic Tissue Pattern | |
|---|---|---|
| Lymphocytic lymphoma | | |
| Well differentiated | Nodular (rare) | Diffuse |
| Moderately well differentiated | Nodular | Diffuse |
| Poorly differentiated (lymphoblastic) | Nodular | Diffuse |
| Reticulum cell sarcoma | | |
| (various cell types) | Nodular | Diffuse |
| Hodgkin's disease | Nodular (rare) | Diffuse |

In general, the nodular pattern carries a better prognosis than the corresponding diffuse pattern. The better the cell differentiation, the better the prognosis, just as in the leukemias.

Reticulum cell sarcoma may be found with different types of reticulum cells, but the various cell types all have roughly the same prognosis. Untreated reticulum cell sarcoma has a comparable prognosis to acute leukemia. The same is true for the poorly dif-ferentiated lymphocytic lymphomas. Treatment is somewhat more effective against these neoplasms than it is for acute leukemia.

The nodular form of lymphoma has been called Brill-Symmers disease, or giant follicular lymphoma. This has been reported to have a relatively good prognosis. However, the prognosis depends as much on the cell type as the architectural pattern, so that the poorly differentiated or more primitive cell types do not have a good prognosis even when they appear in a nodular ("follicular") form.

Hodgkin's disease is usually considered a subgroup of the ma-lignant lymphomas. The basic neoplastic cell is the malignant re-ticulum cell. Some of these malignant reticulum cells take on a bi-nucleated or multinucleated form with distinctive large nucleoli and are called Reed-Sternberg cells. These are the diagnostic cells of Hodgkin's disease.

Other types of cells may accompany the Reed-Sternberg cells. Therefore, Hodgkin's disease is usually subdivided according to the cell types present (Fig. 3). Besides Reed-Sternberg cells (R-S cells), there may be various combinations of lymphocytes, histio-cytes, eosinophils, neutrophils, and reticulum cells. The main histologic forms of Hodgkin's disease are the following (using a classification developed at the Armed Forces Institute of Pathology [AFIP]):

1. Paragranuloma: Lymphocytes only (plus R-S cells).

2. Lymphohistiocytic: Lymphocytes and histiocytes (plus R-S cells).

3. Granuloma: At least 3 different cell types (plus R-S cells).

4. Nodular sclerosing: A peculiar variation of granuloma which occurs in the mediastinum and cervical lymph nodes, charac-terized by a nodular pattern, the nodules separated by bands of fibrous tissue.

5. Sclerosing: Rare—granuloma which is mostly replaced by spontaneous fibrosis.

6. Sarcoma: Predominantly malignant reticulum cells (in-cluding R-S cells).

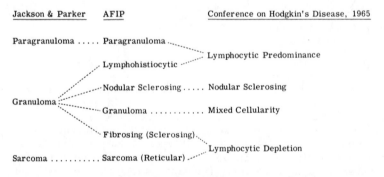

Fig. 3.—Various histologic classifications of Hodgkin's disease.

The prognosis is relatively good for paragranuloma and lym-phohistiocytic Hodgkin's disease (9-15 years average survival), with paragranuloma as a group slightly better than lymphohistiocytic. Granuloma has an intermediate prognosis (average 2-4 years). The nodular sclerosing type as a group falls between paragranuloma and granuloma, with considerable individual variation; a significant num-

ber approaches the paragranuloma survival figures. Hodgkin's sarcoma behaves like reticulum cell sarcoma (as one would expect,
since the cell of origin is the same for both) and therefore has an
average prognosis of 1 year or less. However, life expectancy in
Hodgkin's disease has proved quite variable, and some patients live
for many additional years with the paragranuloma and even the granuloma form. Also of great importance, especially for therapy, is
the degree of spread when the patient is first seen (Table 3). Localized Hodgkin's disease has some possibility of cure by adequate
radiotherapy. Naturally, there is considerable correlation between
the tissue histologic patterns and the clinical stage (degree of localization) that the disease has when first seen.

---

### TABLE 3.—CLINICAL CLASSIFICATION OF THE MALIGNANT LYMPHOMAS

#### (Extended Classification of Peters)

Stage  I:  Localized in one group of lymph nodes.
Stage  II:  Localized in two separate groups of lymph nodes on the
same side of the diaphragm.
Stage III:  Involving components of the lymphoid system (including
spleen) on both sides of the diaphragm, but not other
tissues.
Stage IV:  Involving both lymphoid and nonlymphoid tissue.

---

The diagnosis of malignant lymphoma is made by tissue biopsy,
usually of lymph nodes. As a rule, the peripheral blood and bone
marrow are not involved early in the disease. Later in the disease,
the bone marrow may become infiltrated. In some cases of lymphocytic lymphoma, the lymphoma cells appear in the peripheral blood,
with or without bone marrow invasion. Since lymphocytic leukemia
may, in the later stages, involve and replace lymph nodes, there
occasionally may be a problem in differentiation between lymphocytic leukemia and lymphocytic lymphoma. However, since the two
are equivalent, the differentiation in such cases simply rests on the
peripheral blood and bone marrow findings at the time of first diagnosis. If the marrow is involved, the disease is considered leukemia; if not involved, lymphoma. Reticulum cell sarcoma may
occasionally disseminate malignant cells into the peripheral blood;
this is rare in Hodgkin's disease.

Clinically, malignant lymphoma is more common in males.
The peak incidence for Hodgkin's disease is age 20-40 and for other
malignant lymphomas, age 40-60. Lymph node enlargement is found
in the great majority of cases, but may not become manifest until
later. A palpable spleen is present in about half the cases at some
time during the disease, but is less common with reticulum cell
sarcoma. Fever is present at some time in at least half the cases.

Anemia is found in 33-50%, most commonly in Hodgkin's disease and least commonly in reticulum cell sarcoma. Occasionally, this anemia becomes overtly hemolytic. The platelet count is usually normal unless the bone marrow is extensively infiltrated. The WBC count is usually normal in malignant lymphoma until late in the disease; in Hodgkin's disease, it may be normal, increased, or decreased. WBC differential counts are usually normal in malignant lymphoma unless malignant cells disseminate into the peripheral blood; or, more commonly, if some other condition is superimposed, such as infection. In Hodgkin's disease, lymphopenia is said to be common.

Several diseases may enter into the differential diagnosis of malignant lymphoma. Tuberculosis, sarcoidosis, and infectious mononucleosis all have fever, lymphadenopathy, and, frequently, splenomegaly. The atypical lymphocytes of infectious mononucleosis (p. 191) may simulate lymphocytic lymphoma cells, since both are abnormal lymphocytic forms. Usually, lymphoma cells in the peripheral blood are either more immature or more distorted than the average infectious mononucleosis (virocyte) cell. Nevertheless, since infectious mononucleosis patients are usually younger persons, the finding of lymphadenopathy and a peripheral blood picture similar to infectious mononucleosis in a patient over age 40 would suggest lymphosarcoma (if some other viral illness is not present). This suspicion would be intensified if the Paul-Bunnell (heterophil) test (p. 191) is less than 1:28, or is 1:28-1:112 with a normal differential absorption pattern (two different determinations normal; done 2 weeks apart, to detect any rising titer). Occasionally, the rheumatoid-collagen disease group may cause a clinical picture which might suggest either an occult malignant lymphoma or its early stages. Malignant lymphoma often enters into the differential diagnosis of splenomegaly, especially if no other disease is found to account for the splenomegaly.

As mentioned before, diagnosis of the malignant lymphomas is obtained by tissue biopsy. This usually means lymph node biopsy. The particular node selected is important. The inguinal nodes should be avoided if possible, because they often contain changes due to chronic inflammation which tends to obscure the tissue pattern of a lymphoma. If several nodes are enlarged, the largest one should be selected; when it is excised, the entire node should be taken out intact. This helps to preserve the architectural pattern and allows better evaluation of possible invasion outside the node capsule, one of the histologic criteria for malignancy.

## REFERENCES

Ahmann, D. L., et al.: Malignant lymphoma of the spleen: A review of 49 cases in which the diagnosis was made at splenectomy. Cancer 19:461, 1966.

Bentley, H. P. , et al. : Eosinophilic leukemia, Am. J. Med. 30:310, 1961.

Chikkappa, G. , et al. : Correlation between various blood white cell pools and the serum B12 binding capacities, Blood 37:142, 1971.

Clifford, G. O. : The clinical significance of leukoerythroblastic anemia, M. Clin. North America 50:779, 1966.

Davis, C. S. : Diagnostic value of muramidase, Postgrad. Med. 49:51, 1971.

Escobar, M. A. , and Trobaugh, F. E. : Erythrocythemia, M. Clin. North America 46:253, 1962.

Gilbert, H. S. , and Dameshek, W. : The Myeloproliferative Disorders, in Dowling, H. F. (ed.): Disease-a-Month (Chicago: Year Book Medical Publishers, Inc. , Oct. 1970).

Herbert, V. : Diagnostic and prognostic values of measurement of serum vitamin B12 binding proteins, Blood 32:305, 1968.

Hollander, P. , and Mauer, A. M. : Myeloid leukemoid reactions in children, Am. J. Dis. Child. 105:568, 1963.

Kaplow, L. S. : Leukocyte alkaline phosphatase in disease, CRC Crit. Rev. Clin. Lab. Sc. 2:243, 1971.

Kyle, R. A. , and Pease, G. L. : Basophilic leukemia, Arch. Int. Med. 118:205, 1966.

Linman, J. W. : Differential diagnosis of massive splenomegaly, M. Clin. North America 46:49, 1962.

Lukes, R. J. , et al. : Natural history of Hodgkin's disease as related to its pathologic picture, Cancer 19:317, 1966.

Modan, B. : Polycythemia: A review of epidemiological and clinical aspects, J. Chron. Dis. 18:605, 1965.

Mond, E. : Laboratory tests in leukemia, M. Clin. North America 44:569, 1960.

Pisciotta, A. V. , and Hirschboeck, J. A. : Therapeutic considerations in chronic lymphocytic leukemia, Arch. Int. Med. 99:334, 1957.

Pitcock, J. A. , et al. : A clinical and pathological study of seventy cases of myelofibrosis, Ann. Int. Med. 57:73, 1962.

Prosnitz, L. R. , et al. : Role of laparotomy and splenectomy in the management of Hodgkin's disease, Cancer 29:44, 1972.

Rappaport, H. , et al. : Follicular lymphoma, Cancer 9:792, 1956.

Rebuck, J. W. : Structure of the Lymphocytic Series of Cells in Relation to Disease, in Rebuck, J. W. (ed.): The Lymphocyte and Lymphocytic Tissue (New York: Paul B. Hoeber, Inc. , 1960), p. 260.

Rheingold, J. J. , et al. : Smoldering acute leukemia, New England J. Med. 268:812, 1963.

Rivers, S. L. , et al. : Acute leukemia in the adult male, Cancer 16:249, 1963.

Rosenthal, D. S. , and Maloney, W. C. : Myeloid metaplasia: A study of 98 cases, Postgrad. Med. 45:136, 1969.

Saarni, M. I., and Linman, J. W.: Myelomonocytic leukemia: Dis-
  orderly proliferation of all marrow cells, Cancer 27:1221, 1971.
Sandberg, A. A.: Chromosomes and leukemia, CA 15:2, 1965.
Schwartz, D. L., et al.: Lymphosarcoma cell leukemia, Am. J.
  Med. 38:788, 1965.
Sinn, C. M., and Dick, F. W.: Monocytic leukemia, Am. J. Med.
  20:588, 1956.
Staging in Hodgkin's Disease (Symposium), Cancer Res. 31:1707,
  1971.
Wasserman, L. R., and Gilbert, H. S.: Complications of polycy-
  themia vera, Seminars Hemat. 3:199, 1966.

# CHAPTER 7

# Blood Coagulation

Normally, blood remains fluid within a closed vascular system. Abnormalities of blood coagulation take two main forms—failure to clot normally (and thus to prevent abnormal degrees of leakage from the vascular system) and failure to prevent excessive clotting (and thus maintain the patency of the blood vessels). Most emphasis in clinical medicine has been on diagnosis and treatment of coagulation deficiency. To understand the various laboratory tests designed to pinpoint defects in the coagulation mechanism, it is necessary to outline the most currently accepted theory of blood coagulation (Fig. 4).

The theory states that circulating blood contains two inactive proteins—prothrombin and fibrinogen. When blood comes in contact with an area of damaged blood vessel endothelium, platelets are stimulated to release a coagulation-initiating substance. In conjunction with certain factors present in normal blood (thromboplastin-generating factors) a substance called thromboplastin is formed. With the cooperation of ionized calcium, this thromboplastin catalyzes the conversion of prothrombin to thrombin. The reaction of prothrombin to thrombin is greatly speeded up by certain accelerator factors present in normal blood. Thrombin is a powerful enzyme which acts on the soluble monomer protein fibrinogen and causes it to polymerize to the insoluble product fibrin. Fibrin forms the structural framework of a blood clot. This series of reactions will be discussed in more detail, followed by consideration of laboratory tests which reflect abnormality in the various reactions. Note that many authors use only three stages in their coagulation schemes, combining stage I and II into stage I.

Stage I—The Initiator Reaction: Abnormality in this stage of coagulation concerns defects in platelets, either in number or in

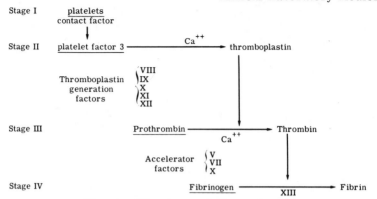

Fig. 4.—Blood coagulation pathway.

functional ability. Also included for purposes of discussion are intrinsic abnormalities of the capillary wall leading to abnormal permeability, either congenital or acquired (although this is not strictly
a part of the blood coagulation sequence itself, it is inseparable
from it clinically).

Stage II—Thromboplastin Generation: The various blood factors involved will be listed and briefly discussed. The biochemistry
of most is obscure, and most have not been isolated in even a relatively pure form. Knowledge of these factors derives mainly from
study of persons who lack one or more of them. They are designated by roman numerals, but other names have been applied to
them in the past and are still frequently used.

Factor VIII (antihemophilic globulin or AHG): Deficiency of
this factor causes classic hemophilia. It is inherited as a sex-
linked recessive gene, so that females with the gene are usually
carriers (heterozygous, xX), and males with the gene have clinical
disease (xY, the hemophilic x gene not being suppressed by a normal X gene as it would be in a female carrier). However, sporadic
cases do occur without known inheritance. Hemophilia can exist in a severe (classic) form or in a mild clinical form, depending on the a-
mount of factor VIII (AHG) the patient has. Classic (severe) hemophil-
iacs show 1-10% of normal factor VIII levels on assay; mild hemo-
philiacs have 10-35% of normal. Carrier females sometimes fall into
the mild group, although usually they are completely asymptomatic.

The major clinical symptom is excessive bleeding. This classically occurs from what would be considered minor trauma or injury (sometimes almost not noticeable) in normal persons. In classic hemophilia, bleeding into joints is a characteristic finding. In
mild hemophilia, there may be only an equivocal history of excessive bleeding or no history at all before severe trauma or surgery
brings the condition to light. Of course, both classic and mild he-
mophiliacs vary somewhat in symptoms, depending on the amount
of AHG they have.

Factor VIII is an unstable substance. Once blood is withdrawn from the body, there begins a slow decay of factor VIII activity which reaches the 50% level at about 1 week. Fresh blood or fresh frozen plasma are the current therapeutic sources of factor VIII. Serum does not contain factor VIII.

Factor IX (plasma thromboplastin component or PTC): Deficiency of this factor creates a condition similar to hemophilia, which has been called Christmas disease (named after the first patient studied in detail). Clinical manifestations may show a severe or mild form, just as in hemophilia. However, although hemorrhage into joints may occur in severe cases, it is not nearly as frequent as in severe hemophilia.

Factor IX is found in both plasma and serum, and is stable in either.

Factor X (Stuart factor): This is the only factor which is equally important in both thromboplastin generation (stage II) and thrombin generation (stage III). Deficiency is rare, and results in a disease similar to hemophilia but somewhat milder, inherited as an incompletely dominant trait. The factor is stable and is present in both serum and plasma.

Factor XI (plasma thromboplastin antecedent or PTA): This is a mild disease. There is usually no history of excessive bleeding, which occurs only after major trauma or during surgery. It occurs in both males and females. The factor is stable and is present in plasma and in serum.

Factor XII (Hageman factor): This is a very strange substance which does not seem to enter into the actual intrinsic blood coagulation mechanisms. Its importance derives from the fact that it is a glass contact factor, and deficiency of factor XII markedly prolongs blood clotting time in glass containers. Since most laboratory tests in hemorrhagic disease are carried out in glass test tubes, a defect in factor XII mimics the effect of the real hemorrhagic stage II factor deficiencies. Factor XII deficiency is detected only on routine laboratory screening tests, since no clinical manifestations are ever produced.

Stage III—Thrombogenesis: This involves conversion of prothrombin to thrombin in the presence of ionized calcium, aided by the accelerator factors.

Prothrombin: This substance is synthesized by the liver. Vitamin K is necessary for its synthesis, although vitamin K is apparently not an actual precursor substance. Vitamin K is a fat-soluble vitamin which is manufactured by small intestinal bacteria from food precursors, but which is itself present in an adequate diet and can be absorbed directly. A deficiency of vitamin K may thus result from malabsorption of fat (such as lack of bile salts in obstructive jaundice, or primary malabsorption of sprue—see Chapter 19); or from failure of the bacteria to synthesize this substance (due to prolonged oral antibiotic therapy). It usually takes more than 3 weeks before the body vitamin K stores are exhausted and thus for deficiency of available vitamin K to become manifest. Dietary lack may be important but ordinarily does not cause a severe enough deficiency to give clinical abnormality unless other factors (such as the anticoagulant vitamin K inhibitors) are present. Assuming normal supplies of available vitamin K, the other main limiting factor in prothrombin formation is the ability of the liver to synthesize it. In severe liver disease (most often far-advanced cirrhosis), enough parenchyma is destroyed to decrease prothrombin formation in a measurable way, eventually leading to a clinical coagulation defect. Whereas a deficiency of available vitamin K responds promptly to administration of parenteral vitamin K, hypoprothrombinemia due to liver parenchymal disease responds little if at all to parenteral vitamin K therapy.

Vitamin K is also necessary for synthesis of factors VII, IX, and X. The greatest effect seems to be on prothrombin and factor VII.

Factor VII (stable factor): As just mentioned, vitamin K is necessary in some way for synthesis, which takes place in the liver. Next to prothrombin, factor VII is affected the most both by lack of vitamin K and by severe parenchymal liver disease. Factor VII is present in serum or plasma, and is stable.

Factor V (labile factor): This substance is apparently also synthesized by the liver, although direct proof is lacking. It is often decreased in severe parenchymal liver disease, although to a somewhat lesser degree than prothrombin and factor VII. Factor V is found in plasma only, and disappears in a few days from stored blood.

Calcium: Ionized calcium is essential for blood coagulation, mainly in stages II and III. Most laboratory anticoagulants, such as oxalate, citrate, and EDTA, take advantage of this by their calcium-binding action. It is very rare to have an ionized (serum) calcium level decreased enough to interfere with clotting; hypocalcemic tetany and death would probably occur first. Massive transfusion of citrated blood rarely makes this "citrate intoxication" a possibility, although when bleeding difficulties are encountered in this situation, it is more likely due to the low platelets or low factor VIII and V levels of bank blood (pp. 87 and 108).

Stage IV—Fibrin Formation: This reaction features the conversion of fibrinogen to fibrin, catalyzed by previously formed thrombin. Besides catalyzing the reaction, some of the thrombin is apparently adsorbed onto the clot as it forms, so that eventually not enough thrombin is left to carry the reaction further. This provides a limiting mechanism to the coagulation process.

Factor XIII is known as fibrin-stabilizing factor. Subclinical deficiency occurs in a variety of conditions, such as severe liver damage; clinically evident defects are rare, and the few cases reported are mostly in newborns. The results of all the usual coagulation tests are normal.

Fibrinogen is a protein which, like so many other coagulation substances, is synthesized in the liver. Apparently the production mechanism is very efficient, because hypofibrinogenemia due to liver disease is extremely uncommon. In some patients with cirrhosis there is a mild degree of fibrinolytic activity, usually not enough to be evident clinically, due to circulating fibrinolysins. Low plasma fibrinogen levels are most often due to certain obstetrical conditions, the most common being premature separation of the placenta. A thromboplastin tissue substance is liberated into the blood stream and causes fibrin deposition (clots) in small blood vessels, thus depleting the plasma of the precursor substance fibrinogen ("defibrination syndrome"). Hypofibrinogenemia may also be due to circulating fibrinolysins—enzymes which destroy fibrinogen. This most often occurs in disseminated prostate carcinoma, although other carcinomas have also been associated. Fibrinolysins have been occasionally reported after extensive surgery, most often pulmonary operations. Fibrinolysin may rarely accompany a wide variety of diseases, and may rarely appear without any apparent cause.

The defibrination syndrome is becoming better known as disseminated intravascular coagulation (DIC). This is a much more frequent cause for hypofibrinogenemia than primary fibrinolysis. Originally considered an obstetrical disease, DIC is now being attributed to a growing list of etiologies, among which are septicemia, surgery complicated by postoperative shock, severe burns or trauma, extensive cancer, and newborn respiratory distress syndrome; and it is occasionally seen in many other conditions. Shock is the best common denominator but is not always present; nor has it been definitely proved to be either a cause or an effect. A wide range of laboratory tests have been advocated for diagnosis of DIC, many of which are being discarded as newer tests are announced or older ones re-evaluated. At present, hypofibrinogenemia and thrombocytopenia are the two best-established lab findings. Cases have been reported in which either fibrinogen or platelet levels are normal. Other lab procedures are discussed in the section on protamine sulfate test (p. 81).

Some persons with dysproteinemia, either multiple myeloma or one of the macroglobulinemias, have interference with conversion of fibrinogen to fibrin despite normal fibrinogen levels. This is manifest by poor clot stability and failure of clot retraction, and may cause a hemorrhagic tendency or purpura.

## INHIBITOR SYSTEMS

Having discussed the blood coagulation substances and the blood factors which are involved in their activation, we should give some attention to inhibitors of various essential substances in this system. These inhibitors retard coagulation, and thus are considered anticoagulants.

Dicumarol and the Coumadin Drugs: These inhibit the utilization of vitamin K by the liver and therefore decrease prothrombin synthesis (as well as the other vitamin K-dependent factors). Dicumarol affects mainly stage III in the coagulation scheme. The most frequent clinical sign of Coumadin toxicity is hematuria.

Heparin: Heparin has both antithrombin and antithromboplastin activity. Therefore, anticoagulation effects are seen in both stage III (which requires thromboplastin) and stage IV (which requires thrombin). Protamine sulfate is a specific neutralizing agent for heparin.

Severe Liver Disease: This was discussed earlier. The main effect is on stage III of coagulation.

The Plasmin System: This is an intrinsic blood fibrinolytic system. Plasmin is a fibrinolytic enzyme which exists in blood as the inactive precursor plasminogen. A trigger mechanism is needed to set off the reaction. This may be accomplished by certain enzymes such as streptokinase or by other means, at present poorly understood. Note that the mechanism involved is very similar to that of coagulation stage IV, except that the activator is streptokinase (or other enzymes) instead of thrombin, and the reaction catalyzed is plasminogen to plasmin instead of fibrinogen to fibrin. There also are inhibitors of the plasmin system, just as antithrombins may inhibit stage IV coagulation development. In the plasmin system, the most effective inhibitor available is a compound called epsilon-aminocaproic acid (EACA). This provides effective therapy for many cases of circulating fibrinolytic anticoagulants. However, note that EACA would not affect a hypofibrinogenemia due to disseminated intravascular fibrin coagulation (most commonly seen in obstetrics, as mentioned earlier), where the plasmin mechanism is not involved.

## TESTS IN HEMORRHAGIC DISORDERS

1. History: History of easy bleeding or easy bruising should lead to further investigation.

2. Platelet Count: Platelet disorders will be discussed later. Using the direct count (normal values 150,000-300,000), a platelet count below 100,000/cu. mm. indicates moderate thrombocytopenia; under 50,000/cu. mm. means severe thrombocytopenia. Platelet number can be estimated with a reasonable degree of reliability from a well-made peripheral blood smear.

3. Clot Retraction: Platelets have a major role in clot retraction. The clot shrinks and pushes out serum which was trapped within as the blood clotted. The shrunken clot is much firmer than it was originally. Normally, clot retraction begins at about 1 hour and is complete by 24 hours. With thrombocytopenia, there is deficient clot retraction.

4. Tourniquet Test: This demonstrates capillary fragility, due either to intrinsic defect in capillary walls (vascular purpura) or to some types of thrombocytopenia. The tourniquet test is usu-

ally positive with idiopathic thrombocytopenic purpura (ITP), immunologic or drug-induced thrombocytopenia. It gives variable,
more often negative, results with thrombocytopenia from other
causes. It is usually negative in stages II, III, and IV defects, but
occasionally may be positive.

5. Bleeding Time: The routine bleeding and clotting times
used for presurgery screening tests have been shown to be highly
inaccurate and inefficient. An Ivy technique bleeding time is preferred when such a procedure is indicated. The bleeding time is
most helpful as an indication of defective capillary wall function.
It is also positive in immunologic thrombocytopenic purpura, and
is positive in most, but not all, cases of severe thrombocytopenia.
It is usually positive in thrombocytopathia (Glanzmann's disease),
whereas the tourniquet test is variable. In stage II defects, it is
variable, often normal in mild cases. In stages III and IV defects,
it is more often normal, but may be positive if the defect is severe.

6. Prothrombin Time (PT Time): A "complete" tissue thromboplastin (which contains a platelet substitute) plus calcium is added
to the patient's plasma. Formation of a fibrin clot is the end point.
The PT time shows mainly defects in stage III, most often prothrombin. Nevertheless, single or multiple stage III (factors V, VII, or
X) defects of sufficient severity will give abnormal results, not just
prothrombin deficiency. Usually, however, factors V and VII defects are accompanied by prothrombin deficiency. Moreover, if defects in stage IV are severe, they will also produce abnormal test
results, since the test depends on an intact stage IV to produce the
clot end point. However, the fibrinogen level usually must be under
100 mg./100 ml. (normal 200-400 mg./100 ml.) before hypofibrinogenemia affects the PT time. Stages I and II defects do not influence
the PT time, because a complete thromboplastin reagent is provided.

7. Partial Thromboplastin Time (PTT): An "incomplete"
thromboplastin reagent plus calcium is added to the patient's plasma
in the same way as the PT time. This incomplete (partial) thromboplastin is essentially only a platelet substitute, with all the other
thromboplastin factors lacking. The PTT is very sensitive to defects in stage II. It may also be abnormal in stages III and IV defects, but only if severe (stages III and IV may influence the test because the test depends on fibrin clot formation as the end point).
The reason that the PTT is not as sensitive to stage III defects as
the PT is that the extrinsic thromboplastin used in the PT is more
powerful than the intrinsic thromboplastin generated in the PTT,
thus enabling the PT to demonstrate relatively smaller defects in
the substrate prothrombin or the accelerator factors. Stage I abnormalities do not influence the PTT. Also, deficiency of factor VII
does not influence the PTT, for unknown reasons.

8. Prothrombin Consumption Test (PCT): This is also called
the serum prothrombin time or the two-stage prothrombin time.
The patient's blood is drawn and allowed to clot. A standard PT
time is then run on the serum left after the clot. $Al(OH)_3$ absorbed

normal plasma without prothrombin is added to provide an end point. If prothrombin was utilized normally when the patient's blood clotted, only a very small amount of prothrombin will remain in the serum unused, and the serum PT time will be considerably prolonged. However, if a defect is present in either stage I or stage II, the utilization of prothrombin will be decreased and a greater amount will be left in the serum, thus shortening the serum PT time. The platelet defect in stage I may be either defect in platelet quantity or a normal quantity but defective function (thrombasthenia). The PCT is thus very sensitive to stage I and stage II defects, but is not influenced by stage III and stage IV defects (unless there was a circulating anticoagulant).

9. Venous Clotting Time (VCT): The Lee-White method is preferred. Technique is extremely important. When the usual three test tubes are used, tube #3 is filled first, since the last blood to enter the syringe is probably least contaminated with tissue juice. With glass syringes, start the test timing as soon as blood enters the syringe. With plastic syringes, one can wait until blood enters tube #3 (the first tube filled) to start the test timing, because clotting time in plastic is prolonged. The VCT is affected mainly by defects in stages II and IV. It is not sensitive to defects in stage I, and is relatively insensitive to defects in stage III, where extremely severe deficiency is required to show significant VCT abnormality. In stages II and IV, the test is only moderately sensitive, requiring considerable quantitative deficiency to cause abnormal test results.

It might be useful to compare the results of the laboratory tests just discussed in the various stages of blood coagulation:

|       | Stage I | Stage II | Stage III | Stage IV |
|-------|---------|----------|-----------|----------|
| PT    | no      | no       | VS        | ins.     |
| PTT   | no      | VS       | ins.      | ins.     |
| PCT   | VS      | VS       | no*       | no*      |
| VCT   | no      | mod. S   | ins.      | mod. S   |

*Unless circulating anticoagulants are present.
VS = very sensitive; ins. = insensitive; mod. S = moderately sensitive.

In hemophilia (factor VIII defect), the various tests have approximately the following sensitivity:

VCT—normal until AHG values are less than 2% of normal.
PCT—normal until AHG values are less than 10% of normal.
PTT—normal until AHG values are less than 30-35% of normal.

Note that normal persons may show 60-100% of "normal" levels on factor VIII assay.

10. Thromboplastin Generation Time (TGT): This is the basic reference test for pinpointing defects in stage II, and can be used to assay the degree of defect. This procedure tests the ability of the patient to generate thromboplastin (stage II). If the patient's platelets are used in the TGT instead of a platelet substitute, a sensitive assay system for stage I is added, which reflects deficiency either

in number or in function of the platelets. The TGT is quite complicated and time consuming, demanding an expert technician and strict attention to a considerable number of technical details in order to provide reliable results. Therefore, only a relatively few research centers do this procedure. The TGT is extremely sensitive to stage II defects, detecting abnormality of AHG when less than 30% of normal levels is present. As mentioned, the TGT can also pinpoint what the stage II defect is. Stages III and IV defects can be detected, but are more easily picked up by other tests.

11. Plasma Fibrinogen: A fibrin clot is precipitated from plasma, either by adding thrombin or calcium. The fibrin clot is then quantitated chemically by one of several indirect methods. Mild cases of circulating fibrinolysins have normal plasma fibrinogen. However, if the fibrinolysin is potent, fibrinogen may be inactivated as well, so that a fibrin clot cannot be produced by ordinary methods and plasma fibrinogen will appear falsely low or absent. True low plasma fibrinogen levels may be due to primary fibrinolysins or to the disseminated intravascular coagulation (DIC) syndrome (p. 77). DIC is by far the more common. A thromboplastin tissue substance or equivalent in action is liberated in the blood stream and causes fibrin deposition (clots) in small blood vessels.

12. Clot Lysis Test: This is a simple yet fairly sensitive and fairly reliable test for circulating fibrinolysins. Normally, a blood clot retracts and forms a solid, firm, hard mass. Circulating fibrinolysin in sufficient quantity attacks and dissolves the clot. This is different from the clot retraction defect of thrombocytopenia, where the clot forms and simply does not retract well, but does not dissolve. In mild cases of circulating fibrinolysins, the patient's own blood will clot, followed by clot lysis. However, if the fibrinolysin is potent, fibrinogen may be inactivated and the blood will not clot; in these cases, plasma fibrinogen level determinations will show a falsely low level, as noted above. The clot lysis test should then be done by adding the patient's plasma to a fresh blood clot from a normal person. The euglobulin lysis test, which is a variation of the clot lysis procedure, is considered more sensitive and accurate. However, it is not as widely available.

13. Protamine Sulfate Test: Normally, thrombin catalyzes conversion of fibrinogen to fibrin monomers; fibrin monomers then polymerize with the assistance of factor XIII. Polymerized (clotted) fibrin is the scaffolding on which a blood clot forms. Fibrinolysins may attack either fibrinogen or fibrin, splitting off fragments ("split products") which in turn are broken into smaller pieces. These split products may form a complex with fibrin monomers and prevent polymerization. Protamine sulfate in low concentration is thought to release fibrin monomers from the split product complex and allow the monomers to polymerize. The test is positive in conditions producing secondary fibrinolysin and is negative with primary fibrinolysin. Primary fibrinolysin will not induce a protamine sul-

fate reaction because the end point of this test depends on the presence of fibrin monomers produced by action of thrombin. Primary fibrinolysin is not ordinarily associated with activation of the thrombin clotting mechanism.

Since DIC is the major condition associated with substantial production of secondary fibrinolysin, recent studies endorse protamine sulfate as the best screening test for DIC. Negative results would be strong evidence against DIC. Various modifications of the protamine sulfate method are being introduced. These vary in sensitivity, so that it is difficult to compare results in diseases other than DIC. Any condition leading to intravascular clotting may conceivably produce secondary fibrinolysin; these conditions include pulmonary embolization, leg vein thrombosis, and postoperative complications. Occasional positive results have been reported without good explanation.

Classic lab findings in DIC include hypofibrinogenemia (leading to abnormal PTT and PT) and thrombocytopenia. In mild cases these tests may be within normal limits. The protamine sulfate test is positive, apparently even in some of the milder cases. The clot lysis test is most often negative.

## WORKUP FOR HEMORRHAGIC PROBLEMS

A basic workup for suspected or actual hemorrhagic problems begins with a good history. Laboratory tests include a bleeding time and a tourniquet test (to rule out capillary fragility), a platelet count (to rule out thrombocytopenia), a PT time (to rule out stage III defects), and a PTT (to rule out stage II defects). For example, a normal PT with an abnormal PTT means a stage II defect only; the opposite results would point toward a pure stage III defect, while finding both tests abnormal would suggest factor X or a stage IV problem (although marked defects in prothrombin or factor V can begin to affect the PTT). Stage IV defects may then be investigated with a plasma fibrinogen level and a protamine sulfate test; if necessary, a clot lysis test may be done. In this manner, one can narrow down the problem to a manageable size. Once the problem area is isolated, the exact defect can be pinpointed using specialized procedures, such as the TGT (or PCT if the TGT is not available), details of which are listed in standard textbooks on the subject. Also, diseases present or drugs which are known to cause difficulty in a certain coagulation area certainly call for the selected tests referable to that problem.

If facilities for specialized coagulation tests are not available, a coagulation defect can be further isolated by means of certain simple correction experiments. Normal serum contains factors VII, IX, X, XI, and XII. Therefore, one can mix an equal quantity of the patient's fresh oxalated plasma with normal serum. If the mixture of patient's plasma and normal serum corrects the coagulation defect, the defect must be due to one of the factors supplied by the normal serum. Similar procedures can be used to further isolate the individual defect, and actually are carried out as part of the TGT; however, they should be left to persons experienced in their performance and interpretation.

Anticoagulation by Coumadin-type drugs is best monitored by the PT time. Therapeutic range varies with each manufacturer's thromboplastin (p. 440); the most commonly desired effect is a reduction to a level of 10-20% of those clotting factors affected by Coumadin. A recent report indicates that the commonly accepted therapeutic range of 2.0-2.5 times control cannot be blindly imposed on all thromboplastins because of variability in composition and thereby in effect on clotting factors. Results in terms of seconds compared to control is preferred to percentage of normal, because percentage must be based on dilution curves which frequently are inaccurate.

Anticoagulation by heparin is monitored by the VCT, because heparin effects on either stage II or stage III tests separately are too variable, and because the desired action of heparin is to decrease whole blood clotting. The therapeutic range is a VCT time of 20-30 minutes. The plasma recalcification time (PRT) can be used instead of the VCT; it offers advantages in terms of better reproducibility and convenience. The "activated" PTT may also replace the VCT. "Activation" consists in adding a substance to the PTT reagent which activates contact factor (XII) swiftly and uniformly and thus eliminates one variable in the clotting process.

Although the coagulation theory outlined in Figure 4 is probably the best sequence to explain coagulation test actions, it very likely is not the actual manner in which blood clots. A current and widely accepted theory is presented in Figure 4a.

Fig. 4a. —Blood coagulation pathway.

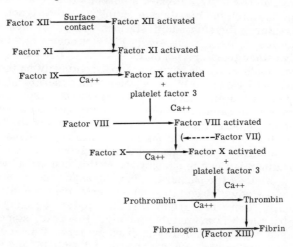

## VASCULAR DEFECTS

A disease that combines platelet abnormality with other defects produces a hemorrhagic disorder, sometimes quite severe. This condition is frequently termed "von Willebrand's disease." It has also been called "pseudohemophilia." Although there is considerable dispute as to just what this disease should include, it is generally restricted to a congenital (hereditary) type of disorder. These patients have an abnormal bleeding time (and, in many cases, a positive tourniquet test) with abnormal platelet adhesiveness. Some investigators have found decreased factor VIII levels in many of these patients; also, there is some evidence that although much of the defect lies in defective platelet adhesiveness, there may be increased rather than intrinsic capillary fragility.

A frequent nonhereditary type of vascular fragility problem is called "senile purpura." Localized purpuric lesions or small bruises develop on the extremities in older people. The only laboratory abnormality is a positive tourniquet test in some of the cases. A somewhat similar clinical condition is the easy bruising found in many younger adult persons, especially women. The reason is unknown, and all results of laboratory tests are usually normal, except for an occasional positive tourniquet test. Also, the exanthems produced by viral infection might be included in this group.

It should be mentioned that continued or intermittent bleeding from a small localized area is most often due to physical agents (such as repeated trauma) or to a local condition (such as scar tissue) which prevents normal small vessel retraction and subsequent closure by thrombosis.

Allergic (anaphylactoid) purpura is characterized by small blotchy hemorrhages over the extremities and bilateral ankle swelling. The cause is allergy, but it may also appear in association with glomerulonephritis. Henoch's purpura is a subdivision of this condition, in which the bleeding is mainly in the GI tract. Schönlein's purpura features the skin manifestations without GI involvement. The tourniquet test is usually positive. Platelet counts and results of other laboratory tests are normal.

Occasional cases of purpura, most commonly on the extremities, have been reported in association with hyperglobulinemia. This may be idiopathic, secondary to various diseases (such as cirrhosis or granulomatous infection) which produce considerably elevated gamma globulin levels, or secondary to one of the "monoclonal gammopathies." These globulins are not macroglobulins, however. It may or may not be accompanied by cryoglobulinemia. "Purpura hyperglobulinemia" is one name given to this condition, which is not a frequent etiology for purpura. The tourniquet test is sometimes positive; most other coagulation defect tests are normal.

Finally, there is a group which simulates capillary fragility defects, but which is primarily embolic. However, some element of increased capillary fragility is often present. These diseases include subacute bacterial endocarditis, fat emboli, and some cases

of septicemia (although other cases of septicemia also have thrombocytopenia). The tourniquet test is often positive, and the bleeding
time is variable. Other coagulation defect tests are normal (except
as mentioned).

## PLATELET DEFECTS

Platelet defects affect stage I of the clotting mechanism. They
may be due to decreased number (thrombocytopenia) or defective
function (thrombasthenia). Defective platelet function (with normal
platelet count) is uncommon, the most famous examples being hereditary thrombasthenia (Glanzmann's purpura). The platelets are large
and do not function normally. In some cases of uremia and occasional
cases of severe chronic liver disease, defective platelet function has
been observed even in the absence of the thrombocytopenia that these
patients may occasionally also develop. Giant platelets may be found
in certain conditions, especially in myeloid metaplasia (less often in
chronic myelocytic leukemia), but platelet function in these other
diseases does not seem to suffer materially. Interestingly enough,
when greatly increased platelet numbers are found (thrombocythemia),
such as occasionally is seen in chronic myelocytic leukemia or polycythemia vera, a bleeding tendency may appear. Very high platelet
counts (over 1 million/cu. mm.) seem to interfere with thromboplastin generation (stage II of coagulation).

Clinically, purpura is the hallmark of platelet defects. Most
other types of coagulation disorders do not produce purpura.

Most platelet problems involve defects in number (thrombocytopenia). In general, such conditions may be classified according
to etiology.

1. Acquired immunologic thrombocytopenia.
2. Idiopathic thrombocytopenic purpura.
3. Hypersplenism.
4. Bone marrow hypoplasia.
5. Toxic or other causes.

1. Acquired Immunologic Thrombocytopenia: This syndrome
occurs due to idiosyncratic hypersensitivity to certain drugs. This
may develop either during initial, continued, or intermittent use of
the drug; once commencing, platelet depression occurs swiftly. The
bone marrow shows most often normal or increased megakaryocytes. Degenerative changes are frequent. The most frequently
associated drugs are quinidine, various sulfonamides, and ristocetin (Spontin), but many other drugs have been incriminated in rare
cases. Of course, even with the relatively frequent offenders, this
effect is very uncommon. Platelet antibodies have been demonstrated in many cases.

2. Idiopathic Thrombocytopenic Purpura (ITP): This syndrome may exist in either an acute or a chronic form. The acute
form is usually seen in children, has a sudden onset, lasts a few
days to a few weeks, and does not recur. The majority of cases

follow infection, most often viral, but some do not have a known precipitating cause. The chronic form is more common, and is not frequent after age 40. There are usually remissions and exacerbations over variable periods of time. No precipitating disease or other factor is usually found. Platelet antibodies have been found in many patients with ITP.

Clinically, there is purpura or other hemorrhagic manifestations. The spleen is usually not palpable, and an enlarged spleen is evidence against the diagnosis of ITP. Bone marrow aspiration shows a normal or increased number of megakaryocytes, although not always.

3. Hypersplenism: This entity was discussed in Chapter 4 (see p. 49). The syndrome may be primary or secondary; if secondary, it is most commonly due to portal hypertension. There may be any combination of anemia, leukopenia, or thrombocytopenia, but isolated thrombocytopenia is a fairly frequent manifestation. The spleen is usually palpable, but not always. Bone marrow megakaryocytes are normal or increased. The thrombocytopenia seen in lupus erythematosus is often secondary to splenic involvement even though the spleen is often not palpable.

4. Bone Marrow Hypoplasia: This condition and its various etiologies was discussed in Chapter 3 (see p. 28). This group forms a large and important segment of the thrombocytopenias, and is the reason why bone marrow examination is nearly always indicated in a patient with thrombocytopenia.

Thrombocytopenia is a very frequent feature of acute leukemia and monocytic leukemia. This is true even when the peripheral blood WBC pattern is aleukemic. It may also occur in the terminal stages of chronic leukemia.

Aplastic anemia and extensive replacement of bone marrow by tumor often includes thrombocytopenia as an accompanying finding.

5. Toxic or Other Causes: A miscellaneous group is left which includes several unrelated disorders:

a) Neonatal thrombocytopenia: This may be due to ITP or idiosyncratic platelet antibodies in the mother, may follow virus infection in utero, or may be idiopathic. Hemorrhagic manifestations are usually not severe, and the symptoms subside spontaneously.

b) Thrombotic thrombocytopenic purpura (Moschcowitz's disease) is a very uncommon disorder which is most frequent in young adults, although it may occur at any age. There is a characteristic triad of severe hemolytic anemia, thrombocytopenia and multiple shifting neurologic symptoms. The WBC count is usually increased, although it may be normal. Fibrin and platelet thrombi occur in capillaries and small arterioles, giving rise to the symptoms. Diagnosis is through biopsy, usually of the kidney,

      although other tissues (even bone marrow sections) have
been used.

c) Megaloblastic anemia: In untreated, well-established
cases, occasionally even when clinically mild, thrombocytopenia occurs as a frequent manifestation of the $B_{12}$
and folic acid deficiency anemias. In chronic iron deficiency anemia, platelets are normal and may at times actually be somewhat increased.

d) Infections: Transient thrombocytopenia may be an uncommon manifestation of a wide variety of severe infections or
septicemia. It occasionally follows various viral infections.

    Massive Transfusions with Stored Bank Blood: If given during
a relatively short period, thrombocytopenia may develop, due to the
low functional platelet content of stored bank blood. This may or
may not be accompanied by a bleeding tendency. However, deficiency
of factors V and VIII (the unstable clotting factors) may contribute to
any bleeding problem from this source. It takes at least 5 units of
blood, and usually over 10, given in 1-2 days' time.

    The etiologic diagnosis of purpura should begin with a platelet
count and a complete blood count (CBC), with special emphasis on
the peripheral blood smear. Investigation of thrombocytopenia
should include a platelet count and a bone marrow examination utilizing preferably both a clot section and a smear technique. The
clot section affords a better estimate of cellularity. The smear allows better study of morphology. This is true for megakaryocytes
as well as other types of cells. Investigation of purpura without
thrombocytopenia should include a bleeding time and tourniquet test,
attempting to demonstrate abnormal capillary fragility. These tests
are not indicated in already known thrombocytopenia, because their
results would not add any useful information. If the platelet count
is normal and thrombasthenia is suspected, a PCT or TGT should
be run (using the patient's platelets in the TGT). The other tests
for hemorrhagic disease must previously rule out abnormality in
other areas. Occasional cases of nonthrombocytopenic purpura are
caused by abnormal serum proteins, which may be demonstrated by
serum protein electrophoresis (then confirmed by other tests, described in Chapter 21).

    Usually, a bleeding tendency does not develop in thrombocyto-
penia until the platelet count is less than 100,000/cu. mm. (direct
method), and most often does not occur until the platelet count is
below 50,000 cu. mm. The 50,000 value is usually considered the
critical level. However, some patients do not bleed even with platelet counts near zero, while occasionally there may be trouble with
those above 50,000. Most likely there is some element of capillary
fragility involved, but the actual reason is not known at this time.

## BLEEDING PROBLEMS IN SURGERY

Bleeding constitutes a major concern to surgeons; problems may arise during operation or postoperatively, and bleeding may be concealed or grossly obvious. The major causes are:

1. Physical defect in hemostasis—improper vessel ligation, overlooking a small transected vessel, or other failure to achieve adequate hemostasis.

2. Unrecognized preoperative bleeding problem—one of the coagulation defects present which was not recognized prior to surgery. This may be congenital (such as the hemophilias), may be secondary to a disease that the patient has (such as cirrhosis), or may be due to drug therapy (such as anticoagulants).

3. Transfusion reactions or complications from massive transfusion.

4. Unexplained bleeding difficulty.

Unusual bleeding has some correlation to the type (magnitude) of the operative procedure, the length of the operation, and the particular disease involved. The more that any of these parameters is increased, the more likely that excessive bleeding might occur. In most cases, the defect can be traced by means of laboratory tests; or, retrospectively, by re-establishing physical hemostasis. However, of category number 4 (unexplained etiology), after thorough investigation, some patients still show no real explanation. Nevertheless, this fact cannot be used as an excuse for inadequate workup, because proper therapy depends on finding the etiology. This is why some knowledge of blood coagulation is necessary.

## REFERENCES

Alami, S. Y., et al.: Fibrin stabilizing factor (factor XIII), Am. J. Med. 44:1, 1968.

Bachman, F.: Paradoxes of disseminated intravascular coagulation, Hosp. Practice 6:113, 1971.

Bleeding and the Surgical Patient (Conference Proceedings), Ann. New York Acad. Sc. 115:1-542, 1964.

Bowie, E. J. W., and Owen, C. A.: The diagnosis of von Willebrand's disease, Ann. Clin. Lab. Sc. 1:85, 1971.

Coleman, R. W., et al.: Statistical comparison of the automated activated partial thromboplastin time and the clotting time in the regulation of heparin therapy, Am. J. Clin. Path. 53:904, 1970.

Conference on Platelet Transfusions, Transfusion 6:1-63, 1966.

Day, H. J., and Holmsen, H.: Laboratory tests of platelet function, Ann. Clin. Lab. Sc. 2:63, 1972.

Deykin, D.: The clinical challenge of disseminated intravascular coagulation, New England J. Med. 283:636, 1970.

Diamond, L. K., and Porter, F. S.: Inadequacies of routine bleeding and clotting times, New England J. Med. 259:1025, 1958.

Friedman, L. L.: Familial Glanzmann's thrombasthenia, Mayo Clin. Proc. 39:908, 1964.

Gurewich, V., and Hutchinson, E.: Detection of intravascular coagulation by a serial-dilution protamine sulfate test, Ann. Int. Med. 75:895, 1971.

Hathaway, W. E.: Bleeding disorders due to platelet dysfunction, Am. J. Dis. Child. 121:127, 1971.

Hemofil and Other Factor VIII Concentrates, Med. Letter Drugs & Therapeutics 11:96 (Nov. 14), 1969.

Karpatkin, M.: Diagnosis and management of disseminated intravascular coagulation, Pediat. Clin. North America 18:23, 1971.

Karpatkin, S.: Autoimmune thrombocytopenic purpura, Am. J. M. Sc. 261:127, 1971.

Marcus, A. J.: Platelet function, New England J. Med. 280:1213, 1278, 1330, 1969.

Miale, J. B., and Kent, J. W.: Standardization of the therapeutic range for oral anticoagulants based on standard reference plasmas, Am. J. Clin. Path. 57:80, 1972.

Post, R. M., and Desforges, J. F.: Thrombocytopenia and alcoholism, Ann. Int. Med. 68:1230, 1968.

Prentice, C. R. M., and Ratnoff, O. D.: Genetic disorders of blood coagulation, Seminars Hemat. 4:93, 1967.

Quick, A. J.: The Minot-von Willebrand syndrome, Am. J. M. Sc. 253:520, 1967.

Ratnoff, O. D.: Hemostatic mechanisms in liver disease, M. Clin. North America 47:721, 1963.

Rossi, E. C. (ed.): Symposium on hemorrhagic disorders, M. Clin. North America 56:3, 1972.

Rozengvaig, S., et al.: Benign purpura hyperglobulinemia, A.M.A. Arch. Int. Med. 99:913, 1957.

Schloesser, L. L., et al.: Thrombocytosis in iron-deficiency anemia, J. Lab. & Clin. Med. 66:107, 1965.

Schulman, I.: Pediatric aspects of the mild hemophilias, M. Clin. North America 46:93, 1962.

Udall, J. A.: Human sources and absorption of vitamin K in relation to anticoagulation stability, J.A.M.A. 194:127, 1965.

Weintraub, R. M., et al.: Rapid diagnosis of drug-induced thrombocytopenic purpura, J.A.M.A. 180:130, 1962.

Willoughby, M. L. N., and Crouch, S. J.: Hemorrhagic tendency in renal failure, Brit. J. Haemat. 7:315, 1961.

Yip, M. L. B., et al.: Nonspecificity of the protamine test for disseminated intravascular coagulation, Am. J. Clin. Path. 57:487, 1972.

Yoshikawa, T., et al.: Infection and disseminated intravascular coagulation, Medicine 50:237, 1971.

Ziegler, F. D., and Kelly, J. H.: The critical evaluation of thromboplastin, Ann. Clin. Lab. Sc. 2:16, 1972.

# CHAPTER 8

# Immunohematology: Antibodies and Antibody Tests

Before discussing this subject, it is useful to give some definitions:

Antigen: Any substance which causes formation of antibodies to it. The most common antigens are protein, but certain carbohydrate polysaccharides may act in a similar manner. Lipid may be combined with either. Each antigen has a certain chemical configuration which gives it antibody-provoking ability. This specific chemical group may become detached from its carrier molecule and temporarily lose antigenic power; it is then called a hapten. Attachment of a hapten to another suitable molecule leads to restoration of antigenic properties.

Antibody: Serum proteins produced by the reticuloendothelial system in response to antigenic stimulation. Antibodies are globulins—most often gamma globulins. They may be specific, combining only with specific antigen molecules, or nonspecific, combining with a variety of antigens. Presumably, nonspecific antibodies attack a variety of molecules because similar hapten groups may be present even though the carrier molecule is different (so-called cross reactivity).

Agglutinogen: Antigen on the surface of a red blood cell.

Agglutinin: Antibody which attacks red blood cell antigens and manifests this activity by clumping the RBC.

Hemolysin: Same as an agglutinin except that lysis of affected erythrocytes takes place.

Isoantibodies: Antibodies produced to antigens coming from outside the body; in other words, to "foreign"antigens. These antibodies do not cause disease unless red cells containing these antigens are subsequently added or exposed to these antibodies.

Autoantibodies: Antibodies produced by the body against one or more of its own tissues. These antibodies are associated with autoimmune disease and may cause clinical difficulty.

There are several types of antibodies, depending on their occurrence and laboratory characteristics:

1. Natural antibody: These appear without any apparent antigenic stimulus.

2. Immune antibody: These appear following introduction of antigen due to disease, transfusion, or other mechanisms.

3. Complete (bivalent) antibody: These usually will directly agglutinate appropriate RBC. In-vitro tests for these antibodies tend to demonstrate better reaction in saline medium at room temperature ($20^O$ C) or lower. They often require complement.

4. Incomplete (univalent) antibody: These usually cannot directly agglutinate appropriate RBC but only coat their surface. In-vitro tests for these antibodies tend to show better reaction at higher temperatures such as $37^O$ C, and in high-protein medium.

5. Warm antibody: Reacts best in vitro at $37^O$ C.

6. Cold antibody: Reacts best at $4-10^O$ C.

There are two methods of detecting and characterizing these antibodies; these are the Coombs test and a group of procedures which demonstrate the action of the antibody under controlled conditions so as to exhibit some of its properties.

To prepare reagents for the Coombs test, human globulin, either gamma, nongamma, or mixed, is injected into rabbits. The rabbit produces antibodies to the injected human globulin. Rabbit serum containing these antihuman globulin antibodies is known as Coombs' serum. Since antibody is globulin, usually gamma globulin, the addition of Coombs' serum (antihuman globulin rabbit antibodies) to any solution containing human antibodies will result in the combination of the Coombs rabbit antibody with human antibody. Incidentally, this can be seen visually if the Coombs rabbit antibody has been tagged with a fluorescent dye.

The Coombs test may be carried out in either direct or indirect form. The direct Coombs test consists of adding Coombs' serum to a preparation of RBC which is coated with antibody. The Coombs reagent will attack this antibody coating the surface of the RBC and will cause the RBC to agglutinate to one another. This is a one-stage procedure. The direct Coombs test demonstrates that in-vivo coating of RBC by incomplete antibody has occurred, but does not identify the antibody responsible other than that. The direct Coombs test may be done by either a test tube or a slide method.

The indirect Coombs test is a two-stage procedure. The first stage takes place in vitro and may be done in either of two ways:

1. RBC of known antigenic makeup are exposed to serum containing unknown antibodies. If the antibody combines with the RBC, as detected by the second stage, this proves that circulating anti-

body to one or more antigens on the RBC is present. Since the RBC antigens are known, this may help to more specifically identify that antibody.

2. Serum containing known specific antibody is exposed to RBC of unknown antigenic makeup. If the antibody combines with the RBC, as detected by the second stage, this identifies the antigen on the RBC.

The second stage consists of adding Coombs' serum to the RBC, after the red cells have been washed to remove nonspecific unattached antibody or proteins. If specific antibody has coated the RBC, the Coombs serum will attack this antibody and cause the cells to agglutinate. The second stage is thus essentially a direct Coombs test done on the products of the first stage.

Therefore, the indirect Coombs test can be used either to detect free antibody in a patient's serum or to identify certain red cell antigens, depending on how the test is done.

The main indications for the direct Coombs test include the following (most of which will be discussed later in detail):

1. For the diagnosis of hemolytic disease of the newborn.
2. For diagnosis of hemolytic anemia in adults. These include many of the acquired autoimmune hemolytic anemias of both idiopathic and secondary varieties. The direct Coombs test at normal temperatures is usually negative with cold agglutinins.
3. For investigation of hemolytic transfusion reactions.

In these clinical situations the indirect test should not be done if the direct test is negative, since, in these situations, one is interested only in those antibodies which are affecting red cells (and thus precipitating clinical disease).

The main indications for the indirect Coombs test are:

1. Detection of certain weak antigens in RBC such as $D^u$ or certain red cell antigens whose antibodies are of the incomplete type, such as Duffy or Kidd (see Chapter 9).
2. Detection of incomplete antibodies in serum, usually for purposes of titration.
3. Demonstration of cold agglutinin autoantibodies.

Therefore, it should be noted that the indirect Coombs test is almost never needed routinely. In most situations, such as cold agglutinins or antibody identification, simply ordering a test for these substances will automatically cause an indirect Coombs test to be done. The indirect Coombs test should be thought of as a laboratory technique rather than as an actual laboratory test.

False positives and false negatives may occur with either of the Coombs tests due to poor technique, contamination, or faulty commercial Coombs' serum. The test must be done on clotted blood or serum, since laboratory anticoagulants may interfere. A false positive direct Coombs test may be given by increased peripheral blood reticulocytes using the test tube method, although the slide technique will remain negative. Therefore, one should know which method the laboratory uses for the direct Coombs test. False positive direct Coombs tests are also reported after Aldomet and cephalosporin therapy and after cardiac operations.

Autoantibodies present an interesting problem both in their clinical manifestations and the difficulty of laboratory detection and identification (p. 46). They may be either warm or cold type, complete or incomplete.

Warm autoantibodies react at body temperature and are most often of the incomplete type. They may be idiopathic or secondary to certain diseases (causing so-called symptomatic hemolytic anemia). The main disease categories responsible are leukemias and lymphomas, particularly chronic lymphocytic leukemia and Hodgkin's disease; collagen diseases, especially disseminated lupus; and uncommonly a variety of other diseases including cirrhosis, carcinomas, and ovarian dermoids. The direct Coombs test is usually, but not always, positive, both in the secondary and the "idiopathic acquired" hemolytic anemias. If the Coombs test is negative it becomes very difficult and often impossible to demonstrate that warm autoantibodies are present.

Cold autoantibodies react at 4-20° C and are found so frequently in normal persons that titers up to 1:64 are considered normal. They are hemagglutinating and are believed due to infection by organisms having antigenic groups similar to some of those on RBC. These antibodies mostly behave as bivalent types and require complement for reaction. In normally low titer they need icebox temperatures to attack RBC. In response to a considerable number of diseases these cold agglutinins are found in high titer, sometimes very high, and may then attack RBC in temperatures approaching body levels, causing hemolytic anemia. High-titered cold agglutinins may be found in viral infections, especially Eaton agent pneumonia (primary atypical pneumonia), influenza, and infectious mononucleosis; in collagen diseases, including rheumatoid arthritis; in malignant lymphomas; and occasionally in cirrhosis. Fortunately, even in high titer there usually is no trouble, and generally only very high titers are associated with in vivo erythrocyte agglutination or hemolytic anemia. This is not always true, however. The direct Coombs test is usually negative. When cold agglutinin studies are ordered, an indirect Coombs test is generally done, with the first stage being incubation of RBC and the patient's serum at 4-10° C.

## REFERENCES

Chaplin, H., Jr.: Antiglobulin (Coombs) testing (1966): How much ignorance is bliss, Transfusion 6:64, 1966.

Dacie, J. V.: The Haemolytic Anemias, Congenital and Acquired (2d ed.; New York: Grune & Stratton, Inc., 1960-1963).

Fayen, A. W., and Miale, J. B.: False positive antiglobulin tests in
    reticulocytosis, Am. J. Clin. Path. 39:645, 1963.
Gralnick, H. R., et al.: Drug-related positive direct Coombs test
    (abstr.), Am. J. Clin. Path. 49:241, 1968.
Griffitts, J. J., et al.: The influence of albumin in the antiglobulin
    crossmatch, Transfusion 4:461, 1964.
Hyland Reference Manual of Immunohematology (2d ed.; Los Angeles:
    Hyland Laboratories, 1964).
Kabat, E. A.: Blood Group Substances: Their Chemistry and Im-
    munochemistry (New York: Academic Press, Inc., 1965).
Mollison, P. L.: Blood Transfusion in Clinical Medicine (4th ed.;
    Philadelphia: F. A. Davis Co., 1967).
Samter, M. (ed.): Immunological Disease (Boston: Little, Brown
    & Company, 1965).
Stratton, F.: Complement in immunohematology, Transfusion 5:211,
    1965.

# CHAPTER 9

# Blood Groups and Isoimmunization

The ABO blood group system is a classic example of agglutinogens and their corresponding isoantibodies.  There are three of
these antigens—A,  B,  and O—whose genes are placed in one locus
on each of two paired chromosomes.  These genes are alleles,
meaning that they are interchangeable at their chromosome location.  Therefore, one chromosome carries any one of the three
antigen genes and likewise for the other chromosome.  This makes
four major phenotype groups possible—A,  B,  AB,  and O—since A
and B are dominant over O.  A and B are strong antigens,  whereas
O is so weak an antigen that for practical purposes it is considered
nonantigenic.  Furthermore,  it is a rule that when either A or B is
present on an individual's RBC, the corresponding isoantibodies
anti-A or anti-B will be absent from his serum; conversely,  if he
lacks either A or B, his serum will contain the isoantibody to the
missing isoantigen.  Therefore, a person who is AA or AO will
have anti-B in his serum; a person who is OO will have both anti-A
and anti-B,  and so on.  Why the body is stimulated to produce antibodies to the missing AB antigens is not definitely understood,  but
apparently antigens similar to ABO substances exist elsewhere in
nature and somehow cause a natural type of sensitization.
     Anti-A and anti-B are bivalent antibodies which react in saline
at room temperature.  Ordinarily,  little difficulty is encountered in
ABO typing.  There is, however,  one potentially serious situation
which arises from the fact that subgroups of agglutinogen A exist.
These are called $A_1$, $A_2$, and $A_3$.  The most common and strongest
of these is $A_1$.  $A_2$ is troublesome because sometimes it is so weak
that some commercial anti-A serums fail to pick it up.  This may
cause $A_2B$ to be falsely typed as B, or $A_2O$ to be falsely typed as O.
Fortunately, this situation is not frequent with present-day potent

95

typing serums.  Group A subgroups weaker than $A_2$ exist, but are
rare.  They are easily missed even with potent anti-A typing serums.  The main importance of the $A_2$ subgroup is that these persons sometimes have antibodies to $A_1$ (the most common subgroup
of A).

The next major blood group is the Rh system.  There is considerable controversy over nomenclature of the genetic apparatus
involved, between advocates of the English Fisher-Race CDE-cde
and the American Wiener's Rh-Hr labeling (Fig. 5).

According to Wiener, the Rh group is determined by single
genes, each chromosome of a pair containing one of these genes.
In most situations, each gene would be expected to determine one
antigen, to which there may develop one specific antibody.  In
Wiener's Rh system theory, each gene does indeed control one

Fig. 5.—Comparison of the Fisher-Race and Wiener nomenclatures.  (From Hyland Reference Manual of Immunohematology
(2d ed. ; Los Angeles:  Hyland Division of Travenol Laboratories,
Inc., 1964), pp. 38-39.)

SIMPLIFIED REPRESENTATION OF WIENER AND FISHER-RACE THEORIES
(schematic)

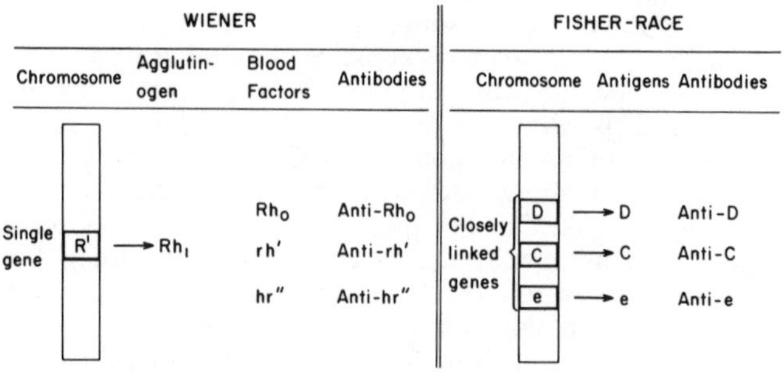

COMPARISON OF THE WIENER MULTIPLE ALLELE THEORY
AND THE FISHER-RACE LINKED GENE THEORY

| | WIENER | | | FISHER-RACE | |
| Gene | Corresponding agglutinogen | Blood factors | Genes | Corresponding antigens |
|---|---|---|---|---|
| $r$ | rh | hr' and hr" | cde | c,d,e |
| $r'$ | rh' | rh' and hr" | Cde | C,d,e |
| $r''$ | rh" | rh" and hr' | cdE | c,d,E |
| $r^y$ | $rh_y$ | rh' and rh" | CdE | C,d,E |
| $R^0$ | $Rh_0$ | $Rh_0$, hr' and hr" | cDe | c,D,e |
| $R^1$ | $Rh_1$ | $Rh_0$, rh' and hr" | CDe | C,D,e |
| $R^2$ | $Rh_2$ | $Rh_0$, rh" and hr' | cDE | c,D,E |
| $R^z$ | $Rh_z$ | $Rh_0$, rh' and rh" | CDE | C,D,E |

antigen. However, each of these antigens (agglutinogens) gives rise
to several different antibodies (blood factors), and it is these antibodies which are the serologic components of the Rh system. There
are eight of these agglutinogens, and each is associated with certain
specific blood factors. In most situations, specific antibodies are
produced when a person is stimulated by a specific antigen which he
lacks. In the Rh system, most people respond in the usual manner
to stimulation by specific Rh-system agglutinogens by producing
certain specific blood factors. In a few persons, a blood factor
different from the expected ones may be produced along with some
or all of the expected blood factor antibodies to one of the specific
agglutinogens. Since this rare factor is inherited as one of a specific group of factors dependent on a specific agglutinogen, new
antibodies can be added to Wiener's Rh system and assigned to one
of the agglutinins by statistical computation of inheritance patterns.

According to the Fisher-Race theory, there are supposed to
be three sets of two allelic genes, Cc, Dd, Ee, of which one gene
from each of the three pairs is linked together in one single locus
on each of two paired chromosomes. Therefore, the result is CDE,
each letter of which can be either big or little, on each of the two
chromosomes.

Therefore, in the Fisher-Race system, a single gene controls
one single antigen, which controls one single antibody. Moreover,
this means that three genes would be present on each chromosome
of a chromosome pair, and that the three-gene group is inherited as
a unit. New antibodies are assumed to be due to mutation or defective separation of the genes (comprising the gene group) during
meiosis ("crossover" rearrangement).

At present, the majority of experts believe that Wiener's theory fits the actual Rh situation better than the Fisher-Race theory.
The main drawback to the Wiener theory is its cumbersome terminology. Actually, in the great majority of situations, the much
simpler Fisher-Race terminology works very adequately, because
the antibodies which it names by its special letters are the same as
the basic blood factors of Wiener's system. It is only when the unusual or rare situations develop that the Wiener system becomes indispensable. In other words, the Fisher-Race terminology has persisted because, for most practical work, one can use this terminology even though its underlying theory of gene inheritance is ignored.
In the literature, one often finds both the Fisher-Race and the Wiener
nomenclatures, one of them being given in parentheses.

Of the Rh antigens, D ($Rh_0$) is by far the most antigenic and
when it is present on at least one chromosome the patient types as
Rh positive. Only 20% of the population lacks D ($Rh_0$) completely
and is considered Rh negative. Of the other antigens, c (hr') is the
next strongest, although nowhere near D.

Rh antigens lack corresponding naturally occurring antibodies
in the serum. Therefore, when antibodies appear, they are of im-

mune type, and are the result of sensitization by having received Rh antigen stimulation from the red cells of another person. This may occur by transfusion or in pregnancy. It is now well documented that red cells from the fetus escape the placenta into the blood stream of the mother. In this way the mother can develop Rh antibodies against the Rh antigen of the fetus. One exception to this occurs when the mother's serum contains antibodies against the ABO group of the fetus; for example, if the mother were group O and the fetus group B. In these cases the fetal RBC are apparently destroyed in the maternal circulation before Rh sensitization can proceed to a significant extent, although this does not always happen. The syndrome of Rh-induced erythroblastosis will be discussed later. Rh incompatibility was a major cause of incompatible blood transfusions, although the incidence is now much less than ABO transfusion reactions. Rh antibody transfusion reactions may occur by transfusion of donor blood containing Rh antibodies, or by previous sensitization of a recipient, who now will have the antibodies in his own serum.

Rh antigen may be typed using commercial antiserum. Preliminary screening is only for antigen D, which establishes a person as Rh positive or negative. If a person is Rh negative, further studies with antiserum to other components of the Rh group may be done, depending on the situation and the individual blood bank. In particular, there recently has been found a weak subgroup of D ($Rh_0$) called $D^u$ ($Rh_0$ variant) which is analogous to the weak $A_2$ subgroup of A in the ABO system. $D^u$ blood often fails to give a positive reaction with some commercial Rh anti-D typing serums, and thus may falsely type as Rh negative. Therefore, many large blood banks screen Rh negative red cells for $D^u$ as well as for c (hr') and E (rh''), the most antigenic of the minor Rh antigens.

Rh antibodies are usually univalent and react best in vitro at $37^0$ C in high-protein medium. Large blood banks screen donor serum for these antibodies using a variety of techniques. When Rh antibodies attack RBC in vivo, whether in transfusion or in hemolytic disease of the newborn, they coat the surface of the red cells in the usual manner of univalent antibodies and are then positive with the direct Coombs test (until the affected RBC are destroyed).

Besides the ABO and the Rh systems there are a considerable number of other unrelated antigenic systems which have some importance, either from medicolegal parenthood studies or from sensitization leading to transfusion reactions or hemolytic disease of the newborn. The most important of these systems is Kell (K), a well-recognized blood bank problem. The Kell antibodies are similar in characteristics and behavior to the Rh system D ($Rh_0$) antibody. Fortunately, only about 10% of whites and 2% of Negroes have the Kell antigen and are thus Kell-positive, so that opportunities for sensitization of a Kell-negative person are not great. Kell antibody is univalent and acts best in vitro using high-protein media at $37^0$ C just as Rh does. If reactions due to Kell antibodies occur, the direct Coombs test is positive (until the affected RBC are destroyed). A similar situation exists for the rare Duffy (Fy) and Kidd (jK) systems. There are other systems which resemble ABO in their antibody characteristics, and these include the MN, P, Lewis (Le), and Lutheran (Lu) systems. They are primarily bivalent antibodies, best reacting in vitro with saline media at room temperature or below. They are rare causes for transfusion reactions, and even when difficulty arises are clinically milder than the univalent antibody systems. They may, however, be dangerous, and cannot be ignored.

Even if major blood group typing has been done, transfusion reactions may occur due to antibodies other than ABO or $Rh_0$ (D). To prevent this, the concept of a crossmatch has evolved. There are two basic procedures: the major crossmatch, involving the serum of the recipient and the cells of the donor, and the minor crossmatch, involving the cells of the recipient and the serum of the donor. Some blood banks replace the minor crossmatch with antibody screening procedures using the donor's serum and a panel of different RBC containing various blood group antigens. Theoretically, even if the serum of the donor contains antibodies to one or more of the red cell antigens of the recipient, the relatively large blood volume of the recipient should dilute the relatively small volume of the donor serum to a point at which it is harmless. This is the rationale for using O negative blood in emergencies without crossmatch as so-called universal donors. Even so, there is risk involved, since the recipient may possess antibody to some other blood group antigen of the donor (such as anti-Rh or anti-Kell). A crossmatch would pick this up. Moreover, sometimes the anti-A or anti-B in group O blood is in high titer, and transfusion reactions may occur when these bloods are used in recipients of other ABO groups. Many blood banks maintain a certain amount of low-titer O negative blood for use in emergencies. Titers over 1:50 are considered too high for this purpose. In addition, A and B group specific substance (Witebsky substance) may be added to the donor blood to partially neutralize anti-A and anti-B. Those substances are A and B antigen manufactured from animal sources and, being foreign antigens, may possibly sensitize the patient.

Therefore, the purpose of crossmatch compatibility tests is to detect antibodies of either person. It incidentally serves as a check on ABO typing, since antibodies to the ABO system occur naturally. The procedure will not detect errors in Rh typing if no Rh antibodies are present in donor or recipient. Since Rh antibodies do not occur naturally, either donor or recipient would have to be previously sensitized before Rh or similar antibodies would appear. Without antibodies present the crossmatch does not demonstrate antigens, and thus will not prevent immunization (sensitization) of the recipient by Rh or similar groups. This can be done only by proper typing of the donor and recipient cells beforehand.

The crossmatch is usually carried out in several steps using several techniques so as to pick up groups of antibodies which have different temperature and reaction media requirements. Occasionally, the laboratory is asked to do an "emergency crossmatch." There is no such thing. Certain procedures may be eliminated in order to gain speed, but this correspondingly increases the risk of missing those antibodies which they are designed to detect. It must be realized that emergency crossmatch blood has not been properly screened.

A word must also be said regarding a few patients whose blood presents unexplained difficulty in crossmatching. The laboratory should be allowed to solve the problem, possibly to obtain aid from a reference laboratory. Blood products, such as plasma or packed cells, may temporarily assist the patient during this time. Otherwise, blood is given at a calculated risk.

If blood is needed for emergency transfusion without crossmatch, a frequent decision is to use group O Rh negative blood. A better method would be to use blood of the same ABO and Rh type as the patient's. ABO and Rh typing can be done within five minutes using anticoagulated specimens of the patient's blood. This would avoid interpretation problems produced by putting group O cells into a group A or B patient and subsequently attempting crossmatches for more blood.

When repeated transfusions are needed, a new specimen should be drawn from the patient (recipient) for crossmatching purposes if blood had been given over 24 hours previously. Some patients demonstrate marked anamnestic responses to red cell antigens which they lack, and may produce clinically significant quantities of antibody in a few hours. This antibody would not be present in the original specimen from the patient.

In summary, red cell typing is designed to show what antigens are on the RBC, and thus what blood group red cells can be given to a recipient without either being destroyed by antibodies the recipient is known to possess, or without danger of sensitizing the recipient by introducing antigens that he might lack and thus against which he might produce antibodies. The crossmatch procedure (comprising major and minor techniques) is designed to demonstrate unexpected antibodies in the serum (of donor or recipient) which may destroy RBC which were otherwise considered compatible by the results of RBC blood group typing.

## REFERENCES

Griffitts, J. J., and Schmidt, P.: Effectiveness of techniques in
    demonstrating the isohemagglutinins, Transfusion 2:385, 1962.
Grove-Rasmussen, M.: Routine compatibility testing, Transfusion
    4:200, 1964.

Grove-Rasmussen, M. : Selection of "safe" group O blood, Trans-
  fusion 6:331, 1966.
Hyland Reference Manual of Immunohematology (2d ed. ; Los Angeles:
  Hyland Laboratories, 1964).
Jennings, E. R. , and Hindmarsh, C. : The significance of the mi-
  nor crossmatch, Am. J. Clin. Path. 30:302, 1958.
Mollison, P. L. : Blood Transfusion in Clinical Medicine (4th ed. ;
  Philadelphia: F. A. Davis Co. , 1967).
Race, R. R. , and Sanger, R. : Blood Groups in Man (4th ed. ; Phila-
  delphia: F. A. Davis Co. , 1962).
Simmons, A. , et al. : Effect of varying the crossmatch procedure
  upon detection of anti-D and anti-Kell, Am. J. M. Tech. 37:83,
  1971.
Stern, K. : Unusual blood types as a cause of disease, M. Clin.
  North America 46:277, 1962.
Wiener, A. S. , and Wexler, I. B. : Heredity of the Blood Groups
  (New York: Grune & Stratton, Inc. , 1958).

# CHAPTER 10

# Immunohematologic Reactions

Transfusion reactions occur in a certain percentage of blood transfusions. The three main types are: hemolytic, pyrogenic, and allergic.

Pyrogenic reactions are the most frequent transfusion complication. They are due to contamination by bacteria, dirt, or foreign proteins. Their symptoms begin during or shortly after transfusion and consist of sudden chills and fever. In addition, the more serious cases often have abdominal cramps, nausea, and diarrhea. Very severe reactions due to heavy bacterial contamination lead to shock. If such a situation occurs, a smear should be made from the remaining bank blood and gram-stained without waiting for culture results. Since early symptoms of hemolytic reactions are similar to those due to pyrogens, transfusion should be discontinued and routine transfusion reaction studies done before continuing with another unit of blood.

Allergic types of reaction are presumably due to substances in the donor blood to which the recipient is allergic. Symptoms are localized or generalized hives or urticaria, although occasionally severe asthma or even laryngeal edema may occur. There is usually excellent response to antihistamines or epinephrine.

Transfusion reactions may be caused by either complete or incomplete antibodies. In those resulting from complete antibodies such as occur in the ABO system, there is usually intravascular hemolysis. The amount of hemolysis depends on several factors, such as quantity of incompatible blood, antibody titer, and the nature of the antibody involved. However, there is an element of individual susceptibility, for some die from less than 100 ml. of incompatible blood, whereas others survive after several times this amount. The direct Coombs test is often positive, but this depends on whether all

102

the RBC attacked by the complete antibody have been lysed, whether more antibody is produced, and to some extent on how soon the test is obtained. If the sample is drawn more than 1 hour after the ABO transfusion reaction is completed, the chance of a positive direct Coombs test begins to become less and less. Also, a "broad-spectrum" Coombs reagent is needed; most laboratories use this type routinely nowadays. Free hemoglobin is released into the plasma (thence into urine via the kidney), and indirect bilirubin then rises also. In reactions caused by incomplete-type antibodies such as the Rh system, there is sequestration of antibody-coated cells in organs such as the spleen, with subsequent breakdown by the reticuloendothelial system. Thus, RBC breakdown is extravascular; in small degrees of reaction, plasma free hemoglobin may not rise, although indirect bilirubin eventually will. In more extensive reactions, plasma hemoglobin is often elevated, although sometimes delayed in onset. The direct Coombs test is naturally positive in reactions due to incomplete antibodies (unless all the affected RBC have been destroyed).

Hemolytic reaction is usually caused by incompatible blood, although occasionally it may be due to partial hemolysis of the red cells before transfusion. The great majority of cases result from human error, usually mislabeled crossmatch specimens or administration to the wrong patient. Symptoms include chills, fever, and pain in the low back or legs. Jaundice may appear later. Severe reactions lead to shock. Renal shutdown is common, due either to shock or to precipitation of free hemoglobin in the renal tubules. Therefore, oliguria and often hemoglobinuria develop, manifested by red urine or nearly black coffee-ground acid hematin urine color.

Tests for severe intravascular hemolysis include plasma hemoglobin ("free hemoglobin") immediately and at 6 hours, and serum indirect bilirubin at 6 and 12 hours. The best immediate test for plasma hemoglobin is simple visual inspection of plasma. Most complete-antibody transfusion reactions produce enough hemolysis to be grossly visible (artifact hemolysis from improperly drawn specimens must be ruled out). If chemical tests are to be done, plasma hemoglobin is preferred to serum hemoglobin because less artifact hemolysis takes place before the specimen reaches the laboratory. The urine should be examined for hemoglobin, hemoglobin casts, red cells, and proteinuria. Although hemolytic reactions due to incomplete antibodies such as Rh have clinical symptoms similar to those of ABO, direct signs of hemolysis (such as free plasma hemoglobin) are more variable or may be delayed for a few hours, although they become abnormal if the reaction is severe. Another drawback in the interpretation of plasma hemoglobin values is the effect of the transfusion itself. The older erythrocytes stored in bank blood die during storage, adding free hemoglobin to the plasma. Therefore, although normal values are usually stated in the range of 1-5 mg./100 ml., values between 5-50 mg./100 ml.

are equivocal if stored bank blood is given.  Besides tests for
hemolysis, a direct Coombs test should be done, as well as crossmatch recheck studies, which are to be described next.

Transfusion should be stopped at the first sign of possible reaction, and complete studies done to recheck compatibility of the
donor and recipient blood.  If these are still satisfactory, and if the
direct Coombs test and the studies for intravascular hemolysis are
negative, a different unit can be started on the assumption that the
symptoms were pyrogenic rather than hemolytic.  Naturally, whatever unused blood remains in the donor bottle, the donor bottle pilot
tube, and a new specimen drawn from the patient must all be sent to
the blood bank for the recheck studies.  Especially dangerous situations exist in transfusion during surgery, where anesthesia may
mask the early signs and symptoms of a reaction.  A development
during surgery of a marked bleeding tendency at the operative site
is an important danger signal.  A transfusion reaction requires immediate mannitol therapy to protect the kidneys.

The other major area where blood banks meet immunohem-
atologic problems is that of hemolytic disease of the newborn.  This
may be due to ABO, Rh, or rarely minor group incompatibility between fetal and maternal red cells.  Basically, the situation results
from fetal red cell antigens which the maternal red cells lack.  These
fetal RBC antigens provoke maternal antibody formation when fetal
red cells are introduced into the maternal circulation after escaping
from the placenta.  The maternal antibodies eventually cross the
placenta to the fetal circulation and attack the fetal red cells.

Hemolytic disease of the newborn due to Rh incompatibility
varies in severity from subclinical status through mild jaundice
with anemia to the dangerous and often fatal condition of erythroblastosis fetalis.  The main clinical findings are anemia and rapidly
developing jaundice.  Reticulocytosis over 6% accompanies the anemia, and the jaundice is mainly due to unconjugated (indirect) bilirubin released from the reticuloendothelial sequestration and destruction of red blood cells.  The direct Coombs test is positive.  In
severe cases there are usually many nucleated RBC in the peripheral blood.  Jaundice is not present at birth, but develops several
hours later or even after 24 hours in mild cases.  Diseases which
cause jaundice in the newborn, often accompanied by anemia and
sometimes a few peripheral blood nucleated RBC include septicemia,
cytomegalic inclusion disease, toxoplasmosis, and syphilis.  Physiologic jaundice of the newborn is a frequent benign condition which
may be confused with hemolytic disease or vice versa.  There is,
however, no significant anemia.  A normal newborn has an (average)
hemoglobin value of 18 Gm./100 ml., and less than 15 Gm./100 ml.
indicates anemia.

Fifty per cent or more of hemolytic disease is due to ABO incompatibility between mother and fetus.  Anti-A and anti-B production begins between 3 and 6 months of age.  At birth and until this

time, ABO antibodies in the infant's serum come from the mother.
If the infant's ABO isoagglutinogens are compatible with the ABO
group of the mother, everything is fine. If, however, the mother
possesses antibodies to the A or B red cell antigens of the fetus,
hemolytic disease of the newborn may result, just as if the newborn
had received a transfusion of serum with antibodies against his red
cells. This being the case, it is surprising to find that 20-25% of
all pregnancies have maternal-fetal ABO incompatibility and yet the
great majority of these infants seem perfectly healthy. Only a small
minority develop various degrees of hemolytic disease. This may
be due to the fact that ABO hemolytic disease as a group is usually
milder than its counterpart caused by Rh incompatibility, which was
discussed earlier. In fact, many cases of ABO disease may have
degrees of hemolysis too small to be detected clinically and are apparently well. The incidence of clinically evident disease is about
the same as that from Rh, although, as just said, even severe cases
are relatively milder than the comparable Rh cases. Some infants,
however, will die or suffer cerebral damage if treatment is not
given. Therefore, the diagnosis of ABO disease and its differential
diagnosis from the other causes of jaundice and anemia in the newborn are of great practical importance.

There are two types of ABO antibodies—the naturally occurring
complete saline-reacting type discussed earlier, and an immune univalent (incomplete) type produced in some unknown way to fetal A or
B antigen stimulation. Most cases of clinical ABO disease have a
group O mother and a group A or B infant. The immune anti-A or
B antibody, if produced by the mother, may cause ABO disease, because it can pass the placenta. Maternal titers of 1:32 or more are
considered dangerous. The saline antibodies do not cross the placenta and are not significant in hemolytic disease of the newborn.

The direct Coombs test done on the infant with ABO hemolytic
disease is sometimes positive but not often. Spherocytes are often
present. Good evidence for ABO disease is detection of immune
anti-A or anti-B in the cord blood of a newborn whose RBC belong
to the same blood group as the antibody. Detection of these antibodies only in the serum of the mother does not conclusively prove
ABO disease in the newborn.

Hemolytic disease caused by Rh sensitization occurs usually
in a mother who is Rh negative with a fetus who is Rh positive. The
direct Coombs test on the cord or infant blood is usually positive
and should be done in all cases of possible hemolytic disease of the
newborn, because incomplete antibodies occasionally may coat the
surface of the fetal RBC to such an extent as to interfere with proper
Rh typing. Maternal serum contains immune antibodies to the Rh
factor whose titer usually rises if serial studies are done during
pregnancy. The first child is usually not affected, but the mother
becomes sensitized during that pregnancy. Subsequent pregnancies
may show fetal hemolytic disease, although not always. For the

sake of prognosis in future pregnancies, the husband should get a complete Rh typing to see if he is homozygous or heterozygous for the Rh factor involved.

Infants with hemolytic disease of the newborn can usually be saved by exchange transfusion. The indications for this procedure are:

1. Infant serum indirect bilirubin above 20 mg./100 ml. or premature infant 15 mg./100 ml.

2. Cord blood indirect bilirubin over 4 mg./100 ml.

3. Hemoglobin less than 13 Gm./100 ml.

4. Maternal Rh antibody titer of 1:64 or greater, although this is not an absolute indication if the bilirubin does not rise very high.

Routine prenatal tests should include ABO and Rh typing of the mother. If the mother is Rh negative, the father should be Rh typed also. If an Rh incompatibility exists, follow-up should include maternal Rh antibody titration at 3 months and 6 months, then bimonthly to detect any rising titer.

Serum bilirubin levels are considered the main parameter of severity in hemolytic disease of the newborn. Recently, amniocentesis has been advocated as a means of estimating fetal risk while still in utero. A long needle is introduced into the amniotic fluid cavity of the fetus by means of a suprapubic puncture approach in the mother. The amniotic fluid is subjected to spectrophotometric estimation of bilirubin pigments. Markedly increased bilirubin pigment strongly indicates significant degrees of hemolytic disease in the fetus. If necessary, delivery can then be induced prematurely once the 32d week of gestation has arrived. Before this, or, in cases with severe disease in utero, intrauterine exchange transfusion has been attempted, using a transabdominal approach. The indications for aminocentesis are development of significant titer of Rh antibody in the mother, or a history of previous erythroblastosis. Significant maternal antibody Rh titers do not always mean serious fetal Rh disease, but absence of significant titer nearly always indicates a benign prognosis. Also, if initial amniocentesis at 32 weeks does not suggest an immediately dangerous situation, even though mild or moderate abnormalities were present, a fetus could be allowed to mature as long as possible (being followed by repeated studies) so as to avoid the danger of premature birth.

Even more recently, studies suggest that some mothers who had potential or actual Rh incompatibility problems could be protected against sensitization by the fetus. A "vaccine" composed of gamma globulin with a high titer of anti-Rh antibody (anti-D or $Rh_0$) is given to the patient in the 1-3 days following delivery of the first child with red cell Rh antigen incompatibility to the mother. This exogenous antibody seems to suppress maternal endogenous antibody production in many cases. Subsequent pregnancy in these cases would not provoke anamnestic antibody response.

## REFERENCES

Alter, A. A., et al.: Direct antiglobulin test in ABO hemolytic disease of the newborn, Obst. & Gynec. 33:846, 1969.

Baker, R. J., et al.: Diagnosis and treatment of immediate transfusion reaction, Surg., Gynec. & Obst. 130:665, 1970.

Bohnen, R. F., et al.: The direct Coombs test: Its clinical significance, Ann. Int. Med. 68:19, 1968.

Bowman, J. M.: Hemolytic disease of the newborn, Obst. & Gynec. 40:217, 1966.

Chan, A. C., et al.: ABO hemolytic disease, J. Pediat. 61:405, 1962.

Davidsohn, I., and Stern, K.: Diagnosis of hemolytic transfusion reactions, Am. J. Clin. Path. 25:381, 1955.

Fink, D. J., et al.: Serum haptoglobin. A valuable diagnostic aid in suspected hemolytic transfusion reactions, J. A. M. A. 199:615, 1967.

Freda, V. J.: Placental transfer of antibodies in man, Am. J. Obst. & Gynec. 84:1756, 1962.

Freda, V. J.: The control of Rh disease, Hosp. Practice 2:54, 1967.

Jandl, J. H., and Tomlinson, A. S.: The destruction of red cells by antibodies in man. II. Pyrogenic, leukocytic, and dermal responses to immune hemolysis, Medicine 43:207, 1964.

Javid, J.: Human serum haptoglobins—A brief review, Seminars Hemat. 4:35, 1967.

Jennings, E. R.: Recent Advances in Diagnosis, Treatment, and Prevention of Hemolytic Disease of the Newborn, in Stefanini, M. (ed.): Advances in Clinical Pathology (New York: Grune & Stratton, Inc., 1966), Vol. 1, p. 458.

McConnell, R. B.: The Prevention of Rh Hemolytic Disease, in DeGraff, A. C., and Creger, W. P. (eds.): Annual Review of Medicine (Palo Alto, Calif.: Annual Reviews, Inc., 1966), Vol. 17, p. 291.

Mollison, P. L.: Blood Transfusion in Clinical Medicine (4th ed.; Philadelphia: F. A. Davis Co., 1967).

Odell, G. B., et al.: Exchange transfusion, Pediat. Clin. North America 9:605, 1962.

Polesky, H. F., et al.: Positive antiglobulin tests in cardiac surgery patients, Transfusion 9:43, 1969.

Unger, L. J.: Medicolegal aspects of blood transfusion, New York J. Med. 60:237, 1960.

# CHAPTER 11

# Blood Transfusions

Blood transfusions may consist of whole blood or various blood fractions.

Whole blood at present is ordinarily collected in a citrate preservative and anticoagulant called ACD. Acceptable storage life is 21 days at $4^{\circ}$ C; at the end of this time there is approximately 70% red cell survival in the patient. There are certain problems involving stored bank blood. After approximately 2 weeks' storage, some of the RBC lose vitality and become spherocytes. Since spherocytosis is a feature of certain isoimmune and autoimmune hemolytic anemias, transfusion of such blood prior to diagnostic investigation may cause confusion. Potassium concentration slowly rises during storage as it escapes from devitalized RBC. After 15 days' storage, blood levels reach approximately 25 mEq./L. This may become undesirable if the patient already has elevated serum potassium, as seen in uremia or renal shutdown. Three units of blood equal about 1 liter of plasma, remembering that normal plasma (or serum) potassium levels are 4.0-5.5 mEq./L. Ammonium levels of stored blood also increase, and may reach values of 10-15 times normal. Large volumes of such blood may be dangerous in severe liver disease. The citrate anticoagulant may cause difficulty with really massive transfusions. Its calcium-binding actions may lead to hypocalcemia if substituted for a large portion of the blood volume. This is the so-called citrate intoxication and fortunately is rare. In addition, citrate in large quantities does have a depressant effect on the myocardium. Platelets disintegrate rapidly on storage and are physiologically useless after 1-2 days. Bank blood, therefore, essentially has no platelets. This may cause difficulty in massive transfusions using old bank blood, although there is usually no difficulty with the usual size of transfusion. In massive rapidly administered transfusions, reports indicate that a high incidence of cardiac arrest can be reduced by warming stored blood to body temperature just before or during administration. Blood transfusion of ordinary quantities at the usual slow rate does not require this precaution.

A new anticoagulant named CPD recently has been introduced which is said to extend whole blood storage time to 28 days. Stored blood may carry the organisms of hepatitis, syphilis, and malaria. The spirochete of syphilis will die in 4-5 days under usual storage conditions, but the others survive.

Whole blood is used for restoration of blood volume due to simultaneous loss of both plasma and red blood cells. This is most frequently seen in hemorrhage, both external and internal. Stored blood is adequate for this in most cases.

Fresh whole blood is used within 2 days and preferably 1 day after collection. Platelets are still viable and certain other substances such as factor VIII (antihemophilic globulin) and factor V are still at least partially active. The other disadvantages of prolonged storage are absent. Obviously, donor and administrative problems greatly limit use and availability of fresh blood.

Since the use of blood transfusion has increased dramatically over the years, maintenance of adequate donor sources has been a constant problem. In Russia, cadaver blood has apparently been utilized. If collected less than 6 hours post mortem, it does not differ significantly from stored (bank) blood, except that anticoagulation is not required. A few experimental studies have been done in the United States, with favorable results. Another recent development is the use of freezing to preserve packed red cells. Glycerol is added to packed red cells to protect the red cells during freezing; this substance prevents intracellular fluid from becoming ice. The blood is slowly frozen, and is maintained at below-zero temperatures until ready for use. Thereafter it must be thawed, after which the glycerol is removed (to avoid osmotic hemolysis) and the cells are resuspended in saline. This technique will maintain packed red cells for up to 18 months. At present, this method is not widely available.

Packed red cells consist of bank blood with about two thirds of the plasma taken out. Packed cells help avoid the problem of overloading the patient's blood volume and throwing him into pulmonary edema. This is especially useful in anemias due to destruction or poor production of red cells, where the plasma volume does not need replacement. In fact, when anemia is due to pure red cell deficiency, plasma volume becomes greater than usual, because extracellular fluid tends to replace the missing RBC volume in order to maintain total blood volume. Packed cells are sometimes used when the donor red cells type satisfactorily but antibodies are present in donor plasma. Packed cells administration also helps diminish some of the other problems of stored blood, such as elevated plasma potassium or ammonium.

Plasma alone may be either fresh frozen or stored. The fresh frozen variety is used mainly as a source of coagulation factor VIII. This is currently the treatment of choice for hemophilia. Stored plasma, until recently, was the treatment of choice for blood volume depletion in burns and proved very useful as an initial temporary measure in hemorrhagic shock while whole blood was being typed and crossmatched. It was also useful in some cases of shock not due to hemorrhage. Stored plasma may be either from single donors, in which case it must be crossmatched prior to transfusion, or more commonly from a pool of many donors. Pooled plasma dilutes any dangerous antibodies present in any one of the component plasma units, so that pooled plasma may be given without cross-match. For many years it was thought that hepatitis virus in plasma would be inactivated after storage for 6 months at room temperature. For this reason, pooled stored plasma was widely used. Recently, a study has reported a 10% incidence of subclinical hepatitis even after prescribed lengths of storage. The National Research Council Committee on plasma and plasma substitutes now recommends that 5% albumin solution be used instead of plasma whenever possible. A method of concentrating factor VIII has been devised. If this concentrate (cryoprecipitate) is available it would avoid some of the problems inherent in giving large amounts of plasma in hemophilia.

Fibrinogen is a blood fraction which is essential for clotting. It is decreased in two ways, both relatively uncommon: by intravascular deposition of fibrin in the form of small clots (disseminated intravascular coagulation, DIC) and by inactivation in the presence of primary fibrinolysin. DIC is seen most commonly in the obstetric condition of premature placental separation (abruptio placentae) and in medical or surgical conditions associated with shock. Primary fibrinolysins are rare; they occasionally are seen with widespread cancer, especially prostatic. The most useful diagnostic tests are plasma fibrinogen level, protamine sulfate test, and clot lysis test. These conditions and laboratory tests are discussed more extensively in Chapter 7. The treatment for circulating fibrinolysins is transfusion with fibrinogen solution and the use of epsilon-amino-caproic acid, a fibrinolysin antagonist. Treatment of DIC (disseminated intravascular clotting) syndrome is fibrinogen administration and, in the early stages, the use of heparin to prevent further clotting. Fibrinogen solution brings with it an even greater risk of viral hepatitis than plasma.

The most frequent indication for transfusion therapy is to replace depleted blood volume. This most commonly arises in association with surgery or from nonsurgical blood loss, acute or chronic. Immediately after an acute bleeding episode, the hemoglobin and hematocrit are unchanged (because whole blood has been lost), even though total blood volume may be greatly reduced, even down to the point of circulatory collapse (shock). With the passage of time, extracellular fluid begins to diffuse into the vascular system in order to partially restore total blood volume. Since the hematocrit is simply the percentage of red cells compared to total blood volume (total blood volume being the red cell mass plus the plasma volume), this dilution of the blood by extracellular fluid means that the hematocrit begins eventually to decrease even while total blood volume is being increased (by extracellular fluid increasing plasma volume). Hemodilution (and thus the hematocrit drop) may be hastened if the patient was receiving intravenous fluids. Serial hematocrit determinations (once every 2-4 hours) may thus be used as a rough indication of blood volume changes. It usually takes at least 2 hours after an acute bleeding episode for a significant drop in hematocrit to be demonstrated. Sometimes it takes longer—even as long as 6-12 hours. The larger the extracellular blood loss, the sooner a significant hematocrit change (over 2%) is likely to appear.

Previous dehydration and/or low plasma protein level will tend to delay a hematocrit drop. Besides the uncertainty of time lag, other conditions may affect the hematocrit and thus influence its interpretation as a parameter of blood volume. Anemias due to red cell hemolysis or blood factor deficiencies such as iron may decrease red cell mass without decreasing plasma or total blood volume. Similarly, plasma volume may be altered in many situations involving fluid and electrolyte imbalance without changing the red cell mass. Obviously, a need exists for more accurate methods in measuring blood volume.

The method most widely used until recently has been Evans blue dye (T-1824). This is a dilution technique in which a measured amount of the dye is injected intravenously and allowed to equilibrate; then serial blood samples are drawn and the rate of dye dilution is calculated. From this, an estimation of plasma volume may be obtained. This technique was reasonably good, but had many technical and clinical drawbacks. More recently, radioisotopes have taken over this field. These also are based on the dilution principle. Chromium-51 can be used to tag RBC; a measured amount of the tagged red cells is then injected into the patient. After equilibration for 15 minutes, a blood sample is obtained and counted for radioactivity. Since the tagged RBC have mixed with the patient's RBC, comparison of the radioactivity in the patient's RBC with the original isotope specimen that was injected gives the amount that the original isotope specimen has been diluted by the patient's red cells, and thus the patient's total RBC mass (RBC volume) may be calculated. Knowing the RBC mass, plasma volume and total blood volume may be obtained using the hematocrit value of the patient's blood. Another widely used method is that using serum albumin labeled with radioactive iodine (RISA). This substance circulates in the plasma along with the other plasma proteins. Again, a measured amount is injected, a blood sample is withdrawn after a short period of equilibration, and the dilution of the original injected specimen is determined by counting the radioactivity of the patient's plasma. RISA gives plasma volume; red cell volume must be calculated using the patient's hematocrit. There is no doubt that isotope techniques are much more accurate than hematocrit for estimating blood volume. Nevertheless, there are certain limitations to isotope techniques in general and specific limitations to both $Cr^{51}$ and RISA. The main drawback of blood volume techniques is the lack of precise normal values. Attempts have been made to establish normal values for males and females in terms of height, weight, or surface area, or from lean body mass. Unfortunately, when one tries to apply one of these formulas to an individual patient, there is never any guarantee that the patient fits whatever category of normal persons that the formula was calculated from. The only way to be sure is to have a blood volume measurement when the patient was healthy, or prior to the bleeding episode. Unfortunately, this information is usually not available. Another drawback is the fact that any dilution method will not detect bleeding which is going on during the test itself. This is true because whole blood lost during the test contains the isotope in the same proportion as the blood remaining in the vascular system (a diminished isotope dose in a diminished blood volume) contrasted to the situation which would prevail if bleeding were not going on, where the entire isotope dose would remain in a diminished blood volume. Fortunately, such active bleeding would have to be severe before test results are materially affected. Another problem is dependence on hematocrit when results from RISA are used to calculate RBC mass or data from $Cr^{51}$ are used to obtain plasma volume. It is well established that hematocrits from different body areas or different size vessels can vary considerably—and disease may accentuate this variation. The venous hematocrit may therefore not be representative of the average vascular hematocrit.

All authorities in the field agree that blood volume determination combining independent measurement of RBC mass by $Cr^{51}$ and plasma volume by RISA is more accurate than the use of either isotope alone. Nevertheless, because both isotopes must be counted separately with special equipment, most laboratories use only a single isotope technique. $Cr^{51}$ is conceded by most to have a slightly better over-all accuracy than RISA. However, most $Cr^{51}$ techniques call for an extra venipuncture to obtain RBC from the patient for tagging, plus an extra 30-minute wait for the actual tagging of the cells. In addition, the tagged RBC (and their radioactivity) remain in the circulation during the life span of the cells. The main advantages of RISA are the need for one less venipuncture than $Cr^{51}$, and the fact that RISA procedures can be done in less than half the time of $Cr^{51}$. However, the majority of blood volume workers feel that RISA does not have the over-all accuracy of $Cr^{51}$, although some dispute this strongly. The expected error with RISA blood volume reaches 300 ml. in some studies, although the majority of determinations come much closer to double isotope results. In patients with markedly increased vascular permeability, significant quantities of RISA may be lost from blood vessels during the test, and thus lead to even greater errors. Severe edema is an example of such a situation. Nevertheless, even under adverse conditions RISA (and $Cr^{51}$) represent a decided advance over use of hematocrits for estimating blood volume.

## REFERENCES

Boyan, C. P. : Cold or warmed blood for massive transfusions, Ann. Surg. 160:282, 1964.

Dagher, F. J., et al.: Blood Volume Measurement: A Critical Study, in Welch, C. E. (ed.): Advances in Surgery (Chicago: Year Book Medical Publishers, Inc. , 1965), Vol. I, p. 69.

Davidsohn, I. : Calcium and citrate intoxication, J. A. M. A. 196:130, 1966.

Gump, F. E. : Physiological measurements and their interpretation, M. Clin. North America 55:1141, 1971.

Hershgold, E. J., et al. : The potent antihemophilic globulin concentrate derived from a cold insoluble fraction of human plasma: Characterization and further data on preparation and clinical trial, J. Lab. & Clin. Med. 67:23, 1966.

Huggans, C. E. : Frozen blood, J. A. M. A. 193:169, 1965.

Ingram, G. I. C. : The bleeding complications of blood transfusion, Transfusion 5:1, 1965.

Jacobs, R. G., et al.: Serial microhematocrit determinations in evaluating blood replacement, Anesthesiology 22:342, 1961.

LeVeen, H. H., et al. : Hemorrhage and transfusion as the major cause of cardiac arrest, J. A. M. A. 173:770, 1960.

Medical News: Pooled plasma may transmit hepatitis, J. A. M. A. 204:21, 1968.

Merritt, J. A. : Complications related to blood replacement, Am. J. Surg. 116:333, 1968.

Milles, G., et al. : Experiences with autotransfusion, Surg., Gynec. & Obst. 115:689, 1962.

Mollison, P. L. : Blood Transfusion in Clinical Medicine (4th ed. ; Philadelphia: F. A. Davis Co., 1967).

Moore, C. J., et al. : Present status of cadaver blood as transfusion medium, Arch. Surg. 85:364, 1962.

Schecter, D. C., and Swan, H. : Biochemical alterations of preserved blood. Results in two different citrate solutions (ACD and CPD). Arch. Surg. 84:269, 1962.

Symposium on Blood Volume, Am. Surgeon 30:347, 1964.

Thistlethwaite, J. R., et al.: Blood volume fluctuations determined by radioisotopes of chromium and radioactive iodinated serum albumin, Surg., Gynec. & Obst. 105:34, 1957.

Tullis, J. L., and Lionetti, F. J.: Preservation of blood by freezing, Anesthesiology 27:483, 1966.

Zucker, M. B. : Unexplained bleeding in operations for neoplasias, Ann. New York Acad. Sc. 115:225, 1964.

# CHAPTER 12

# Urinalysis and Renal Disease

## A. URINALYSIS

Urinalysis is an indispensable part of clinical pathology. It may reveal pathology anywhere in the urinary tract. Also, it may afford a semiquantitative estimate of renal function, and furnish clues to the etiology of dysfunction. Finally, systemic diseases may be revealed by quantitative or qualitative alterations of urine constituents or by the presence of abnormal substances, quite apart from direct effects on the kidneys. Contrariwise, urinary tract disease may produce striking systemic symptoms.

The standard urinalysis includes: Appearance of the specimen, pH, specific gravity, protein semiquantitation, presence or absence of glucose and ketones, and microscopic examination of the centrifuged urinary sediment.

1. Appearance: Usually reported only if abnormal.

   Red color: blood; porphyria; occasionally urates, phenophthalein or Dorbane (laxative use).

   Brown color: blood (acid hematin); alkaptonuria (urine turns brownish on standing); melanin (may be brown and turn black on standing).

   Dark orange color: bile, pyridium (a urinary tract disinfectant).

2. pH: A determination of little importance in the usual case. Normal urine is usually acid; it may be alkaline in alkalosis or in those rare instances when the acidifying mechanism of the kidney fails (renal acidosis syndrome) or is poisoned (carbonic anhydrase inhibitors). Proteus infections characteristically alkalinize. Finally, urine standing at room temperature will slowly become alkaline due to bacterial growth.

114

3. Specific gravity will be considered also under renal function. It is important for several reasons: (1) As one parameter of renal tubular function. (2) Inability to concentrate may accompany certain diseases with otherwise relatively normal tubular function — such as diabetes insipidus or occasionally in severe hyperthyroidism and sickle cell anemia. (3) It affects other urine tests: a concentrated specimen may give higher results (for protein, etc.) than a dilute specimen, since the amount excreted per 24 hours is usually quantitatively the same in both cases; that is, the same amount of substance tested in a small quantity of fluid (high specific gravity) may appear more than if present in a larger dilute urine volume (low specific gravity).

4. Protein: In health, the glomerular membrane prevents most of the relatively large protein molecules of the blood from escaping into the urine. A small amount does get through, of which a small fraction is reabsorbed by the tubules and the remainder (up to 0.1 Gm./24 hours) is excreted. These amounts are normally not detected by routine clinical methods. One of the first responses of the kidney to a great variety of clinical situations is an alteration in glomerular filtrate. To a lesser extent, mere increase in glomerular filtration rate may increase normal protein excretion. Since albumin has a relatively small molecular size, it tends to become the dominant constituent in proteinuria, but rarely so complete as to justify the term "albuminuria" in a pure sense. Depending on the clinical situation, the constituents of "proteinuria" may or may not approach the constituents of plasma. Besides excess of normal plasma proteins, at times abnormal proteins may appear in the urine, notably Bence Jones (up to 50% of multiple myeloma patients).

To interpret proteinuria, one needs to know not only the major conditions responsible, but also the reason for production of excess urine protein. A system such as the following one is very helpful in this respect; proteinuria is classified according to the relationship of its etiology to the kidney and also to the mechanism involved.

a) Functional: Not associated with easily demonstrable systemic or renal damage.
   1) Severe muscular exertion.
   2) Pregnancy (p. 134).
   3) Orthostatic proteinuria. (This term designates slight to mild proteinuria associated only with the upright position; the exact etiology is poorly understood, with usual explanations tending to revolve around local factors causing renal passive congestion when in the upright position. It is easily diagnosed by an early morning urine specimen produced entirely while asleep, compared with one taken late in the day. This is probably the most common cause of "functional" proteinuria.)

b) Organic: Associated with demonstrable systemic disease or renal pathology.
   1) Prerenal proteinuria; not due to primary renal disease.

a. Fever, or a variety of toxic conditions (this is the most common etiology for "organic" proteinuria and is quite frequent).
b. Venous congestion (this is most often produced by chronic passive congestion due to heart failure; also, occasionally, by intra-abdominal compression of the renal veins).
c. Relative anoxia. (Such situations may be produced by severe dehydration, shock, severe acidosis, acute cardiac decompensation, severe anemias—all leading to a decrease in renal blood flow or possibly hypoxic renal changes. Very severe hypoxia, especially if acute, may lead to renal tubular necrosis.)
d. Hypertension (moderate or severe chronic hypertension; malignant hypertension; eclampsia).
e. Myxedema.
f. Bence Jones protein of multiple myeloma.

2) Renal proteinuria: primarily kidney disease.
a. Glomerulonephritis.
b. Nephrotic syndrome, primary or secondary.
c. Destructive parenchymal lesions (tumor, infection, infarct).
d. Poisoning with certain nephrotoxic drugs or chemicals.

3) Postrenal proteinuria: protein added to the urine at some point farther down the urinary tract from the renal parenchyma.
a. Infection of the renal pelvis or ureter.
b. Cystitis.
c. Urethritis or prostatitis.
d. Contamination with vaginal secretions.

Postrenal proteinuria is usually relatively small. Thus, by testing the supernate of a centrifuged specimen for protein, it can tentatively be assumed that pus mainly originated in the lower urinary tract, if pyuria occurs in the absence of proteinuria.

There are several clinically acceptable methods for semiquantitative protein testing. Those most used are heat with acetic acid, sulfosalicylic acid (3, 10, or 20%), and Robert's reagent. Sulfosalicylic acid is slightly more sensitive than the heat and acetic acid method. Sulfosalicylic acid false positive reactions may occur, notably with Orinase (tolbutamide); urates; hemoglobin (RBC or hemolysis); massive penicillin dose; dextran; occasionally salicylates; and various radiopaque x-ray substances. Bence Jones protein is also positive. Results are expressed as $1^+$ to $4^+$; this correlates very roughly to the amount of protein present (Table 4).

The Kingsbury-Clark procedure is a quantitative sulfosalicylic acid method using a series of permanent standards, each representing a different but measured amount of protein. After adding sulfosalicylic acid to the unknown specimen, a precipitate is formed which is compared with the standards and reported as the amount in the

TABLE 4.—RELATIONSHIP OF QUALITATIVE AND QUANTITATIVE
URINE PROTEIN RESULTS

| Qualitative | Protein | Rough Quantitative Correlation |
|---|---|---|
| Light cloud | Trace | 0.1- 0.5 Gm./liter |
| Medium cloud | $1^+$ | 0.5- 1.0 Gm./liter |
| Heavy cloud | $2^+$ | 3.0 Gm./liter |
| Light coagulum | $3^+$ | 5.0 Gm./liter |
| Heavy coagulum | $4^+$ | 10.0 Gm./liter (or more) |

particular standard that it matches. Besides these traditional
methods, there are two newer tests which are widely used. One is
a tablet procedure (Albutest) and the other is a paper dipstick (Albustix). The sulfosalicylic acid method is sensitive to as little as
10 mg./100 ml. protein. Albutest and Albustix are not reliable for
less than 25-30 mg./100 ml. Both will react with hemoglobin, but
will not give the other false positives occasionally found with sulfosalicylic acid and listed earlier. Behavior with Bence Jones is erratic; many cases are positive, but some unaccountably give negative test results. Urine with very alkaline pH may give false positives with the dipstick, but not the tablet test. In addition, the readings are often difficult to quantitate, especially with the dipstick,
and vary widely when the amount of protein is large.

Because individuals often vary in their interpretations, it is
sometimes useful to determine 24-hour urine protein excretion. It
should also be noted that degree of concentration may influence results on random urine specimens; a 24-hour specimen may also be
affected, but to a lesser extent.

In summary, not all proteinuria is pathologic (p. 115); even if
so, it may be transient; often the kidney is only indirectly involved;
individual interpretations of turbidity tests may vary widely; and occasionally protein may be added to the urine beyond the kidney.

5. Glucose: The most common and important glucosuria occurs in diabetes mellitus. A normal renal threshold is usually about
180 mg./100 ml. blood glucose level; beyond that, enough glucose is
filtered to exceed the usual tubular transfer maximum for glucose
reabsorption, and the surplus remains in the urine. However, individuals vary in their tubular transfer reabsorptive capacities, and,
if this happens to be low, that individual may spill sugar at lower
blood levels than the average person ("renal" glucosuria). Certain
uncommon conditions may elevate blood sugar levels in nondiabetic
persons. A partial list of the more important conditions associated
with glucosuria includes the following (discussed more fully in
Chapter 27):

a) Glucosuria without hyperglycemia.
   1) Renal glucosuria.
   2) Glucosuria of pregnancy (lactosuria may occur as well as
      glucosuria).

3) Certain inborn errors of metabolism (Fanconi syndrome).
4) After certain nephrotoxic chemicals (carbon monoxide, lead, mercuric chloride).

b) Glucosuria with hyperglycemia.

1) Diabetes mellitus.
2) Alimentary glucosuria (hyperglycemia is very transient).
3) Increased intracranial pressure (tumors, intracerebral hemorrhage, skull fracture).
4) Certain endocrine diseases or hormone-producing tumors (Cushing's disease; pheochromocytoma).
5) Hyperthyroidism (Graves' disease) occasionally.
6) Occasionally, transiently, after myocardial infarction.
7) After certain types of anesthesia, such as ether.
8) Emotional (infrequent).

The most commonly used tests are Benedict's method and Clinitest, which depend on copper sulfate reduction of potentially reducing substances and, therefore, are not specific for glucose or even sugar; and glucose oxidase enzyme papers (Clinistix and Tes-Tape) which are specific for glucose. In several reported comparisons of these tests, Tes-Tape proved most sensitive, but also gave occasional false positives. Clinistix gave few false positives, but also gave equivocal results or missed a few that Tes-Tape picked up. The copper reduction tests included about 10% positive results from reducing substances other than glucose. Clinitest is a copper reduction tablet test which seemed to have median sensitivity, whereas Benedict's, which is a standard type of chemical procedure, was least, missing 10-15% positive by glucose oxidase, but with very few false positives apart from other reducing substances. Some feel that Benedict's is equally as sensitive; the difficulty seems to lie in different criteria for what constitutes a trace reaction as opposed to a negative reaction. Although Benedict's method has been the traditional reference procedure of the past, it is time-consuming and is not commonly used today, since the tablet and dipstick tests are much faster and easier.

Although specific and relatively sensitive, the enzyme papers are not infallible. False positive results have been reported due to hydrogen peroxide and to hypochlorites (found in certain cleaning compounds). These substances give negative copper reduction test results. False negative results using Clinistix (but not Tes-Tape) have been reported from homogentisic acid (alkaptonuria), L-dopa, and large doses of aspirin. Also, the enzyme papers may unaccountably miss an occasional positive result which is picked up by the copper reduction techniques.

Reducing sugar (copper reduction) false positives include sugars besides glucose (galactose, lactose); also homogentisic acid (alkaptonuria). Other potentially troublesome substances are para-aminosalicylic acid (PAS), Aldomet, heavy salicylate therapy (salicyluric acid excreted), heavy concentrations of urates, and high doses of streptomycin or Keflin and occasionally of penicillin and terramycin.

An important technical consideration is to keep Clinitest tablets (and the enzyme papers) free from moisture before use.

   6. Microscopic: This examination is routinely done on centrifuged urine sediment. There is no widely accepted standardized procedure for this, and the varying degrees of sediment concentration which result make difficult any strict interpretation of quantitative reports. It is fairly safe to say, however, that normally so few cellular elements are excreted as to fall within normal clinical values no matter how much the specimen is centrifuged. Normal range means fewer than 1 red blood cell (RBC) or 5 white blood cells (WBC) per high-power field and only an occasional cast.

   The main pathologic elements of urinary sediment include RBC, WBC, casts, and other less important findings such as yeast, crystals or epithelial cells.

a) RBC

   Gross urinary bleeding is usually associated with stones, tumors, tuberculosis, and acute glomerulonephritis, although these may less often present only as microscopic hematuria. There are conditions which usually give significant microscopic hematuria, but occasionally approach gross bleeding, and some of the more important include: bleeding and clotting disorders (such as purpura or anticoagulants); blood dyscrasias (including sickle cell anemia or leukemia); renal infarction; malignant hypertension; subacute bacterial endocarditis (SBE); collagen diseases (especially lupus and periarteritis nodosa); Weil's disease; and various bladder, urethral, and prostatic conditions, including necrotizing cystitis and acute prostatitis. RBC casts are the only means of localizing the source of bleeding to the kidney. In the female, vaginal blood or leukocytes may contaminate ordinary voided specimens; finding significant numbers of squamous epithelial cells in the urinary sediment suggests such contamination. Yeast may simulate RBC (discussed later).

b) WBC

   These may be from any point in the urinary tract. Hematogenous spread of infection to the kidney usually first localizes in the renal cortex. Isolated cortical lesions may be relatively silent. Retrograde invasion from the bladder tends to involve calyces and medulla initially. Urinary tract obstruction is often a factor in retrograde pyelonephritis. Generally speaking, pyuria of renal origin is usually accompanied by significant proteinuria. That originating from the lower urinary tract may have proteinuria but it tends to be relatively slight.

   Urinary tract infections tend to be accompanied by bacteriuria. Tuberculosis of the kidney, besides producing hematuria, is said to characteristically have pyuria without bacteriuria. Naturally, ordinary urine cultures would be negative in tuberculosis. WBC casts are definite evidence localizing WBC to renal origin (discussed later). WBC in clumps are strongly suggestive, but are not conclusive.

c) Casts
   1) Casts are protein conglomerations outlining the shape of the
      renal tubules in which they were formed. Factors involved
      in cast formation include:
      a. pH: Protein casts tend to dissolve in alkaline medium.
      b. Concentration: Casts tend to dissolve in considerably di-
         lute medium. Concentration also has a considerable role
         in formation of casts; it favors precipitation out of protein.
      c. Proteinuria: Protein is necessary for cast formation, and
         significant cylindruria (cast excretion) is most often ac-
         companied by proteinuria. Proteinuria may be of varied
         etiology (p. 115). The post-renal type is added beyond
         the kidneys, and obviously cannot be involved in cast
         formation.
      d. Stasis: Stasis is usually secondary to intratubular ob-
         struction and thus allows time for protein precipitation
         within tubules.

   2) Mechanisms of cast formation are better understood if one
      considers the normal physiology of urine formation. The sub-
      stance filtered at the glomerulus is essentially an ultrafiltrate
      of plasma. In the proximal tubules, up to 85% of filtered so-
      dium and chloride is reabsorbed, with water passively ac-
      companying these ions. In the thick ascending loop of Henle,
      sodium is actively reabsorbed; but since the membrane here
      is impermeable to water, an excess of water ("free water")
      remains. As water passes along the distal tubules, some
      may be reabsorbed with sodium ions; and in the collecting
      tubules, up to 5% of the glomerular filtration rate is osmoti-
      cally reabsorbed due to the relatively high osmolarity of the
      renal interstitial cells. Water reabsorption in distal and col-
      lecting tubules is under the control of antidiuretic hormone
      (ADH). At this point, the urine reaches its maximum con-
      centration and proceeds to the bladder relatively unchanged.
          Thus, cast formation takes place ordinarily in the distal
      and collecting tubules, where acidification takes place and
      concentration reaches its height.

   3) There are two main types of casts, depending on their main
      constituents—cellular and hyaline.
      a. Cellular: Either RBC, WBC, desquamated renal epithe-
         lial cells, or any combination of these may conglomerate
         together in a protein matrix. The cast is basically cellu-
         lar in content (Fig. 6).
             As the cellular cast moves slowly down the nephron,
         the cells begin to disintegrate. Eventually, all that is left
         of the cells are relatively large fragments, chunks, or
         granules. This has now become a coarsely granular cast.
         The cast is now composed entirely of large irregular or
         coarse solid granules.

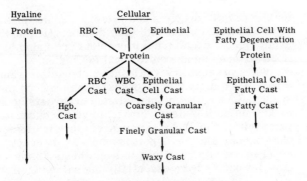

Fig. 6.—Formation of casts.

If disintegration is allowed to continue, the coarse granules break down to small granules, and a relatively homogeneous finely granular cast is formed.

The end stage of this process is the production of a homogeneous refractile material still in the shape of the tubule, known as waxy cast. Now the cast is translucent, without granules, and reflects light, giving a somewhat shiny or solid appearance. What stage of cast finally reaches the bladder depends on how long the cast takes to traverse the nephron and thus how long it remains in the kidney, where the forces of disintegration may work. A waxy cast is thus indicative of fairly severe localized stasis in the renal tubules.

b.  Hyaline: Hyaline casts are composed almost exclusively of protein alone. They pass almost unchanged down the urinary tract. They are dull, nearly transparent material and reflect light poorly in contrast to waxy casts; thus, hyaline casts are often hard to see, and the microscope condenser usually has to be turned down in order to give better contrast.

   Sometimes cellular elements may be trapped within hyaline casts; if hyaline material still predominates, the result is considered a hyaline cast with cellular inclusions. Degenerative changes can take place just as with regular cellular casts, with the production of hyaline coarsely and hyaline finely granular casts.

c.  Fatty casts: These are a special type of cellular cast. In certain types of renal tubular damage, fatty degeneration of the tubular epithelial cells takes place. These cells desquamate and are incorporated into casts. The epithelial cells contain fatty droplets; as the cells themselves degenerate, the fatty droplets remain and even may coalesce somewhat. The end result is a cast composed mainly of fatty droplets and protein. Sometimes either renal epithelial cells with fatty degeneration or the remnants thereof containing fat droplets are found in the urine floating free and are called oval fat bodies.

When present in significant number, this kind of picture is seen mainly in diseases which produce the nephrotic syndrome, such as primary lipoid nephrosis or secondary to Kimmelsteil-Wilson, lupus, amyloid, subacute glomerulonephritis, the nephrotic stage of chronic glomerulonephritis, certain tubule poisons such as mercury, and rare hypersensitivity reactions to such things as insect bites. Oval fat bodies have essentially the same significance as fatty casts. Fat droplets have a "Maltese Cross" appearance in polarized light, but are identifiable without this.

d.  In cases where severe stasis takes place, irrespective of the type of cast involved, cast formation may take place in the larger collecting tubules, where large ducts drain several smaller collecting tubules. If this occurs, a broad cast is formed, several times wider than ordinary sized casts. This is always indicative of severe localized renal stasis, and is most often found when the kidney is bordering on renal shutdown. These broad casts may be of any cast type, and due to their peculiar mode of formation are sometimes spoken of as "renal failure casts." This is not entirely accurate, for the kidney may often recover from that particular episode.

e.  Hemoglobin casts: These are derived from RBC casts which degenerate into granular (rarely even waxy) material but still have the peculiar orange-red color of hemoglobin. Not all casts derived from RBC retain this color. Strongly acid urine changes the characteristic color of hemoglobin to the nonspecific gray-brown color of acid hematin. Also, one must differentiate the brown or yellow-brown coloring derived from bile or other urine pigments from the typical color of hemoglobin.

4)  The significance of casts in the urine is a difficult question. Fatty casts, RBC and WBC casts are always significant. In all honesty, the only general statement one can make about ordinary hyaline or granular casts is that their appearance in significant numbers has some correlation with the factors involved in cast formation—proteinuria, concentration, and stasis. Of these, the most general correlation is with stasis, although one cannot even tell whether this is generalized or merely localized. It is common for showers of casts to clear dramatically once the underlying cause for their formation is corrected. On the other hand, significant numbers of casts which persist for some time despite therapeutic efforts may

suggest serious intrarenal derangement. In this respect, granular casts in the late stages of their development will be seen. Generally speaking, hyaline casts alone are of little practical importance and are usually only an acute, mild, and temporary phenomenon. Thus, to have any meaning, appearance of casts must be correlated with other findings and to the clinical situation. A few hyaline or granular casts in themselves have no importance.

d) Crystals: These are often overemphasized in importance. They may, however, be a clue to calculus formation and certain metabolic diseases. Crystals tend to be pH-dependent:

Acid urine: uric acid; cystine; calcium oxalate.

Alkaline urine: phosphates, as triple phosphate (magnesium ammonium phosphate) which comprises many staghorn calculi.

Note: Alkaline urine is most often produced by (Proteus) infection.

Amorphous crystalline sediment: If pH is acid, urates; if alkaline, phosphates. Rarely one might find sulfa crystals in acid urine, since sulfadiazine is still sometimes used. Most sulfas resemble needle-like crystals in bunches; but this appearance can be mimicked by certain nonpathologic crystals.

e) Miscellaneous:
Trichomonas is fairly common; often associated with slight proteinuria, WBC, and epithelial cell sediment. Diagnosis is by motility (and thus, a fresh specimen is essential); when nonmotile, it resembles a large WBC or small tubular epithelial cell. Trichomonas is found occasionally in the male. Spermatozoa may appear in the urine of males and, occasionally, in females.

Yeasts are important; the most usual type is Candida (Monilia). Yeast cells are often misdiagnosed as RBC. Differential points are: budding (not always present without careful search); ovoid shape (not always pronounced); yeasts appear slightly more opaque and homogeneous than RBC, and are insoluble in both acid and alkali. If the cells are numerous and still in doubt, a chemical test for blood is recommended.

Note: The most common mistake in microscopic examination is failure to mix the specimen sufficiently before putting it into the centrifuge tube. This is most important.

7. Other Examinations:

a) Bile (direct-acting bilirubin) typically appears secondary to hepatic obstruction, either extrahepatic (common duct obstruction) or intrahepatic (obstruction phase of hepatitis). Typically in infectious hepatitis, bile appears in urine a few days before the icteric stage, clearing swiftly once this begins.

In pulmonary infarction, there often occurs some elevation in serum (indirect-acting) bilirubin but not in the urine.

Tests for bile include Fouchet's reagent or Ictotest. The simple foam test (yellow foam after shaking) may be all that is necessary (false positive: pyridium). The commercial tablet test, Ictotest, is fairly sensitive, detecting as little as 0.1 mg./100 ml. It also is reasonably specific.

b) Urobilinogen appears classically as a secondary product from increased RBC breakdown (hemolytic processes). It may also be present in hepatitis, presumably due to inability of damaged hepatic parenchyma to handle normal amounts of urobilinogen produced by the intestine.

Tests for urobilinogen include an Ehrlich's reagent semiquantitative method, or a 24-hour quantitative determination.

For routine specimens, it is of the greatest importance that the test be done within one half hour after voiding. Urobilinogen rapidly oxidizes in air to nondetectable urobilin, and, without special preservatives, will decrease significantly after about one half hour. It is probably this unrecognized fact that accounts for the test's poor reputation. If the procedure cannot be done relatively soon after voiding, it is probably better to get a 24-hour specimen with preservatives.

c) Acetone and diacetic acid (also called ketone bodies) are classic findings of diabetic acidosis. However, acetonuria may also be found in starvation, many normal pregnancies, and especially in severe dehydration from many causes (vomiting, diarrhea, severe infections). In children, ketone bodies are prone to appear on what, by adult standards, would be very slight provocation. A weakly positive test for acetone is usually of little significance.

In fatty acid metabolism, acetyl-COA formed from fat breakdown may, under appropriate conditions, condense together to form acetoacetic (diacetic) acid, thence convert to acetone.

There are some reports that acetone formation from diacetic acid does not take place as much as is generally thought, and that even in only moderate degrees of ketonuria, the amount of diacetic acid in the urine is several times that of the acetone. This evidence supports the fact that, clinically, there is little need to distinguish between acetone and diacetic acid. Both have essentially the same significance. Most tests for acetone employ a nitroprusside reagent, and since nitroprusside will detect both, there seems no real reason to test for diacetic separately. Among widely used tests, Acetest tablets will detect concentrations of 5 mg./100 ml. of diacetic acid as well as react with acetone, and can be used with either urine, serum, or plasma. There is a new dipstick-type method called Ketostix, which is specific for diacetic acid, as low as 10 mg./100 ml. This method is incorporated into certain multiple-test dipsticks from the same manufacturer. These give false positive results with L-dopa. For the reasons just mentioned, the Acetest tablet is preferable. Finally, it must be em-

phasized that diabetes is practically the only disease in which
ketonuria has real diagnostic importance. Slight to moderate
degrees of ketonuria are fairly common in other conditions, as
mentioned earlier, but are only incidental. In diabetes, the
presence of large amounts of ketones is one of the major indications of diabetic acidosis or impending acidosis. In real diabetic
acidosis, the serum or plasma acetone test will always be positive (however, rare cases of hyperosmolar or lactic acidosis
coma do occur). In fact, the amount of ketones present, estimated by testing dilutions of plasma, is a good indication of the
severity of acidosis and the amount of insulin which is needed.
In the urine of diabetic acidosis, nitroprusside tests usually will
be strongly positive. In most cases, there will be glycosuria as
well as strong ketonuria. The only major exception is the presence of renal insufficiency with oliguria, either due to severe renal disease, shock, or exceptionally severe acidosis with secondary renal shutdown. The BUN is frequently elevated in diabetic acidosis; even so, there usually will be strong ketonuria.
If there is any question, a plasma or serum acetone test should
be done. In summary, the urine ketone level in diabetic acidosis
usually is very strongly positive and the plasma acetone is positive. However, if symptoms of diabetic acidosis are present,
lack of strongly positive urine ketones does not rule out the diagnosis, since a few patients with renal shutdown may be unable to
filter the elevated blood ketones through the kidney.

d) Calcium is tested in urine with Sulkowitch reagent; it is a semiquantitative method reported $0-4^+$ (normal being $1^+$), or as negative, moderately positive, and strongly positive. (For intepreta-
tion, see Chapter 28.) Excessively concentrated or diluted urine
may produce unreliable results, just as it will for protein.

e) Porphobilinogen is diagnostic of acute porphyria (p. 240) (episodes of abdominal crampy pain with vomiting and leukocytosis,
etc.). Porphobilinogen is colorless, and is easily identified by
rapid screening tests.

f) Urinary coproporphyrins show increased urinary excretion in
lead poisoning (p. 241), providing a relatively simple means to
help detect this condition. Type III is the coproporphyrin involved
(actually it is not specific for lead poisoning alone).

g) Phenylpyruvic acid is excreted in phenylketonuria (p. 397). A
ferric chloride test is the classic means of detection. There is
a dipstick ("Phenistix") method for the diagnosis of phenylketonuria, which depends on the reaction between ferric ions and
phenylpyruvic acid, much like the classic ferric chloride test.
It is more sensitive than ferric chloride, detecting down to
8 mg./100 ml. or trace amounts of phenylpyruvic acid in urine.
False positives occur if large amounts of ketone bodies are present. Reactions will take place with salicylates, PAS, and pheno-

thiazine metabolites, but the color is said to be different from
that given by phenylpyruvic acid.

h) Blood: Three simple procedures are on the market for detecting
hemoglobin in urine. Occultest is an orthotolidine tablet test
whose sensitivity has been adjusted to approximately 1:100,000
(which is about that of the old benzidine method). This is reported
to detect less than 5 RBC/HPF. Hematest is another tablet test
with the same basic reagents, but adjusted to approximately
1:20,000 sensitivity—slightly more than the guaiac method. Ex-
perimentally, this will not reliably detect less than 200 RBC/HPF
unless some of the cells have hemolyzed. It is much more sensitive to free hemoglobin, where it can detect amounts produced
by hemolysis of only 25-30 RBC/HPF. It can be used for feces
as well as urine, since, at this sensitivity, there are few false
positives. Hemastix is a dipstick method which is otherwise
identical to Hematest. The usefulness of these tests lies in their
ability to detect hemoglobin even after some or all of the RBC
have disintegrated and are no longer visible microscopically.
Red cell lysis is particularly likely to occur in dilute urine.
However, these tests cannot be used as a substitute for microscopic examination.

Points to remember when interpreting results of a urinalysis:

1. Laboratory reports usually err in omission, rather than
commission (except occasionally in RBC vs. yeast). If technicians
cannot identify something, they usually will not mention it at all.

2. Certain diagnostic findings such as RBC casts may not appear in every high-power (or even every low-power) field. If one
finds hematuria, one should look for them, and, similarly, for WBC
casts and other such structures in the appropriate sediment settings.

3. If the laboratory knows what you are after, they usually
will give more than a routine glance. Otherwise, the pressure of
routine work may result in examination which is not sufficient to
pick up important findings.

4. In many laboratories, reports will include only items specifically requested, even when other abnormalities are grossly visible (such as bile).

5. One fact that should be stressed when using commercial
tests of any type is to follow all the directions exactly. Many dipstick methods require a certain length of time in contact with the
specimen; when this is true, a quick dip-and-read technique may
lead to false results. The time interval of reading may be crucial
in tablet tests or other procedures.

## B.  THE KIDNEY IN DISEASE

1. Glomerulonephritis

a) Acute glomerulonephritis (AGN): In the classic form, this is

considered a hypersensitivity reaction, and usually is associated with concurrent or recent infection. The most common organism incriminated is the beta hemolytic Lancefield
group A streptococcus. Only a relatively small number of
specific group A strains are known to cause AGN, in contrast
to the large number which may initiate acute rheumatic fever.
Clinically, onset of the disease is usually manifested by hematuria. The urine may be red or may be "coffee-ground" in
color (due to breakdown of hemoglobin to brown acid hematin).
In mild cases, gross hematuria may be less evident, or hematuria may be microscopic only. Varying degrees of peripheral
edema, especially of the upper eyelids, are often present.
Varying degrees of hypertension are frequent initially. Laboratory features are a usually elevated erythrocyte sedimentation rate, and frequently a mild-to-moderate normocytic
normochromic (or slightly hypochromic) anemia. There is
mild-to-moderate proteinuria (0.5-3.0 Gm./24 hours). The
urinary sediment contains varying degrees of hematuria, often with white blood cells also present. RBC casts are characteristic, and are the most diagnostic laboratory finding.
They may be present only intermittently, sometimes may be
few in number, and may be degenerated enough to make recognition difficult. RBC casts are not specific for AGN. However, the number of diseases which are consistently associated with RBC casts are relatively few. They include AGN,
subacute and occasionally chronic glomerulonephritis, subacute bacterial endocarditis, some of the collagen diseases
(especially lupus), and hemoglobinuric ("lower nephron")
nephrosis. Significant prolonged azotemia is not common in
AGN (5-10% of cases) despite hypertension, although as many
as 50% have some BUN elevation initially. Renal function
tests are said to be essentially normal in nearly 50%; the remainder have varying degrees of impairment for varying time
intervals, and a small percentage show renal insufficiency
with uremia. Urine concentrating ability is generally maintained for the first few days; in some, it may then be impaired for considerable time intervals. Function tests in
general tend to reflect (although not exclusively) the primarily glomerular lesion found in AGN, histologically manifested by increased glomerular cellularity, swelling, and
proliferation of capillary endothelial cells. In addition to
urinalysis, the antistreptolysin-O (ASL or ASO) titer may be
helpful, since a significant titer (over 200 Todd units) means
recent or relatively recent group A streptococcal infection.
However, a negative ASL titer does not rule out the diagnosis;
nor does a "positive" titer guarantee that the condition is indeed AGN.

It is interesting that AGN is a relatively benign disease in childhood; the mortality is only about 1%, and fewer than that seem to develop permanent damage. In adults, the incidence of the disease is much less, and 25-50% of the cases develop chronic renal disease.

b) Subacute glomerulonephritis: This may follow the acute stage, but much more commonly appears without any previous clinical evidence of AGN. The term "subacute" is somewhat misleading; it refers to the duration of the clinical course, which is longer than that of the average AGN patient but much shorter than chronic glomerulonephritis. Histologically, the glomeruli show marked epithelial cell proliferation with resultant filling in of the space between Bowman's capsule and the glomerular tuft ("epithelial crescent"). The urine sediment includes many casts of hyaline and epithelial series; RBC are present in varying numbers, often with a few RBC casts. There is moderately severe to marked proteinuria, and both the degree of proteinuria and the urinary sediment may sometimes be indistinguishable from the nephrotic syndrome, even with fatty casts present. However, subacute glomerulonephritis is essentially a more severe form of acute glomerulonephritis and generally leads to death in weeks or months. It is not the same process as the nephrotic episodes that may form part of chronic glomerulonephritis. In addition to urinary findings, anemia is usually present. Renal function tests demonstrate both glomerular and tubule destruction, although clinically there is usually little additional information gained by extensive renal function studies.

c) Chronic glomerulonephritis: This infrequently is preceded by AGN, but usually has no antecedent clinical illness or etiology. It most often runs a slowly progressive or intermittent course over several or many years. During the latent phases there may be very few urinary abnormalities, but RBC are generally present in varying small numbers in the sediment. There is almost always proteinuria, generally of mild degree, and rather infrequent casts of the epithelial series. Progression is documented by slowly decreasing ability to concentrate the urine, followed by deterioration in clearance or PSP tests. Intercurrent streptococcal upper respiratory infection or other infections may occasionally set off an acute exacerbation. There may be one or more episodes of the nephrotic syndrome, usually without much, if any, hematuria. The terminal or azotemic stage produces the clinical and laboratory picture of renal failure. Finely granular and waxy casts predominate, and broad casts are often present. There is moderate proteinuria.

2. Nephrotic Syndrome

   The criteria for diagnosis of the nephrotic syndrome include: high proteinuria (over 3.5 Gm./24 hours), edema, hypercholesterolemia, and hypoalbuminemia. However, one or occasionally even more of these criteria may be absent. The level of proteinuria is said to be the most consistent criterion. In addition, patients with the nephrotic syndrome often have a characteristic serum protein electrophoretic pattern, consisting of greatly decreased albumin and considerably increased alpha$^2$ globulin. However, in some cases, the pattern may not be marked enough to be characteristic. The nephrotic syndrome is one of a relatively few diseases in which the serum cholesterol may add a substantial contribution toward establishing the diagnosis, especially in borderline cases.

   The nephrotic syndrome has nothing to do with hemoglobinuric nephrosis (so-called lower nephron nephrosis), despite the unfortunate similarity in names. Hemoglobinuric nephrosis is a distinct clinical entity seen in some cases of acute renal shutdown, most commonly due to marked intravascular hemolysis. The term "nephrotic syndrome" as it is currently used is actually a misnomer, and dates from the time when proteinuria was thought primarily due to a disorder of renal tubules. The word nephrosis was then used to characterize such a situation. It is now recognized that various glomerular lesions form the actual basis for proteinuria in the nephrotic syndrome, either of the primary or secondary type. The nephrotic syndrome as a term is also confusing because it may be of two types:

   a) Primary (or "lipoid") nephrosis: This is the idiopathic form, usually found in childhood. The etiology of primary (idiopathic or "lipoid") nephrosis is still not definitely settled. Renal biopsy has shown various glomerular abnormalities, classified most easily into basement membrane and proliferative varieties. The basement membrane changes may be so slight as to be certified only by electron microscopy (manifested by fusion of the footplates of epithelial cells applied to the basement membrane) or may present a diffuse "wire-loop" basement membrane thickening of varying severity which has been termed "membranous glomerulonephritis." Animal experiments suggest that an autoimmune process may be responsible, although at present this concept is not regarded as proved. The proliferative changes are also etiologically uncertain; many regard such cases as being a stage of chronic glomerulonephritis.

   In primary nephrosis, the urine shows mostly proteinuria; the sediment may or may not contain relatively small numbers of fatty and granular casts, and there may or may not be small numbers of RBC. Greater hematuria or cylindruria suggests greater severity, but not necessarily a worse prognosis. Renal function tests are normal in most; the remainder have various degrees of impairment.

b) Nephrotic syndrome: This is secondary to a variety of diseases, of which the most common are chronic glomerulonephritis, Kimmelsteil-Wilson, lupus, amyloid, and renal vein thrombosis. In the urine, fat is the most characteristic element, appearing in oval fat bodies and fatty casts. Also present are variable numbers of epithelial and hyaline series casts. RBC are variable—usually not frequent, but sometimes considerable. Significant hematuria suggests lupus; the presence of diabetes and hypertension, Kimmelsteil-Wilson; a history of previous proteinuria or hematuria, chronic glomerulonephritis; and the presence of chronic long-standing infection, amyloid. About 50% of cases are associated with chronic glomerulonephritis. Renal function tests in lupus, Kimmelsteil-Wilson, and amyloid generally show diffuse renal damage. The same is true for chronic glomerulonephritis in the later stages; however, if the nephrotic syndrome occurs relatively early in the course of this disease, changes may be minimal, reflected only in impaired concentrating ability. Histologically, renal glomeruli in the nephrotic syndrome exhibit lesions which vary according to the particular disease responsible.

3. Malignant Hypertension (Accelerated Arteriolar Nephrosclerosis)
This disease is most common in middle age, the great majority of patients being between ages 30 and 60. There is a tendency toward males, and an increased incidence in Negroes. The majority of patients have a history of preceding mild or "benign" hypertension, most often for 2-6 years, although the disease can begin abruptly. The syndrome may also be secondary to severe chronic renal disease of several varieties. Clinical features are marked systolic and diastolic blood pressure levels, the presence of papilledema, and evidence of renal damage. Laboratory tests show anemia to be present in most cases, even in relatively early stages. Urinalysis in the early stages shows most often a moderate proteinuria and hematuria, usually without RBC casts. It thus may mimic to some extent the sediment of acute glomerulonephritis. Later, the sediment may show more evidence of tubular damage. There usually develops a moderate-to-high proteinuria (which uncommonly may reach 5-10 Gm./24 hours), accompanied by considerable microscopic hematuria and often many casts, including all those of the hyaline and epithelial series—even fatty casts occasionally. In the terminal stages, later granular or waxy casts and broad renal failure casts predominate. The disease produces rapid deterioration of renal function tests; most cases terminate in azotemia. Nocturia and polyuria are common due to the progressive renal damage. If

congestive heart failure is superimposed, there may be decreased urine volume plus inability to concentrate.

4. Pyelonephritis

Acute pyelonephritis often elicits a characteristic syndrome (spiking high fever, costovertebral angle tenderness, dysuria, back pain, etc.). Proteinuria is mild, rarely exceeding 2.0 Gm./24 hours. Pyuria (and often bacteriuria) develops. WBC casts are diagnostic, although they may have to be carefully searched for, and may be absent. Urine culture may establish the diagnosis of urinary tract infection, but cannot localize the area involved. Hematogenous spread of infection to the kidney tends to localize in the renal cortex and may give fewer initial urinary findings; retrograde ascending infection from the lower urinary tract reaches renal medulla areas first and shows early pyuria.

In chronic low-grade pyelonephritis, the urine may not be grossly pyuric, and sediment may be scanty. In some cases, even random urine culture may be negative. Very frequently, however, there is a significant increase in pus cells, often, but not invariably, occurring in clumps when the process is more severe. Casts other than the WBC type are usually few or absent in pyelonephritis until the late or terminal stages, and WBC casts themselves may be absent.

A urine culture should be obtained in all cases of suspected urinary tract infection, to isolate the organism responsible and determine antibiotic sensitivity.

Tuberculosis is a special type of renal infection. It involves the kidney in possibly 25% of patients with chronic or severe pulmonary tuberculosis, although the incidence of clinical disease is much less. Hematuria is frequent; it may be gross or only microscopic. Pyuria is also common. Characteristically, pyuria should be present without demonstrable bacteriuria (of ordinary bacterial varieties), but this is not reliable due to a considerable frequency of superinfection by ordinary bacteria in genitourinary tuberculosis. Dysuria is also present in many patients. If hematuria (with or without pyuria) is found in a patient with tuberculosis, genitourinary tract tuberculosis should be suspected. Urine cultures are said to be positive in about 7% of cases with significant pulmonary tuberculosis. At least three specimens, one each day for 3 days, should be secured, each one collected in a sterile container. A fresh early morning specimen has been recommended rather than 24-hour collections. If suspicion of renal tuberculosis is strong, an IVP should be done in order to assess the extent of involvement.

Renal papillary necrosis should be mentioned here as a possible complication of acute pyelonephritis, particularly in diabetics.

5. Renal Papillary Necrosis (Necrotizing Papillitis)
   As the name suggests, this condition results from necrosis of
a focal area in one or more renal pyramids. Papillary necrosis
is most frequently associated with infection, but may occur without known cause. It is much more frequent in diabetics. A
small minority of cases are associated with sickle-cell hemoglobin diseases or phenacetin toxicity. The disease usually is
of an acute nature, although some patients may have relatively
minor symptoms, or symptoms overshadowed by other complications or disease. Especially when renal papillary necrosis is
associated with infection, the patients are usually severely ill
and manifest pyuria, hematuria, and azotemia. A drip-infusion
intravenous pyelogram is the diagnostic test of choice. Naturally,
urine culture should be done.

6. Renal Embolism and Thrombosis
   Renal artery occlusion or embolism most often affects the
smaller renal arteries or the arterioles. Such involvement
produces renal infarction in that vessel's distribution; usually
manifested by hematuria and proteinuria. Casts of the epithelial series may also appear.

7. Acute Tubular Necrosis ("Lower Nephron Nephrosis")
   This syndrome may result from acute or sudden renal shutdown from any cause, although marked intravascular hemolysis
from blood transfusion reactions is probably the most famous
etiology. It begins with a period of oliguria or near anuria, and
manifests subsequent diuresis if recovery ensues. Urinalysis
demonstrates considerable proteinuria with desquamated epithelial cells, epithelial and hyaline casts. There are usually
some RBC, occasionally many, and often large numbers of
broad and waxy casts (indicative of severe urinary stasis in
the renal parenchyma). Hemoglobin casts are usually present
in those cases due to intravascular hemolysis. Specific gravity
is characteristically fixed at 1.010 after the first hours, and the
BUN begins rising shortly after onset. In those cases not due
to intravascular hemolysis, the pathogenesis is that of generalized tubular necrosis, most often anoxic.

8. Congenital Renal Disease

   a) Polycystic kidney: There are two clinical forms, one fatal in early infancy, and the other ("adult type") usually asymptomatic until the third or fourth decade. The urinary sediment
is highly variable; microscopic intermittent hematuria is common, and gross hematuria may occasionally take place. Cysts
may become infected and produce symptoms of pyelonephritis.
In general, the rate of proteinuria is minimal or mild, but may

occasionally be higher. Symptoms may be those of hypertension (50-60% cases) or renal failure. If the condition does progress to renal failure, the urinary sediment is nonspecific, reflecting only the presence of end-stage kidneys of any etiology.
Diagnosis may be suggested by family history and the presence
of bilaterally palpable abdominal masses, and confirmed by
radiologic procedures such as the IVP.

b) Renal developmental anomalies: This category includes
horseshoe kidney, solitary cysts, reduplication of a ureter,
renal ptosis, etc. There may be no urinary findings, or sometimes a slight proteinuria. In children, urinary tract anomalies are a relatively frequent predisposing cause for repeated
urinary tract infection. Recurrent urinary tract infection, especially in children, should always be investigated for the possibility of either urinary tract obstruction or anomalies. Diagnosis is by IVP.

9.  Renal Neoplasia
    The most common sign of carcinoma anywhere in the urinary
tract is hematuria. A neoplasm should be suspected if this
finding is not explained by other conditions known to frequently
produce hematuria. Even if such diseases are present, this
would not rule out genitourinary carcinoma. The workup of a
patient with hematuria is discussed elsewhere (p. 146). The
detection of renal cell carcinoma is included in Chapter 32.

10. Lupus Erythematosus or Periarteritis Nodosa
    About two thirds of lupus patients show renal involvement.
Generally, there is microscopic hematuria; otherwise, there
may be a varying picture. In the classic case of lupus (much
less often in periarteritis), one finds a "telescoped sediment,"
containing the characteristic sediment elements of all three
stages of glomerulonephritis (acute, subacute, chronic—manifested by fatty, late granular, and RBC casts). Usually, hematuria is predominant, especially in polyarteritis. RBC casts
are more commonly found in lupus. About one third of lupus
patients develop the nephrotic syndrome.

11. Embolic Glomerulonephritis represents scattered small focal
    areas of necrosis in glomerular capillaries, most often due to
subacute bacterial endocarditis. There is some uncertainty
whether the lesions are embolic, infectious, or allergic in origin. Since the glomerular lesions are sharply focal, there
usually is not much pyuria. Hematuria usually is present and
may be pronounced. If localized tubular stasis occurs in addition, RBC casts may appear with resultant simulation of latent or acute glomerulonephritis. The rate of proteinuria often
remains relatively small, frequently not over 1.0 Gm./24 hours.

12. Dirst="diabetes">Diabetes</u>: The kidney may be affected by several unrelated disorders.

   a) High incidence of pyelonephritis; sometimes renal papillary
   necrosis.

   b) High incidence of arteriosclerosis with hypertension.

   c) Kimmelsteil-Wilson disease (intercapillary glomerulo-
   sclerosis); urinary findings may produce the nephrotic
   syndrome in late stages; otherwise, only varying degrees
   of proteinuria are manifest, perhaps with a few granular
   casts.

13. Pregnancy: Several abnormal urinary findings are associated
with pregnancy:

   a) "Benign" proteinuria: Proteinuria may appear in up to 30%
   of otherwise normal pregnancies during the time of labor. Of
   these, only about 3% are reported to surpass 100 mg./100 ml.
   It is unclear whether proteinuria must be considered pathologic
   if it occurs in uncomplicated pregnancy before labor. Some
   authorities believe that proteinuria is not found in normal pregnancy; others report an incidence of up to 20%, which is ascribed
   to abdominal venous compression.

   b) Eclampsia: This condition, also known as toxemia of
   pregnancy, denotes a syndrome of severe edema, proteinuria,
   hypertension, and convulsions associated with pregnancy. This
   syndrome without convulsions is called pre-eclampsia. In most
   cases, onset occurs either in the last trimester or during labor,
   although uncommonly the toxemic syndrome may develop after
   delivery. The etiology is unknown, despite the fact that delivery usually terminates the signs and symptoms. Pronounced
   proteinuria is the rule; the most severe cases may have oval
   fat bodies and fatty casts. Other laboratory abnormalities include principally an elevated serum uric acid in 60-70% of
   cases and a metabolic acidosis. The BUN is usually normal.
   Diagnosis at present depends more on the physical examination,
   including ophthalmoscopic observation of spasm in the retinal
   arteries and blood pressure changes, than on the laboratory (except for proteinuria). Gradual onset of eclampsia may be confusing, since some degree of edema is common in pregnancy,
   and proteinuria (although only slight or mild) may appear during
   labor.

   c) Glucosuria: Glucosuria is found in 5-35% of pregnancies,
   mainly in the last trimester. Occasional reports state an even
   higher frequency. It is not completely clear whether this is due
   to increased glucose filtration due to increased glomerular fil-

tration rate, decreased renal tubular transport maximum (reabsorptive) capacity for glucose, a combination of the two, or some other factor. As noted elsewhere, lactosuria may also occur in the last trimester, and may be mistaken for glucosuria using copper sulfate reducing tests for urine sugar.

d) Renal function tests: Glomerular filtration rate is increased during pregnancy. Because of this, BUN is apparently somewhat decreased, and clearance tests somewhat increased. Concentration tests may be falsely decreased because of edema fluid excretion that takes place during sleep. Since ureteral dilatation usually occurs in the last trimester, PSP excretion may be falsely decreased because of stasis in the dilated upper urinary tract.

e) Infection: Bacteriuria has been reported in 4-7% of pregnant patients, whereas the incidence in nonpregnant healthy women is approximately 0.5%. It is believed that untreated bacteriuria strongly predisposes to postpartum pyelonephritis.

## C. URINALYSIS IN MISCELLANEOUS DISEASES

1. Fever is the most common cause of proteinuria (up to 75% of febrile patients). If severe, it may be associated with an increase in hyaline casts (etiology unknown; possibly dehydration?).

2. Cystitis-Urethritis: These are lower urinary tract infections, often hard to differentiate from renal infection. Clumping of WBC is suggestive of pyelonephritis, but not absolutely specific, as WBC casts are. Necrotizing cystitis may cause hematuria. The two-glass urine test helps to differentiate urethritis from cystitis. After cleansing the genitalia, the patient voids about 10-20 ml. into container #1 and the remainder into container #2. Significant increase in container #1 cell count suggests urethral origin.

3. Genitourinary Tract Obstruction (neuromuscular disorders of the bladder; congenital urethral strictures and valves; intrinsic or extrinsic ureteral mechanical compressions; intraluminal calculi) produces no specific urinary changes, but predisposes to stasis and infection. Obstruction (whether partial or complete) is a frequent etiology for recurrent GU infections.

4. Amyloidosis: Renal involvement usually leads to proteinuria. In a minority of cases, when the process severely affects the kidney, there may be high proteinuria and sediment typical of the nephrotic syndrome. The urinary sediment, however, is not specific, and RBC casts are not present. Renal amyloidosis is usually

associated with chronic diseases such as long-standing osteomyelitis or infection, or multiple sclerosis.

5. Urinary Calculi often cause hematuria of some type and may be associated with excess excretion of calcium, uric acid, cystine, phosphates, or urates in the urine even when calculi are not clinically evident. Frequent complications are infection or obstruction, and infection may occur even in the absence of definite obstruction. Ureteral stone passage gives hematuria, often gross. An IVP is the best means of diagnosis; some types of calculi are radiopaque, and others may be localized by finding a site of ureteral obstruction.

6. Sickle-Cell Anemia: Kidney lesions may result from intracapillary RBC plugs, leading to congestion, small thromboses, and infarctions. Also, at times of hematologic crises, hematuria is frequent. Hematuria may be present even without crises in sickle-cell disease or sickle-cell variants. Sickle-cell patients may lose urine-concentrating ability for unknown reasons—less commonly, even with sickle-cell variants.

7. Chronic Passive Congestion (CPC) results from cardiac failure or inferior vena caval obstruction. It produces mild diffuse tubular atrophy and hyperemia, leads to proteinuria (usually mild to moderate) and hyaline casts, and sometimes also elicits epithelial casts and a few RBC. Occasionally, but not commonly, severe CPC may simulate the nephrotic syndrome to some extent, including desquamated epithelial cells containing fat plus many casts of epithelial series. In CPC of strictly cardiac origin without significant previous renal damage, there is decreased urine volume but usually retained ability to concentrate. No anemia is present unless due to some other systemic etiology.

8. Benign Arteriosclerosis involves the renal parenchyma secondarily to decreased blood supply. In the majority of cases in the earlier stages, there are few urinary findings, if any; later, there is often mild proteinuria (0.1-0.5 Gm./24 hours) and a variable urine sediment, such as a few hyaline casts, epithelial cells, and perhaps occasional RBC. If the condition eventually progresses to renal failure, there will be significant proteinuria and renal failure sediment with impaired renal function tests.

9. Weil's Disease is a classic combination of hepatitis and hematuria. Characteristically, there are also high fever and severe muscle aching, and there may be associated symptoms of meningitis.

10. Infectious Mononucleosis produces renal involvement with hematuria in 5-6% of cases.

11. Purpura and Hemorrhagic Diseases should be recognized as a cause of hematuria, either by itself or in association with glomerular lesions. The Henoch-Schönlein syndrome (anaphylactoid purpura) is a rare condition which often is concurrent with hematuria and nephritis.

12. Hypersensitivities may lead to proteinuria (usually slight) with hematuria and perhaps a moderate increase in casts. Kidney involvement may occur due to mercurials, sulfas, etc.

13. Fat Embolism is most commonly found after trauma, especially with fractures. Cerebral or respiratory symptoms develop in the second or third day after injury, associated usually with a significant drop in hemoglobin values. Fat in the urine is found in 50% or more of patients and is a very valuable diagnostic test (p. 238). Unfortunately, an order for a test of fat in the urine will usually produce microscopic examination of the sediment. Whereas this is correct procedure for nephrotic syndrome, where fat is located in renal epithelial cells and casts, this is worthless for fat embolism diagnosis, where free fat is the item to be located. Since free fat tends to float, a simple procedure is to fill an Ehrlenmeyer (thin-neck) flask with urine up into the thin neck, agitate gently to allow fat to reach the surface, skim the surface with a bacteriologic loop, place the loop contents on a slide, and then stain with a fat stain such as Sudan IV.

14. Hemochromatosis presents hepatomegaly, gray skin pigmentation, and proteinuria in a diabetic patient. Proteinuria may exceed 1.0 Gm./24 hours, but sediment may be scanty, and fat is absent. Yellow-brown coarse granules of hemosiderin in severe cases are seen in cells, in casts, and lying free. Prussian blue (iron) stains in this material are positive. Distal convoluted tubules are the areas primarily involved. Since hemochromatosis does not invariably involve the kidney until late, a negative urine does not rule out the diagnosis. False positives (other types of urinary siderosis) may occur in pernicious anemia, hemolytic jaundice, and in patients who have received many transfusions.

15. Thyroid Dysfunction:
   a) Myxedema: Proteinuria is said to occur without other renal disease; its incidence is uncertain, especially since some reports state that proteinuria is actually not common, and usually persists after treatment.
   b) Hyperthyroid: The kidney may lose its concentrating ability so that specific gravity may remain low even in dehydration; this is reversible with treatment and return to euthyroid. Glucosuria occurs in occasional patients.

## REFERENCES

Adams, E. C., et al.: Hemolysis in hematuria, J. Urol. 88:427, 1962.

Berman, L. B., and Schreiner, G. E.: Clinical and histologic spectrum of the nephrotic syndrome, Am. J. Med. 24:249, 1958.

Beskow, A.: A survey of tuberculosis of the kidney in relation to tuberculosis in general, Acta tuberc. scandinav., supp. 31, 1952.

Brough, A. J., and Zuelzer, W. W.: Renal vascular disease, Pediat. Clin. North America 11:533, 1964.

Caulfield, J. B.: Application of the electron microscope to renal disease, New England J. Med. 270:183, 1964.

Danowski, T. S., and Nabarro, J. D. N.: Hyperosmolar and other types of nonketoacidotic coma in diabetes, Diabetes 14:162, 1965.

deWardener, H. E.: The Kidney (3d ed.; Boston: Little, Brown & Company, 1968).

Free, A. H., et al.: Studies with a new colorimetric test for proteinuria, Clin. Chem. 3:716, 1957.

Gifford, H., and Bergerman, J.: Falsely negative enzyme paper tests for urinary glucose, J.A.M.A. 178:423, 1961.

Kimmelsteil, P., et al.: Chronic pyelonephritis, Am. J. Med. 30:589, 1961.

Kushner, D. S.: Natural History and Therapy of Acute Glomerulonephritis, in Dock, W., and Snapper, I. (eds.): Advances in Internal Medicine (Chicago: Year Book Medical Publishers, Inc., 1962), Vol. XI, p. 75.

Lee, C. T., Jr.: Renal disease in diabetes mellitus, M. Clin. North America 47:1069, 1963.

Letteri, J. M.: The urinary sediment in renal disease, M. Clin. North America 47:887, 1963.

Levitt, J. I.: The prognostic significance of proteinuria in young college students, Ann. Int. Med. 66:685, 1967.

Lippman, R. W.: Urine and the Urinary Sediment (2d ed.; Springfield, Ill.: Charles C Thomas, Publisher, 1957).

Maxon, W. T.: Benign proteinuria of childhood and adolescence: A survey, Clin. Pediat. 2:662, 1963.

Mostofi, F. K., et al.: Lesions in kidneys removed for unilateral hematuria in sickle cell disease, Arch. Path. 63:336, 1957.

O'Sullivan, J. B., et al.: Comparative value of tests for urinary glucose, Diabetes 11:53, 1962.

Pollak, V. E., et al.: Renal vein thrombosis, Postgrad. Med. 40:282, 1966.

Pollak, V. E., and Kark, R. M.: The toxemias of pregnancy and the renal lesion of pre-eclampsia, Am. J. Med. 30:181, 1961.

Reikers, H., and Miale, J. B.: Ketonuria: An evaluation of tests and some clinical implications, Am. J. Clin. Path. 30:530, 1958.

Reynolds, T. B., and Edmondson, H. A.: Chronic renal disease and heavy use of analgesics, J.A.M.A. 184:435, 1963.

Salomon, M. I., et al.: Renal lesions in hepatic disease, Arch.
    Int. Med. 115:704, 1965.
Strauss, M. B., and Welt, L. G. (eds.): Diseases of the Kidney
    (Boston: Little, Brown & Company, 1963).
Wells, B. B.: Diseases of the Kidney and Urinary Tract, in Wells,
    B. B.: Clinical Pathology: Application and Interpretation (4th ed.;
    Philadelphia: W. B. Saunders Company, 1967).
Wilson, R. M., et al.: Lupus nephritis, Arch. Int. Med. 111:429
    1963.

# CHAPTER 13

# Renal Function Tests

The measurement of renal function is fully as evasive as that of hepatic function. In both the kidney and the liver, a multiplicity of enzyme and transport systems coexist—some related, others both spatially and physiologically quite separate. Processes going on in one section of the nephron may or may not directly affect those in other segments. Like the liver, the kidney has not one but a great many "functions" which may or may not be affected in a given pathologic process. By measuring the capacity to perform these individual functions, one hopes to extrapolate anatomic and physiologic information. Unfortunately, the tests available to the clinical laboratory are few and gross compared to the delicate network of systems at work. It is often difficult to isolate individual functions without complicated research setups, and even more so to differentiate between localized and generalized damage, between temporary or permanent malfunction, and between primary and secondary derangements. One can measure only what passes into and out of the kidney. What goes on inside is all-important, but must be speculated on by indirect means. One can accurately interpret renal function tests only by keeping these facts in mind, by learning the physiologic basis for each test, and by careful correlation with other clinical and laboratory data.

Proteinuria almost invariably accompanies serious renal damage. Its severity does not necessarily correlate with the amount of damaged renal parenchyma or the status of any one renal function or group of systems. Its presence and degree may, in association with other findings, aid in the diagnosis of certain syndromes or disease entities whose renal pathologic findings are known. Its presence may be secondary to benign or even extrarenal etiologies.

1. Tests predominantly of glomerular function: Urea and Creatinine Clearance Tests.

Clearance: Clearance is a theoretical concept defined as that volume of plasma from which a measured amount of substance could be completely eliminated ("cleared") into the urine per unit time. This depends on the plasma concentration and excretory rate, which in turn involve the glomerular filtration rate (GFR) and renal plasma flow (RPF). Clearance tests in general are the best available for estimating mild-to-moderate diffuse glomerular damage (e.g., acute glomerulonephritis). Serum levels of urea or creatinine reveal only extensive renal disease. Note, however, that many "extrarenal" conditions cause vasoconstriction and will reduce RPF (shock, hyponatremia, etc.), and thus possibly reduce clearance values.

a) Urea Clearance: Urea is filtered at the glomerulus, and approximately 40% is reabsorbed in the tubules by passive back-diffusion. Thus, under usual conditions, urea clearance values parallel the true GFR at about 60% of it. However, several factors may adversely influence this situation: (1) The test is dependent on rate of urine flow. At low levels (less than 2 cc. per minute), the values are very inaccurate, even with certain "correction" formulas. (2) Levels of blood urea vary considerably during the day and according to diet and other conditions.

b) Creatinine Clearance: Creatinine is a metabolic product of creatine-phosphate dephosphorylation in muscle. It has a relatively constant hourly and daily production, and fairly stable blood levels. Excretion is by a combination of glomerular filtration and tubular secretion (20-30%). It usually parallels true GFR by $\pm$ 10%. However, at low filtration rates (less than 30% of normal), creatinine rates become increasingly inaccurate due to the relatively higher proportion of the secreted fraction. Advantages are constancy of production, allowing larger time interval collections— also freedom from dependence on urine flow. The main disadvantage is the moderate technical difficulty of laboratory analysis which may magnify small errors when dealing with the small amounts of substance usually present. In general, creatinine clearance is definitely a better test than urea clearance, and, for clinical purposes, affords adequate estimation of GFR.

2. Tests reflecting either severe glomerular or tubular damage, or both: BUN, NPN, Serum Creatinine.

Azotemia: BUN and NPN are equally satisfactory in most cases. BUN is easier to perform technically. In chronic diffuse types of renal disease, significant azotemia usually heralds the end-stage kidney. In other renal diseases, azotemia may be only transient, or permanently reversible. It may occur in many conditions:

a) Prerenal Azotemia
  1) Traumatic shock (head injuries; postsurgical hypotension).
  2) Hemorrhagic shock (varices, ulcer, postpartum hemorrhage, etc.).

3) Severe dehydration or electrolyte loss (severe vomiting, diarrhea, diabetic acidosis, Addison's disease).
4) Acute cardiac decompensation (especially after extensive infarction).
5) Overwhelming infections or toxemia.
6) Excess intake of proteins or extensive protein breakdown (usually other factors are also involved, such as the normally subclinical slight functional loss from aging).

b) Renal
1) Chronic diffuse bilateral kidney disease or bilateral severe kidney damage (e. g. , chronic glomerulonephritis or bilateral chronic pyelonephritis).
2) Acute tubular necrosis (lower nephron nephrosis): primarily tubular disease; due to shock with renal shutdown, crush injuries, transfusion or allergic reactions, certain poisons, and precipitation of uric acid or sulfa crystals in renal tubules.
3) Severe acute glomerular damage (e. g. , acute glomerulonephritis).

c) Postrenal (Obstruction)
1) Ureteral or urethral obstruction, by strictures, stones, external compression (pelvic tumors, etc.).
2) Obstructing tumors of bladder; congenital defects in bladder or urethra.
3) Prostatic obstruction (tumor or benign hypertrophy; a very common cause in elderly males).

In azotemia due to excess protein, some of the more common clinical situations are high protein tube-feedings or gastrointestinal tract hemorrhage (where protein is absorbed from the GI tract); a low-calorie diet (as in patients on intravenous fluids, leading to endogenous protein catabolism); and adrenocortical steroid therapy (since these substances have a catabolic action).

Thus, in general, prerenal azotemia etiologies can be divided into two main categories: (1) decreased blood volume or renal circulation, and (2) increased protein intake or endogenous protein catabolism.

In primary renal disease, azotemia may be due to either primarily glomerular or tubular obstructive conditions, or to diffuse parenchymal destruction. It must be remembered that rarely would one get glomerular damage to the point of severe azotemia (5-10% of AGN cases) without some effect on the tubules and vice versa. BUN must, therefore, be correlated with other clinical observations before its significance can be estimated. There is nothing etiologically distinctive about the terminal manifestations of chronic kidney disease, and it is most important to rule out treatable diseases which may simulate the uremic laboratory or clinical picture. Especially, complete anuria always suggests urinary obstruction.

Terminal azotemia, sometimes to uremic levels, occurs in the last hours or days of a significant number of seriously ill patients

with a variety of diseases, including cancer. Often no clinical or
pathologic cause, even microscopically, is found. Urine specific
gravity may be relatively good.

Two screening methods for BUN, called Urograph and Azostix,
are commercially available. Evaluations to date indicate that both
of these methods are useful as emergency or office screening procedures to separate normal persons (BUN less than 20 mg./100 ml.)
from those with mild azotemia (20-50 mg./100 ml.) and those with
considerable BUN elevation (over 50 mg./100 ml.). If accurate
quantitation is desired, one of the standard quantitative BUN procedures should be done.

Serum creatinine determination has much the same significance as BUN but tends to rise later. Significant elevations thus
suggest, without being diagnostic of, chronicity. It has been reported that ketone bodies may give false elevation of creatinine in
serum or urine.

3. Tests of predominantly tubular function: Phenolsulfonph-
thalein (PSP), Concentration and Dilution.

a) PSP: Over 85% is actively excreted by proximal tubular epithelium; less than 5% is filtered at the glomerulus, and the remainder
is excreted by the liver. Thus, PSP excretion is a measure of
one tubular "function" and indirectly of tubular health. The 15-
minute measurement is the most important in this respect, but a
2-hour specimen should also be done. It is most important to hydrate the patient beforehand and to have some urine in the bladder
when dye is injected; this volume of urine is not a factor in the results, but helps to recover all the excreted dye. Also essential
is accurately timed specimen collection, and care taken to insure
complete bladder emptying at the collection periods even if catheterization is necessary (however, catheterization for this test
alone is not justified clinically because of the risk of introducing
infection). Normal values are 25% or greater excretion at 15
minutes; 40-60% at 1 hour, and 60-80% at 2 hours. The importance of the 15-minute specimen lies in the fact that relatively
early or mild bilateral renal disease may decrease function enough
to influence the early collection specimen, whereas the later
specimens may still fall within the normal range, since they represent an additive or cumulative effect over the longer time intervals.

b) Specific Gravity is important in the evaluation of chronic diffuse
parenchymal disease (chronic glomerulonephritis, chronic pyelonephritis, etc.). As such conditions progress, tubular ability to
concentrate urine is often affected relatively early, and slowly
decreases until the urine has the same specific gravity as the
plasma ultrafiltrate—1.010. This usually, but not always, occurs
in advance of final renal decompensation. Concentration tests, to
be accurate, must deprive the patient of water over a long period
to exclude influence from previous ingestion. The usual test

should run 16-17 hours; after previous forced fluids, longer may be necessary. This may be impossible in cardiacs, renal failure, aged persons, or those with electrolyte problems. Under these test conditions, the average person should concentrate to 1.025; at least to 1.020. Concentration tests are also impaired in diabetes insipidus, diuretic phase of acute tubular necrosis, and occasionally in hyperthyroidism, severe salt-restricted diets, and sickle cell anemia; these diseases may result in failure to concentrate without the presence of irreversible renal tubular damage. Abnormal urinary substances may raise specific gravity to a small extent; for 10 Gm. protein/L. subtract .003; for 1% glucose, subtract .004. In addition, the radiopaque contrast media used for intravenous pyelograms (IVP) considerably increase urine specific gravity; this effect may persist for 1-2 days. Ability to concentrate urine does not rule out many types of active kidney disease, nor does inability to concentrate necessarily mean closely approaching renal failure. Adequate ability to concentrate is, however, decidedly against the diagnosis of chronic severe diffuse renal disease. Beginning of impairment of concentrating ability (on a concentration test) often is a relatively early manifestation of chronic diffuse bilateral renal disease, and often becomes manifest before changes in other function tests (this refers to beginning impairment, not to fixation of specific gravity).

Clinically, fixation of specific gravity is usually manifested by nocturia and a diminution of the day-night ratio (normally 3 or 4:1) approaching 1:1. Other causes must be considered: diabetes mellitus and insipidus, hyperparathyroidism, renal acidosis syndrome, beginning of congestive heart failure, and occasionally hyperthyroidism. True nocturia or polyuria must be distinguished from urgency, incontinence, or enuresis.

One improvement on the standard concentration procedure is to substitute for water deprivation a single injection of Pitressin tannate in oil. Five units of this long-acting preparation are given intramuscularly in the late afternoon, and urine collections for specific gravity are made in the early morning and two times thereafter at 3-hour intervals. One danger of this procedure is the possibility in certain patients, such as infants on liquid diet, of water intoxication.

A relatively recent innovation is to measure the urine osmolality (sometimes incorrectly called osmolarity) instead of conventional specific gravity. Osmolality is a measure of the osmotic strength or number of osmotically active ions or particles present per unit of solution. Specific gravity is defined as the weight or density per unit volume of solution compared to water. Since the number of molecules present in a solution is a major determinant of its weight, it is obvious that there is a relationship between osmolality and specific gravity; since the degree of ionic dissociation is very important in osmolality but not in specific gravity, values of the two for the same solution may not always correspond closely. The rationale for using this concept is that specific gravity is a rather empirical observation and does not measure the actual ability of the kidney to concentrate electrolytes or other molecules relative to the plasma concentration; also, certain substances are of relatively large molecular weight and tend to disproportionately affect specific gravity. The quantity of water present may vary even in concentration tests and influence results. Osmolality is defined in terms of milliosmoles per kilogram of solution and can be easily and accurately measured by determining the freezing point depression of a sample in a specially designed machine (in biologic fluids such as serum or urine, water makes up nearly all of the specimen weight; since water weighs 1 Gm./ml., osmolality may be approximated clinically by values reported in terms of milliosmoles per liter rather than per kilogram). Normal values for urine osmolality after 14-hour test dehydration are 800-1300 milliosmoles/liter. Most osmometers are accurate to less than 5 milliosmoles, so the answer thus has an aura of scientific exactness which is lacking in the relatively crude specific gravity method. Unfortunately, having a rather precise number and being able to use it clinically are often two different things. Without reference to the clinical situation, osmolality has as little meaning as specific gravity. In most situations, they have approximately the same significance. Both vary and depend on the amount of water excreted with the urinary solids. In some cases, however, such as when the specific gravity is fixed at 1.010, osmolality after dehydration may still be greater than that of the serum, suggesting that it is a more sensitive measurement. Also, osmolality does not need correction for glycosuria, proteinuria, or urine temperature.

c) Intravenous Pyelogram (IVP): This radiologic technique uses iodinated contrast media, most of which are tubular secreted. In order to appear radiographically, once secreted they must also be concentrated. Thus, incidental to delineating calyceal and urinary tract outlines and revealing postrenal obstruction, IVP also affords some information as to kidney concentrating ability or ability to excrete the dye—two tubular "functions." These are not sufficient for visualization with BUN over 50 mg./100 ml. using ordinary (standard) IVP technique. New methods ("drip-infusion IVP") can be used with higher BUN levels, but these are not routine and usually must be specifically requested.

d) Another renal tubule activity is the handling of electrolytes such as sodium (p. 284); this may be of clinical value in certain situations (pp. 152, 288) and can be estimated by measurement of the urine levels of these electrolytes. A variety of research techniques not generally available can measure one or another of the many kidney "functions," such as tubular secretion of various substances, glomerular filtration of nonreabsorbed materials such as inulin, and renal blood flow by clearance of substances such as PAH which are both filtered and secreted.

Next will be discussed the interpretation of certain tests and also some suggestions on how to select them. Most of the time, only a few tests are needed to get all the useful information available.

One question which continually arises is the significance of small degrees of proteinuria. Textbook normal values are usually stated as 10 mg./100 ml. (0.1 Gm./liter). Generally speaking, values of up to 30 mg./100 ml. are within normal range; 30-40 mg./ 100 ml. may or may not be significantly abnormal. It should be noted that normal values in terms of total urinary protein output per 24 hours may be up to 100 mg. (0.1 Gm.) per 24 hours. Values stated in terms of mg./24 hours may not coincide with values expressed in terms of mg./100 ml., due to varying quantities of diluent water. It must be stressed that duration of proteinuria is even more important than quantity, especially at low values. As an example, 60 mg./100 ml. or even more may have minor or little importance on an admission urine if this subsequently clears up, whereas 40 mg./100 ml. may possibly be significant if this level persists. This becomes clear by examining the list of possible causes of proteinuria. Intrinsic renal disease usually has proteinuria which persists, whereas many of the extrarenal types will quickly disappear if the primary disease is successfully treated. However, this does not always hold true, and one must remember that a single disease may cause permanent damage to more than one organ. In arteriosclerosis or hypertension, for example, functioning kidney tissue may be reduced or destroyed to varying degrees by arteriolar nephrosclerosis, although cardiac symptoms due to heart damage may overshadow the clinical picture.

The problem of hematuria is somewhat different from that of proteinuria. One must always remember that hematuria is the most frequent symptom of urinary tract cancer—often the only one. If no disease is present to account for the hematuria, which can be either gross or microscopic, the patient should get an IVP. If this is negative, and if the hematuria persists or there is some other reason to suspect a neoplasm, the IVP should be followed by cystoscopy to detect bladder carcinoma. It must also not be forgotten that the patient may have hematuria due to carcinoma of kidney or bladder and at the same time have other diseases, such as hypertension, which themselves are known causes of hematuria. Generally speaking, however, the diseases which cause significant hematuria are in a minority and can usually be diagnosed and evaluated without too much difficulty. Hypertension most often is at least moderately severe for really significant hematuria (e. g., over 5 RBC per high-power field) to be present. Finding RBC casts means that the hematuria is from the kidney and that the problem is a medical disease rather than a surgical one or cancer. Also, the age of the patient is important; in

a child, a neoplasm of the urinary tract would be very unlikely.   In
adults, most bladder and renal carcinomas develop in patients over
age 40 (many other diseases do likewise, unfortunately).

Clearance tests may be needed occasionally, and this usually
happens in three situations; first, in acute glomerulonephritis (AGN),
to follow the clinical course and as a parameter of therapeutic response; second, to demonstrate the presence of acute strictly glomerular disease in contrast to more diffuse chronic structural damage; and third, as a measurement of over-all renal functional impairment.   In AGN, there is frequently, but not always, a decrease
in glomerular filtration due to primary glomerular involvement.
When this is true, the clearance tests have been used to evaluate the
length of time bed rest and other therapy is necessary.   However,
the erythrocyte sedimentation rate gives the same information in a
manner which is cheaper, simpler, and probably more sensitive.
Therefore, the ESR seems preferable in most cases.   Concerning
the second category, it is not so easy to demonstrate strictly glomerular disease because many diseases will reduce renal blood flow
and thus glomerular filtration rate.   Also, some patients with AGN
may have some degree of tubular damage.   One situation in which
clearance tests may be used to diagnostic advantage is the rare case
of a young person with sudden gross hematuria but without convincing
clinical or laboratory evidence of AGN.   Since, in a young person,
one would expect normal clearance values, finding reduced creatinine
clearance would be in favor of nephritis.   Clearance as a measurement of over-all renal function impairment demonstrates roughly
the same information as is obtained from the PSP.   Clearance tests
are reliable in detecting mild-to-moderate diffuse renal disease, but
depend on completely collected specimens and accurate recording
of the time the specimens were collected, and presuppose adequate
renal blood flow.   If a patient is incontinent of urine, one must use
either a short period of collection or a catheter, or else use some
other test.   Of course, if a Foley catheter is already in place, there
is no problem.   The clearance range of 60-80% of normal is usually
taken to represent mild diffuse renal function impairment.   Values
between 40 and 60% of normal are considered moderate decrease,
and between 20 and 40% of normal is severe, since about half the
patients in this group have elevated BUN.

The PSP, as mentioned, gives similar information to clearance procedures over much of the same area.   It is not quite as dependent on renal blood flow, although this is a factor; also, it takes
a total of 2 hours, during which most patients can hold their urine.
Disadvantages are that the patient is not always able to void accurately for the 15-minute specimen, which is often the most important value, or even for the other specimens.   A certain constant
percentage of the PSP dye is excreted into the urine on each cycle
of blood flow to the kidney.   Therefore, the 15-minute value may be
low although over a prolonged period the total values for 2 hours

when added together may be almost within normal range, as noted previously. However, when kidney function is moderately to considerably decreased, the 2-hour value also starts falling. Obviously, it is necessary to be sure that the urine collection is complete so that all the PSP dye is recovered. If the patient has significant residual urine, the test may be falsely low.

In summary, both the PSP and the creatinine clearance give roughly similar information in chronic renal disease; to do both is not necessary. In chronic diffuse renal disease with an elevated BUN, both these tests will almost always be markedly abnormal. When there is a considerably elevated BUN and renal shutdown due to prerenal causes, both these tests are usually abnormal until the kidney recovers. Therefore, as long as the BUN is significantly elevated, these tests usually are not helpful—definitely not the clearance tests.

In the classic case of chronic diffuse bilateral renal disease, the first demonstrable test abnormality is a decrease in the ability to concentrate using the concentration test. As the disease progresses, the creatinine clearance and 15-minute PSP start to become reduced. Then, the specific gravity becomes fixed and the creatinine clearance, followed by the 2-hour PSP, both show considerable decrease. Finally, both these tests show a marked decrease and the BUN starts to rise, followed shortly by the blood creatinine (Fig. 7).

Renal function tests may be useful in the evaluation of hypertension. There are many causes of hypertension and the kidneys are involved in several (discussed further in Chapter 29). The kidney is damaged secondarily by essential hypertension. The kidney may itself be the primary source, since a small but significant number of hypertension cases are due to unilateral renal disease, most commonly renal artery stenosis, and these can often be cured by removal of the ischemic kidney or surgical repair of the stenotic renal artery. The first step in diagnosis is an IVP, but the standard IVP is not very satisfactory for this purpose, and a special modification called the "minute-sequence" IVP should be ordered. Films are made every minute for 5 minutes after injection of the contrast medium, whereas the standard IVP has films at only 5, 10, and 15 minutes after injection. Unilateral lack of dye concentration or a small kidney on one side only is strongly suspicious. The minute-sequence IVP is reported to pick up 70-90% of cases. However, a positive minute-sequence IVP means only that the patient has unilateral renal disease, and does not tell the etiology or whether any hypertension is actually due to the renal disease. For example, it cannot differentiate unilateral renal disease due to renal artery stenosis from unilateral renal disease due to chronic pyelonephritis; and if the patient has hypertension, it cannot show whether the hypertension is due to the renal lesion or to some other cause. Therefore, the minute-sequence IVP is classed as a screening test.

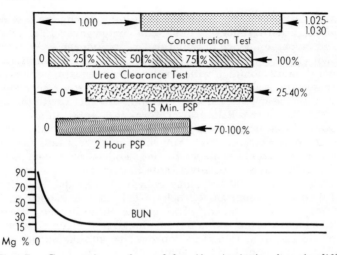

Fig. 7.—Comparison of renal function tests in chronic diffuse bilateral renal disease.

Another good screening test for unilateral renal disease is the radiorenogram (a similar procedure called the chlormerodrin uptake is equally as good). These procedures measure renal blood flow and tubular function after injection of $I^{131}$-labeled hippuran (in the radiorenogram) or labeled mercury chlormerodrin (in the chlormerodrin uptake test), by means of special radiation detectors placed over the kidney areas. The radiorenogram demonstrates significant differences in renal function between the two kidneys. It is said to detect 80-90% of patients with hypertension due to unilateral renal disease. Just as with the minute-sequence IVP, the radiorenogram is not a specific test, does not demonstrate the anatomic site of the lesion or the etiology of the dysfunction (except in cases of ureteral obstruction), and does not measure renal function in a quantitative manner. It also cannot prove that hypertension present is due to the renal disease rather than some other cause, or if the hypertension is potentially curable. Therefore, just as with the minute-sequence IVP, there will be some "positive" results in patients with renal disease, but hypertension from some other etiology.

A third procedure useful to demonstrate unilateral renal disease is the Howard test. The Howard test (or one of its modifications, such as the Stamey test) uses the fact that renal water and electrolyte excretion may be utilized to diagnose and pinpoint the affected kidney in hypertension due to unilateral renal disease. Bilateral ureteral catheters are placed, and the urine from each kidney is analyzed separately for electrolyte content and volume. In the

Howard test, unilateral reduction in volume during the test period over 50%, and/or reduction of sodium content over 15%, is considered strong evidence of unilateral renal disease. Again, this does not exactly pinpoint the type of lesion present, although this pattern is more common with renal artery stenosis. Some believe that this pattern allows an ability to predict whether nephrectomy will benefit the hypertension. The main drawback with the test is technical difficulty. Bilateral ureteral catheterization is not a simple procedure, and proper wedging of the catheters so that no urine escapes is somewhat difficult. For screening purposes, the Howard test has been largely replaced by the radioisotope techniques, which by comparison are relatively simple to perform.

The other useful technique in hypertension due to unilateral renal disease is renal angiography. This is a diagnostic test for renal artery stenosis, since, when technically well done, it will not only demonstrate the lesion but will localize it anatomically. This involves direct injection of radiopaque dye into the abdominal aorta or renal arteries and photographing its passage through the renal arteries with x-ray techniques. Again, this is not a simple procedure and carries with it some risk, although not great. Also, some people with renal artery stenosis do not have hypertension, so that demonstration of a lesion does not in itself prove that the lesion is affecting the kidney. Because of this, most use the renal arteriogram as a confirmatory test for proving renal artery stenosis after screening tests have demonstrated renal abnormality.

Hypertension due to unilateral renal disease is often curable and it should be ruled out as a cause of hypertension when the patient is relatively young or the hypertension is of recent onset. A suggested sequence of action is to obtain a minute-sequence IVP and, if available, a radioisotope procedure such as the renogram. If the results of both are negative, chances that the patient has unilateral renal disease are very small. If either result is positive, a renal arteriogram should be obtained in order to demonstrate renal artery lesions.

Next is a suggested sequence for proper workup of patients with actual or suspected renal problems of a medical type. One of the most common situations is the patient who has asymptomatic proteinuria, or exhibits it in association with a disease in which it is not expected. The first step is to repeat the test after a couple of days or when the presenting disease is under control, using an early morning specimen to avoid orthostatic proteinuria. If proteinuria persists, the microscopic report should be analyzed for any diagnostic hints. The presence and degree of hematuria suggests a certain number of diseases, and pyuria does likewise; if either is present, there should be a careful search for RBC or WBC casts. A careful history may elicit information of previous proteinuria or hematuria, suggesting chronic glomerulonephritis or previous kidney infection or calculi which would be in favor of chronic pyelonephritis. Uremia due to chronic bilateral renal disease often has an associated hypertension (although, of course, hypertension may itself be the primary disease and cause extensive secondary renal damage). In addition, a low-grade or moderate anemia, either normochromic or slightly hypochromic and without evidence of reticulocytosis or blood loss, is often found with severe chronic diffuse renal disease. The next step is to note the random specific gravities taken. If one is normal (i.e., over 1.020), renal function is probably adequate. If these are all lower, one can proceed to a concentration test or a PSP test, since low random specific gravities may simply mean high water excretion rather than inability to concentrate. If the 15-minute value of the PSP is normal, a concentration test is not really necessary, but could be done to pick up smaller degrees of impairment. If the 15-minute PSP is only slightly or moderately abnormal with a relatively normal 2-hour PSP, the patient most likely has only mild or possibly moderate functional loss. If the 2-hour PSP is markedly abnormal and the BUN is normal with no hypertension or anemia present, this is most likely severe diffuse bilateral renal disease, but not a completely end-stage situation. When the BUN is elevated with these other signs present, the prognosis is generally very bad, although some patients with definite uremia may live for years with proper therapy. There will be exceptions to the situations just outlined, but not too many.

Two other procedures have been advocated for use in renal diagnosis; these are the Addis count and renal biopsy. The Addis count is used in suspected subclinical cases of chronic glomerulonephritis to demonstrate 12-hour abnormally increased rates of RBC and cast excretion too small to exceed the normal range in ordinary random specimen microscopics. If the random urine specimen already shows hematuria or pyuria, and if contamination can be ruled out by catheter or clean catch collection technique, then the Addis count cannot do anything more than show the same abnormality. Addis counts should very rarely be necessary with a good history and adequate workup. Renal biopsy is now widely used. It may be helpful, but should be reserved for specially selected cases; most renal diseases can and should be diagnosed by routine methods. Biopsies, because of their random sample nature, more often than not show only nonspecific changes reflecting the result rather than the etiology of the disease process, and frequently are requested only for academic rather than practical diagnostic or therapeutic reasons. It is certainly true that, in some cases, renal biopsy may be the only way to make the diagnosis, but this procedure can never be accepted as a substitute for a proper workup. It should be the last step in a carefully planned program fully utilizing the history, physical examination, clinical progress, and carefully selected laboratory tests.

The patient with an already elevated BUN often presents a diagnostic problem. Many use the term uremia incorrectly as a

synonym for azotemia, although uremia is a syndrome and should
be defined in clinical terms. A BUN of approximately 100 mg./100
ml. is usually considered to separate the general category of acute
reversible prerenal azotemias from the more prolonged acute episodes and chronic uremias. In general, this holds true, but there
is a small but important minority of cases which do not follow this
rule. Thus, some uremics seem to stabilize at a lower BUN level
until their terminal episode, while a few persons with acute transient azotemia may show a BUN close to 100 mg./100 ml. and rarely
over 125 mg./100 ml., which rapidly falls to normal levels after
treatment of the primary systemic condition responsible. It must
be admitted that easily correctable prerenal azotemia having appreciable BUN level is almost always superimposed on kidneys which
have previous subclinical damage or function loss. While not severe
enough to cause symptoms, their functional reserve has been eliminated by aging changes, pyelonephritis, or similar conditions. The
same is usually true for azotemia of mild levels (30 to 50 mg./100
ml.) occurring with dehydration, high protein intake, cardiac failure,
and other important but not life-threatening situations. After the
BUN has returned to normal levels, a PSP will allow adequate evaluation of the patient's renal status.

A normal urine volume is considered over 1000 ml./24 hours.
Normal range is over 800 ml./24 hours, and less than 500 ml./24
hours is considered oliguria, if all urine produced has actually been
collected. Incomplete collection or leakage around a catheter may
give a false impression of oliguria. Occasionally, a patient develops
oliguria and progressive azotemia, and it becomes necessary to differentiate between prerenal azotemia (which is correctable by im-
proving that patient's circulation) and acute renal tubular necrosis
(which must be promptly treated by mannitol diuresis in order to
preserve tubular function). This problem most frequently occurs
after a hypotensive episode or after surgery. If the patient's renal
function is known to be adequate (because of a previous adequately
concentrated specific gravity reading, or if the patient is relatively
young), then, in the presence of oliguria, if the urine osmolality
(p. 144) is less than 400 mOs./L., acute tubular necrosis is a good
possibility. However, in elderly persons or others who may have
significantly decreased renal function, a low osmolality is not helpful, since it may simply reflect the patient's poor concentrating
ability, which he had before the episode of oliguria. If the urine
osmolality is over 500 mOs./L., this demonstrates a significant
ability to concentrate and would be evidence against acute tubular
necrosis. (A specific gravity over 1.015 would have the same significance, but is affected by other variables, such as proteinuria).

If the urine contained many RBC, and especially if hemoglobin
or RBC casts were present, this would suggest hemoglobinuric
nephrosis. If the serum creatinine is normal or only slightly elevated, this suggests relatively acute onset of the BUN elevation.

The finding of many broad and waxy casts tends to suggest severe prolonged renal damage.

Urine excretion of electrolytes may be utilized as a renal function test. Normally, the kidney is very efficient in reabsorbing urinary sodium which is filtered at the glomerulus. In acute tubular necrosis, renal ability to reabsorb sodium is impaired. Therefore, in severe diffuse bilateral renal damage (acute or chronic), renal excretion of sodium is fixed between 40-100 mEq./L. and chloride between 30-100 mEq./L. Finding urine sodium or chloride concentration more than 10 mEq./L. above or below these limits would be evidence against acute tubular necrosis or renal failure. Evaluation is assisted when serum electrolytes are abnormal. Hyponatremia, for example, normally would force the kidney to reabsorb more sodium ions, dropping the urine sodium to very low values, usually well below the 30 mEq./L. level. Therefore, urine sodium of 40-100 mEq./L. in the presence of hyponatremia would suggest severe renal damage.

Measurement of urinary urea nitrogen may be helpful. In severe diffuse bilateral renal damage (acute or chronic), urine urea nitrogen tends to be fixed at 300-500 mg./100 ml. or 3-10 Gm./24 hours. If the kidneys are able to produce urine concentrations significantly above these values in the presence of elevated serum BUN, this would suggest that prerenal causes (pp. 141-142) may be the etiology rather than primary renal failure. A 24-hour collection is more helpful than a random specimen, since a random specimen is affected more by the amount of water output.

In a patient with uremia (chronic azotemia), there is no good way to measure prognosis by laboratory tests. The degree of azotemia does not correlate well with the clinical course in uremia except in a very general way.

## REFERENCES

Barker, J. N.: The renal countercurrent concentrating mechanism, M. Clin. North America 47:873, 1963.

Bell, E. T., and Knutson, R. C.: Extrarenal azotemia and tubular disease, J. A. M. A. 134:441, 1947.

Blahd, W. H. (ed.): Nuclear Medicine (2d ed.; New York: McGraw-Hill Book Company, 1971).

Chapman, E. M., and Halsted, J. A.: The fractional phenolsulphonphthalein test in Bright's disease, Am. J. M. Sc. 186:223, 1933.

Dosseter, J. B.: Creatinemia versus uremia, Ann. Int. Med. 65:1287, 1966.

Galambos, J. T., et al.: Specific-gravity determination: Fact or fancy? New England J. Med. 270:506, 1964.

Howard, J. E., and Connor, T. B.: Use of differential renal function studies in the diagnosis of renovascular hypertension, Am. J. Surg. 107:58, 1964.

Jacobson, M. H., et al.: Urine osmolality, Arch. Int. Med. 110:121, 1962.

Kirkendal, W. M., et al.: Renal hypertension—Diagnosis and treatment, New England J. Med. 276:479, 1967.

Lyon, R. P.: The measurement of urine chloride as a test of renal function, J. Urol. 85:884, 1961.

Martin, J. F.: Urographic diagnosis of renovascular disease, Postgrad. Med. 40:289, 1966.

Miles, B. E., et al.: Maximum urine concentration, Brit. M. J. 2:901, 1954.

Pullman, T. N.: Kidney function tests in clinical practice, M. Clin. North America 43:469, 1959.

Sargent, F., II, and Johnson, R. E.: The effects of diet on renal function in healthy men, Am. J. Clin. Nutrition 4:466, 1956.

Schwartz, W. B., et al.: Intravenous urography in the patient with renal insufficiency, New England J. Med. 269:277, 1963.

Sharpe, A. R., Jr., et al.: Unilateral renal disease and hypertension, Arch. Int. Med. 118:546, 1966.

Sigler, M. H.: Oliguric renal failure and acute tubular necrosis, M. Clin. North America 47:1023, 1963.

Slotkin, E. A., and Madsen, P. O.: Complications of renal biopsy: Incidence in 5000 reported cases, J. Urol. 87:13, 1962.

Strauss, M. B., and Welt, L. G. (eds.): Diseases of the Kidney (Boston: Little, Brown & Company, 1963).

Taplin, G. V.: Radioisotope renography in renovascular hypertension, Postgrad. Med. 40:302, 1966.

Tobias, G. J., et al.: Endogenous creatinine clearance, New England J. Med. 266:317, 1962.

Viamonte, M., Jr., et al.: Renal angiography, South. M. J. 56:1335, 1963.

Wesson, L. G., Jr.: Clinical evaluation of renal function, M. Clin. North America 47:861, 1963.

Wolf, A. V.: Urinary concentrative properties, Am. J. Med. 32:329, 1962.

# CHAPTER 14

# Bacterial Infectious Diseases

Proper therapy of infectious disease depends on knowledge of the etiologic agent. This is accomplished in two ways: direct isolation and identification by culture, or indirectly, by serologic tests which demonstrate antibodies in the patient's blood against an organism. Certain problems arise when interpreting culture or serologic test results. If a culture is positive, one must determine whether the organism which is reported has actual clinical significance. It may be a fortuitous "contaminant," an ordinarily nonpathogenic species which has become infectious under the prevailing circumstances, or a recognized pathogen which is a normal inhabitant of the area and whose presence may be entirely harmless. If a culture is negative, one must weigh the chances of having missed a diagnosis because the laboratory was not given a proper specimen, the specimen was obtained at an unfavorable moment during the disease, or because special culture techniques or media were needed.

Therefore, to evaluate laboratory data, the clinical situation has at least as much importance as considerations of laboratory methodology. It seems desirable to provide a brief survey of the major infectious agents, the diseases and circumstances in which they are most often found, and the conditions under which the appearance of these organisms may be confusing. There is an element of classification because of the way laboratory reports are usually worded. Techniques of diagnosis in the area of infectious disease are discussed here, in relation to specific organisms, specific clinical situations, or general laboratory methods.

The most useful laboratory classification of bacteria involves a threefold distinction: gram stain characteristics (gram positive or negative), morphology (coccus or bacillus), and growth oxygen requirements (aerobic or anaerobic). Species exist which are morphologic exceptions, such as spirochetes, others are intermediate

in oxygen requirements, and still others are identified by other techniques such as the acid-fast stain.  Gram stain reaction has long
been correlated with bacterial sensitivity to certain classes of antibiotics.  A classic example is the susceptibility of most gram-positive organisms to penicillin.  Morphology, when added to gram stain
reaction, greatly simplifies identification of large bacterial groups,
and oxygen growth requirements narrow the possibilities still further.  The interrelationship of these characteristics also helps to
control laboratory error.  For example, if cocci were seen to be
gram negative instead of gram positive, it would call for a laboratory recheck of the decolorization step in the gram stain procedure;
if the staining technique were verified, the possibility of a small
bacillus (coccobacillus) or a diplococcus would have to be considered.

Streptococci: These are gram-positive cocci which are classified in several ways.  The three most useful depend on bacterial
oxygen requirements, on colony appearance on blood agar, and on
specific carbohydrate within the organism.  Depending on oxygen requirements, streptococci are aerobic, microaerophilic, or anaerobic.  Most streptococci are aerobic.  The microaerophilic organisms sometimes cause a chronic resistant type of skin ulcer, and
occasionally are isolated in deep wound infections.  The anaerobic
streptococci are discussed on page 164.

According to usual colony appearance on sheep blood agar,
streptococci are divided into three types—alpha, beta, and gamma.
Alpha streptococci have an incomplete type of hemolysis surrounding
the colony.  This incomplete hemolysis usually has a green appearance, and streptococci producing green hemolysis are often called
viridans.  The beta type has complete clear hemolysis.  Gamma
streptococci do not produce hemolysis of blood agar.  These groupings have clinical value.  Alpha streptococci of the viridans subgroup are one of the most frequent causes of subacute bacterial
endocarditis.  Beta streptococci produce several different types of
infection and syndromes, as will be discussed later, and account
for the great majority of disease associated with streptococci.
Gamma streptococci are of lesser importance, but some of the so-
called enterococci are this type.  The enterococci comprise a group
with certain common characteristics, including resistance to heating (often called "heat-resistant strep") and growth in certain media
which inhibit other streptococci.  Enterococci may produce either
alpha or beta hemolysis or be gamma nonhemolytic.  Their main
importance is the fact that they are resistant to penicillin and sulfa.

The third classification is that of Lancefield, who discovered
antibodies produced to a somatic carbohydrate of hemolytic streptococcal organisms.  Hemolytic streptococci can be divided into groups
depending on the particular carbohydrate they possess.  These groups
are given a capital letter name.  Lancefield group A organisms are
beta hemolytic, and the particular strains of organisms which cause
acute rheumatic fever and acute glomerulonephritis are all in this

group. Those enterococci which are hemolytic are all in Lancefield group D, which not only demonstrates their common properties but also emphasizes that Lancefield grouping does not depend on type of hemolysis, since the enterococci in group D can have either type. It is an accident that Lancefield group A is all beta hemolytic. This accident is useful clinically, since by identifying an unknown streptococcus as group A, one can know it belongs to a potentially dangerous group known to cause certain important diseases. Lancefield grouping is done with appropriate group-specific antiserum. Clinically, since group A organisms seem to have an unusually marked susceptibility to the antibiotic bacitracin, presumptive identification of group A is accomplished by demonstrating inhibition of growth around a disk impregnated with a standardized concentration of bacitracin. Group A organisms may be further separated into subgroups (strains) using special antiserum against surface antigens (M antigens). Strain typing is mostly useful in epidemiologic work, especially in acute glomerulonephritis, and is not helpful in most clinical situations.

Certain strains of beta streptococci are associated with specific diseases, covered in more detail elsewhere, such as acute glomerulonephritis and acute rheumatic fever. Beta streptococci also produce various infections without any strain specificity. The most common is acute tonsillitis (pharyngitis). Wound infections and localized skin cellulitis are relatively frequent. Other diseases which are much less common, although famous historically, include scarlet fever, erysipelas (vesicular cellulitis), and puerperal fever.

Staphylococci are gram-positive cocci which typically occur in clusters. Staphylococci used to be divided into three groups depending on colony characteristics on blood agar. These were Staphylococcus albus (S. epidermidis), with white colonies; S. aureus, with yellow; and S. citreus, with pale green. In that classification, S. aureus was by far the most important; they were generally hemolytic, and the pathogenic species were coagulase positive. The new classification recognizes the fact that coagulase activity (the ability to coagulate plasma) is a better indication of pathogenicity than colony color, since a few coagulase-positive organisms are not yellow on blood agar. Therefore, all coagulase-positive staphylococci are now called Staphylococcus aureus; all coagulase-negative ones are called Staphylococcus epidermidis. Many species of S. aureus are resistant to antibiotics which normally are effective against gram-positive cocci.

Staphylococci, as well as the enteric gram-negative rod organisms and some of the clostridia gram-positive anaerobes (to be discussed later), are normal inhabitants of certain body areas. In the case of staphylococci, their habitat is the skin. Therefore, a diagnosis of staphylococcic infection should not be made solely on the basis of S. aureus isolation from an external wound; there should be evidence that S. aureus is actually causing clinical disease. Besides the skin, about half of all adults outside the hospital carry staphylococcus in the nasopharynx; this reportedly increases to 70-80% if these persons have cultures performed repeatedly over a long period. More than 50% of hospitalized persons have positive nasopharyngeal cultures. Exactly what factors induce these commensal organisms to cause clinical disease are not completely understood. Staphylococci are typically associated with purulent inflammation, and characteristically are abscess-formers. The most common site of infection is the skin, most frequently confined to minor lesions, such as pustules or possibly small carbuncles, but occasionally producing widespread impetigo in children and infants. The most frequent type of serious staphylococcic disease (other than childhood impetigo) is wound infection or infection associated with hospital diagnostic or therapeutic procedures.

In a small but important number of cases, staphylococci produce certain specific infections. Staphylococcic pneumonia may occur, especially in debilitated persons or following a viral pneumonia. Meningitis and septicemia are also occasionally found; again, more commonly in debilitated persons or those with decreased resistance— often without any apparent portal of entry. Staphylococci are the most common cause of acute (rather than subacute) bacterial endocarditis. They are the most common (but not only) etiology for a serious gastrointestinal infection called pseudomembranous enterocolitis, caused by suppression of normal bacterial flora by oral broad-spectrum antibiotics, with resultant overgrowth of pathogens. Finally, staphylococci may cause a type of food poisoning which is different from the infectious variety; symptoms result from ingestion of bacterial toxins rather than from actual enteric infection by living organisms.

Pneumococci are gram-positive diplococci which are still the most common cause of bacterial pneumonia in adults. They also produce many pediatric cases of middle ear infection and are an important etiology of meningitis, most commonly in debilitated persons. All strains are very sensitive to penicillin. Pneumococci usually produce alpha (green) incomplete hemolysis on blood agar and thus mimic viridans streptococci. Morphologic differentiation from streptococci may be difficult, especially in cultures, since streptococci may appear singly or in pairs (instead of chains), and pneumococci often do not have the typical "lancet" shape or diplococcic pattern. In the laboratory, differentiation is readily made because of the special sensitivity of pneumococci to a compound known as optochin. A disk impregnated with optochin is placed on the culture plate; inhibition of an alpha-hemolytic coccus denotes pneumococci.

Gram-negative diplococci include Neisseria organisms such as the meningococcic and gonococcic families. Meningitis due to meningococci is still the most common type, although the incidence varies with age group (p. 207). Incidentally, nonpathogenic Neisseria organisms are common normal inhabitants of the nasopharynx,

and it takes special subculturing to differentiate these from the meningococcic variety which are not normally present.  Gonococci are
the cause of gonorrheal urethritis and the majority of acute salpingitis, so-called pelvic inflammatory disease ("PID").  Chronic salpingitis ("chronic PID") may occur either as residual effects of one
or more episodes of acute gonorrheal salpingitis or from tubal infection by other organisms (mainly streptococcus or E. coli) after the
original gonorrheal infection has disappeared.  A presumptive diagnosis of gonorrhea can often be made from a cervical smear or male
urethral discharge smear prepared by gram stain.  The organisms
appear as gram-negative intracellular diplococci, located within the
cytoplasm of polymorphonuclear neutrophils.  Extracellular organisms are not considered reliable for diagnosis.  Certain other organisms (Mima species) may have a similar morphologic appearance
to the gonococcus; the Mima bacteria are usually extracellular, but
can be intracellular.  Also, it is sometimes difficult to find gonococcic organisms on smears in the male and often difficult in the female.  Cultures should therefore be taken, both to supplement the
smear as a screening technique and to provide a definitive diagnosis.  A study from the U. S. Communicable Disease Center indicates
that in females the endocervical canal (after removal of mucus) is
the single best site for culture; about 82% of patients will be detected.
Surprisingly, in that study about 50% of patients had positive rectal
cultures (swab culture using an anoscope, taking care to avoid fecal
contamination).  The combination of endocervical and rectal culture
raised the percent detected to 92-94%.  Culture of other sites did
not increase the yield.  The remaining 6-8% of patients were discovered on repeat culture 1 week later.

     All the Neisseria have to be cultured on special media, such
as Thayer-Martin (which is replacing the less selective chocolate
agar), and usually grow best in high carbon dioxide atmospheres.  A
modification of the Thayer-Martin medium, called Transgrow, is
being used for immediate specimen inoculation in order to keep the
organisms alive while transporting the culture to a laboratory.

     Enteric bacilli (Enterobacteriaceae) are a large family of gram-
negative rods.  As their name implies, the majority of these bacteria
are found primarily in the intestinal tract.  These organisms include Salmonella, Shigella, E. coli, Enterobacter, Klebsiella, Proteus, and the paracolons.  Many are normal inhabitants and cause
disease only if they escape to other locations or if certain pathogenic
types overgrow; others are introduced from contaminated food or
water.  Salmonella and Shigella are not normal gastrointestinal inhabitants and always mean a source of infection from the environment.

     Salmonella organisms cause several clinical syndromes.  Ty-
phoid fever is produced by S. typhosa (S. typhi).  The classic symptoms are a rising fever during the first week, a plateau at 103-104⁰
for 1 week, then a slow fall during the third week, plus gastrointes-

tinal symptoms and splenomegaly. There is a mild leukopenia with a lymphocytosis and monocytosis. Despite fever, the pulse rate tends to be slow (bradycardia). This picture is often not present in its entirety. During the first and second weeks of illness, blood cultures are the best means of diagnosis; thereafter, the incidence of positive specimens very rapidly declines. During the latter part of the second week to the early part of the fourth week, stool cultures are the most valuable source of diagnosis. However, stools may occasionally be positive in the first week; in carriers, positive stool cultures may persist for long periods. About 3-5% of typhoid patients become carriers (persons with chronic subclinical infection). Urine cultures may be done during the third and fourth weeks, but are not very effective. At best, blood cultures will miss at least 20% of cases, stool cultures at least 25%, and urine cultures at least 75%. Repeated cultures increase the chance of diagnosis. Besides cultures, serologic tests may be performed. There are three major antigens in the Salmonella organism—the H (flagellar), O (somatic), and Vi (capsule or envelope). Antibody titers against these antigens constitute the Widal test. Most authorities agree that of the three antibodies, only that against the O antigen is meaningful for diagnosis. Vaccination causes a marked increase in the anti-H antibodies; the anti-O antibodies rise to a lesser degree and return much more quickly to normal. The Widal test (anti-O) antibodies begin to appear about 7-10 days after onset of illness. The highest percentage of positive tests is reported to be in the third and fourth weeks. As in any serologic test, a rising titer is more significant than a single determination. There has been considerable controversy over the usefulness of the Widal test in diagnosis of Salmonella infections. It seems to have definite, but limited, usefulness. Drawbacks of the Widal test include the following: (1) antibodies do not develop early in the illness, and may be suppressed by antibiotic therapy; (2) antibody behavior is often variable and often does not correlate with the severity of the clinical picture; (3) an appreciable number of cases (15% or more) do not have a significantly elevated anti-O titer, especially if only one determination is done. To summarize: in typhoid fever, blood cultures during the first and second weeks and stool cultures during the second, third, and fourth weeks are the diagnostic tests of choice. The Widal test may also be helpful.

Paratyphoid fever (enteric fever) is produced by salmonellae other than S. typhosa; the clinical picture is similar to typhoid fever, but milder. S. schottmuelleri and S. paratyphosa are the most common causes in the United States. Diagnosis is similar to that of typhoid fever. In the United States, salmonellae gastroenteritis is probably next in frequency after typhoid or enteric fever. The gastroenteritis syndrome has a short incubation, features abdominal pain, nausea, and diarrhea, and is most commonly produced by S. typhimurium. There is usually a leukocytosis with a minimal in-

crease in neutrophils, in contrast to the usual finding in typhoid fever.  Blood cultures are said to be negative; stool cultures are usually positive.  In addition to these syndromes, salmonellae may
cause other types of disease.  Septicemia may occasionally be found,
and salmonellae may rarely cause focal infection in various organs,
resulting in pneumonia, meningitis, and endocarditis.  Salmonella
osteomyelitis has been associated with sickle cell anemia, for unknown reasons.

Shigella is the next most important intestinal infection after
Salmonella.  Shigella organisms cause so-called bacillary dysentery.  Shigellae usually remain localized to the colon and do not enter the peripheral blood; blood cultures are therefore negative, in
contrast to early Salmonella infection.  Stool culture is the main
diagnostic test.  Besides Salmonella and Shigella, certain other bacteria (such as staphylococci and certain strains of E. coli) may
cause gastrointestinal infection; these will be covered elsewhere.

Enterobacter and Klebsiella are normal gastrointestinal inhabitants.  Nomenclature has been particularly confusing in relation
to these organisms.  Enterobacter was formerly called Aerobacter.
Enterobacter (Aerobacter) and Klebsiella have differences in reaction to certain test media, but are similar enough that previous
classification included both in the same group.  According to previous custom, if infection by these organisms was in the lungs it was
called Klebsiella (or Friedländer's pneumonia); if it was in the urinary
tract, it was called Aerobacter.  Klebsiella produces a resistant
necrotizing pneumonia which often cavitates and which characteristically is found in alcoholics and debilitated patients.  Enterobacter
is one of the more frequent urinary tract infections, often resistant
to therapy, and occasionally produces septicemia.

Present classification differentiates Enterobacter from Klebsiella.  Sources of confusion include the family name Enterobacteriaceae, which is similar to the name of one component genus
Enterobacter.  Enterobacteriaceae is a group of several tribes,
each of which contains a genus or genera (p. 444).  One tribe, Kleb-
siellae, has a similar name to one of its three component genera,
Klebsiella, and also includes the genus Enterobacter.  A further
source of difficulty is that the predominant species of Klebsiella is
K. pneumoniae—which, in spite of the name, is found more frequently in the urinary tract than the lungs.

Escherichia coli is the most common cause of urinary tract infection.  As with any urinary tract pathogen, this organism may occasionally reach the blood stream and cause septicemia.  This is more
frequent with urinary tract obstruction.  E. coli is one of the most
common etiologies for severe infections, especially meningitis, in the
newborn.  In addition, certain strains of E. coli have caused epidemic
diarrhea in infants (see p. 443 ).  However, since E. coli is a normal
intestinal organism, a stool culture growing E. coli is of uncertain
significance unless one of these special subtypes is present.

Proteus is a gram-negative rod which is probably second to
E. coli for frequency in urinary tract infection.

The paracolons comprise a sort of dumping ground for gram-
negative rods which have certain laboratory characteristics similar
to E. coli, although cultural behavior in other respects resembles
that of other enteric bacteria groups.   There are four main subgroups of paracolons; Bethesda (Citrobacter), Providencia, Arizona,
and Serratia.   Originally, it was thought that members of the paracolon group were nonpathogenic and that their importance was only
in the necessity for differentiation from more pathogenic enteric
organisms such as Salmonella.   Now, however, it is recognized that
these organisms produce disease, especially urinary tract infections, septicemia, and pulmonary infections, so that the organisms
have been reclassified according to predominant culture characteristics (p. 444).   Serratia is usually considered the most dangerous
of these organisms.

Pseudomonas is a gram-negative rod which is not classified
with the Enterobacteriaceae, although it may be found normally in the
gastrointestinal tract.   Infection is less common than with any of the
Enterobacteriaceae, but becomes more frequent in certain special
situations.   In human disease, pseudomonas has many aspects similar to "opportunistic fungi," in that infection is most often superimposed on serious underlying disease such as leukemia.   Pseudomonas is relatively resistant to many of the standard antibiotics,
such as penicillin, sulfa, and tetracycline, and thus assumes importance as a secondary invader after antibiotic therapy of the original infection.   This is most frequent in urinary tract infections.
Pseudomonas may be found normally on the skin (as well as in the
gastrointestinal tract), and thus is a very important and frequent
problem in severe burns.   Pseudomonas septicemia is not common,
but is increasing as a complication or a terminal event in the conditions just mentioned.

Granuloma inguinale is a venereal disease caused by a gram-
negative rod bacterium which has some antigenic similarity to the
Klebsiella group.   Infection is transmitted by sexual contact.   After
incubation, an elevated irregular flattened granulomatous lesion develops, usually in or around the medial aspect of the inguinal area
or on the labia.   The organism is difficult to culture and requires
special media, so that culture is not usually done.   Diagnosis is accomplished by demonstration of the organisms in the form of characteristic "Donovan bodies," found in the cytoplasm of histiocytes.
The best technique is to take a punch biopsy of the lesion, crush the
fresh tissue between two glass slides, and make several smears
with the crushed tissue.   These smears are air-dried and stained
with Wright's stain.   It is possible to process a biopsy in the routine manner and do special stains on tissue histologic sections, but
this is not nearly as good.   Granuloma inguinale is sometimes confused with lymphogranuloma venereum, a totally different disease,

because of the similarity in names and the fact that both are venereal diseases.

Hemophilic group: These are small gram-negative bacilli of
which the most important are Hemophilus influenzae and Bordetella
pertussis. H. influenzae infection is not very frequent, but is an important cause of meningitis between the ages of 2 months and 2 years.
Occasionally, H. influenzae may produce a serious type of laryngitis
(croup) known as acute epiglottitis. In the laboratory, these organisms grow better next to staphylococcus colonies because staphylococci produce certain substances which H. influenzae needs and in
which blood agar is deficient (the so-called X and V factors). Therefore, Haemophilus culture plates contain a small area previously inoculated with S. aureus ("staph streak"). Bordetella pertussis is
the etiologic agent of whooping cough. This is best isolated from
nasopharyngeal cultures, preferably on the special Bordet-Gengou
medium ("cough plate").

Clostridia are gram-positive anaerobic rods which include several important organisms. Clostridium perfringens (Cl. welchii) is
the usual cause of gas gangrene. It is a normal inhabitant of the
gastrointestinal tract, and reportedly can be isolated from the skin
in about 20% of patients and from the vagina and female genitalia in
about 5%. Therefore, just as with S. aureus, culture reports of Cl.
welchii from an external wound do not necessarily mean that the
organism is producing clinical infection. Cl. tetani is the etiology
of tetanus. This organism is only rarely found in the human gastrointestinal tract. Clinical disease is produced by release of bacterial
exotoxin after local infection in a manner analogous to diphtheria.
The third important Clostridium is Cl. botulinum. Botulism, a severe food poisoning, is precipitated by ingestion of bacterial endotoxin already formed in contaminated food, rather than from actual
infection of the patient by the bacterium. Canned food, especially
home-canned, is the usual source. Any type of food (meat, fish,
vegetables) may be involved. Clostridial infection, with the exception of Cl. tetani and botulinum, is associated with certain clinical
situations. Wound infection is the most frequent, although in the
majority of cases the clostridia coexist with other organisms and do
not produce gangrene. The other major area of concern is septic
(criminal) abortion.

Botulism is frequently confused with other types of "food
poisoning." Cl. botulinum produces a neurotoxin, so that botulism
symptoms commonly include vomiting and cranial nerve or eye
signs; diarrhea is absent or a very minor component, while diarrhea is prominent in most other types of food poisoning. Staphylococcal contamination of food is much more common than botulism;
symptoms are likewise due to ingestion of endotoxin. However,
botulism symptoms most often occur 12-36 hours after ingestion,
whereas staphylococcus endotoxin symptoms usually begin 1-8 hours
after eating. Clostridium perfringens (Cl. welchii) occasionally may

contaminate food in a manner similar to staphylococcus. Symptoms occur 8-12 hours after eating and are due to ingestion of bacterial exotoxin rather than endotoxin. Salmonella and Shigella are other causative organisms. Symptoms are due to infection, not preformed toxin. Shigella dysentery symptoms ordinarily occur 36-48 hours after infection, but the range is 24-48 hours. Salmonella gastro-enteritis (due to species other than S. typhosa) most often becomes clinically manifest in 8-48 hours, with a tendency to approach 24 hours. This should be differentiated from typhoid or paratyphoid fever, which has a considerably longer incubation and a different emphasis in symptoms.

Anaerobic infections usually center on three groups of organisms—clostridia, Bacteroides, and the anaerobic streptococci. The clostridia are discussed above. Bacteroides species are anaerobic gram-negative rods normally found in the mouth, the intestine, and the female genital tract. Isolation of these organisms often raises the question of their significance or pathogenicity. It seems well established that Bacteroides may occasionally cause serious infection, which frequently results in abscess or gangrene. The most commonly associated clinical situations include septic abortion, aspiration pneumonia, and focal lesions of the gastrointestinal tract (such as carcinoma or appendicitis).

Anaerobic streptococci are frequently associated with Bacteroides infection, but may themselves produce disease. They are normally present in the mouth and gastrointestinal tract. Septic abortion and superinfection of lesions in the perirectal area seem to be the most commonly associated factors. Anaerobic streptococci are also part of the fusiform bacteria-spirochetal synergistic disease known as Vincent's angina.

Besides clostridia, the gram-positive rods include Listeria monocytogenes, an aerobic (rather than anaerobic) organism which sometimes causes stillbirths, as well as septicemia or meningitis in newborns, especially in premature infants. Culture of the mother's lochia has been suggested as an aid in diagnosis, as well as blood cultures from the infant.

Diphtheria is now uncommon, but cases appear from time to time, some of them fatal. Contrary to usual belief, the laboratory cannot make the diagnosis from gram-stained smears. Heat-fixed smears stained with methylene blue are better, but, although helpful in demonstrating organisms resembling diphtheria, still are not considered reliable enough for definite morphologic diagnosis. Non-pathogenic diphtheroids are normal nasopharyngeal inhabitants and may resemble Corynebacterium diphtheriae closely. To be certain, one must culture the organisms on special media and do virulence (toxin production) studies. Direct gram stain and methylene blue smears are of value, since other causes of pharyngeal inflammation and pseudomembrane formation such as fungus and Vincent's angina can be demonstrated. Therefore, two or three pharyngeal swabs should be obtained, if possible, to provide smears and cultures.

Brucellosis is an uncommon disease, but sometimes must be considered in the differential diagnosis of fever of unknown origin. The Brucella organism is a gram-negative coccobacillus usually transmitted to man via infected milk or milk products. However, workers in the meat-processing industry are currently the main source of brucellosis in the United States, rather than milk-borne infection. Blood culture is the best means of isolation, but a special culture medium is required. A serologic slide agglutination test is the most frequent method of diagnosis (p. 173).

Tularemia is another uncommon disease which occasionally should be considered in fever of unknown origin. The organism is a small gram-negative coccobacillus. Small wild animals such as the rabbit constitute the main reservoir of infection, and most of those who acquire tularemia are such persons as hunters who handle raw game. Culture from lymph nodes or local lesions on special media is the best means of isolation but is not ordinarily done because of an unusually high rate of laboratory worker infection. A serologic slide agglutination test is the standard method for diagnosis (p. 173).

Spirochetal diseases comprise a large group, of which only three will be mentioned. Vincent's angina is an infection of the mouth caused by an interesting synergistic group of organisms, including anaerobic streptococci, a fusiform gram-negative bacillus, and a spirochete. Gram-stained smears demonstrating all three organisms are usually sufficient for diagnosis. Syphilis is a very important disease and is discussed separately in Chapter 31. Weil's disease is caused by a spirochete of the Leptospira genus. Transmission is usually through accidental contamination by infected rat urine. The most striking findings are a combination of hepatitis and glomerulonephritis, clinically manifested by jaundice with hematuria. Therefore, the disease is sometimes considered in the differential diagnosis of jaundice of unknown etiology. In the classic cases, after an incubation period there is abrupt onset of high fever, severe malaise, conjunctivitis, headache, and muscle ache. Chills may be present. Toward the end of the first week the fever starts to subside and a new set of symptoms begins to develop, including hepatitis and nephritis. This stage lasts about a week, and is followed by improvement or death. Milder cases may lack one or many of these signs and symptoms. Symptoms of meningitis may occasionally predominate. Laboratory findings include a leukocytosis with a shift to the left. A mild normocytic-normochromic anemia usually develops by the second week. Platelet counts are normal. After jaundice develops, liver function test results are similar to those in viral hepatitis. After onset of kidney involvement, the BUN is often elevated, and hematuria is present with proteinuria. Cerebrospinal fluid examination shows normal sugar but increased cell count which varies according to the severity of the case; initially, these are mainly neutrophils, but later on the lymphocytes predominate. Cultures on ordinary bacterial media are negative.

Diagnosis often depends on isolating the organisms, or demonstrating specific antibodies in the serum. During the first week (days 1-8), spirochetes may be found in the blood by darkfield in about 8% of the cases and can be cultured from the blood in many more. Instead of ordinary blood cultures, 1-3 drops of blood are inoculated into a special culture medium (Fletcher's), since larger quantities of blood inhibit the growth of leptospires. The cerebrospinal fluid may be cultured toward the end of the first week. During the second week the blood quickly becomes negative. During the third week (days 14-21) the spirochetes may often be recovered from the urine of those patients with nephritis. Animal inoculation is the most successful method. Antibodies start to appear at about the seventh day and are present in the majority of cases by the twelfth day. Antibodies persist for months and years after cure. A titer of 1:300 is considered diagnostic, although, without a rising titer, past infection could not be ruled out completely. If a significant titer has not developed by the twenty-first day it would be very rare to do so later. In summary, blood cultures during the first week and serologic tests during the second and third weeks are the diagnostic methods of choice.

Tuberculosis is still very important and common despite advances in drug therapy. The disease usually begins in the chest; in this location the most important symptoms are cough, fever, and hemoptysis (the most important diseases to rule out are lung carcinoma and bronchiectasis). The kidney is involved in a significant percentage of advanced cases, with the main symptom being hematuria (p. 131). The laboratory findings in tuberculosis depend to some extent on the stage and severity of the disease.

1. Chest x-rays: these are often the first evidence to suggest tuberculosis, and provide a valuable parameter of severity, activity, and response to therapy. Depending on the situation, there are a variety of possible roentgen findings. These may include one or more of the following:

    a) Enlargement of hilar lymph nodes.

    b) Localized pulmonary infiltrates. These occur characteristically in upper lobe apical location or, less commonly, the superior segment of the lower lobes. Cavitation of lesions may occur.

    c) Miliary spread (small punctate lesions widely distributed). This pattern is not common, and occasionally may be missed on routine chest films.

    d) Unilateral pleural effusion. The most common causes are tuberculosis, carcinoma, and congestive heart failure. Tuberculosis causes 60-80% of so-called idiopathic pleural effusions.

2. Sputum smear: These provide a rapid presumptive diagnosis. They are stained by one of the acid-fast (AFB) procedures (usually the Ziehl-Neelsen method). The more advanced the infection, the more likely it is to yield a positive smear. Therefore, the rate of positive findings is low in early, minimal, or healing tuberculosis. A substantial minority of advanced cases may also be negative. Culture is more reliable for detection of tuberculosis, and also is necessary for confirmation of the diagnosis, for differentiation of M. tuberculosis from the "atypical" mycobacteria, and for sensitivity studies of chemotherapeutic agents. Sputum specimens should be collected (for culture and smear of the concentrated specimen) once a day for at least 3 days. If the smear is definitely positive, it would not be necessary to have more smears done. Also, this means a probable positive culture on the specimens already collected, and it would not be necessary to collect more than three specimens or to proceed to more complicated diagnostic procedures. If smears are negative, then one has to consider the possibility that the culture may also be negative, and cultures take from 3 to 8 weeks to demonstrate growth. Therefore, other procedures may be considered for diagnosis so as not to lose so much time.

3. Culture: Sputum is preferred for pulmonary tuberculosis (gastric aspiration if sputum is not satisfactory); urine for renal involvement; bone marrow in miliary tuberculosis. Reports indicate that an early morning specimen produces as many positive results as a 24-hour specimen, either of sputum or urine, and has much less contamination. Special culture media are needed. The necessity for adequate sputum culture specimens, regardless of the concentrated smear findings, has already been mentioned. Several reports indicate that aerosol techniques will produce a significantly greater yield of positive culture than will ordinary sputum collection. The aerosol mixture irritates the bronchial tree and stimulates sputum production. At any rate, it is necessary to get a "deep cough" specimen; saliva will not be adequate. If sputum cultures are negative, or the patient is unable to produce adequate sputum samples, gastric aspiration may be used. Note that gastric contents are suitable for culture only; nontuberculous acid-fast organisms may be found normally and cannot be distinguished from M. tuberculosis on AFB smear. If renal tuberculosis is suspected, urine culture should be done (this is discussed in Chapter 12). Even with urine specimens on 3 consecutive days, only about 30% of cases are positive.

4. Skin test (Mantoux test): This is performed with PPD or Old Tuberculin (Table 5). A positive result is an area of induration at least 5 mm. in diameter by 48 hours. A positive skin test is a manifestation of hypersensitivity to the tubercle bacillus. This reaction usually develops about 6 weeks after infection, although it may take several months. A positive reaction means previous contact and infection with tuberculosis; the positive reaction does not

itself indicate whether the disease is currently active or inactive. However, in children under 3 years of age it usually means active tuberculosis infection. Apparently, once positive, the reaction persists for many years or life, although there is evidence that a significant number of persons revert to negative if the infection is completely cured early enough. A few apparently never develop a positive test. The Mantoux test may revert to negative or fail to become positive in the following circumstances:

a) Occasionally but not frequently in old age or cachexia.
b) High percentage of cases of miliary tuberculosis.
c) High percentage of cases of overwhelming pulmonary tuberculosis.
d) A considerable number of patients who are on steroid therapy.
e) Many persons who also have sarcoidosis or Hodgkin's disease.

The standard procedure for skin testing is to begin with an intermediate-strength PPD (or the equivalent). If the person has serious infection, it is wise to begin with a 1st strength dose, to avoid necrosis at the injection site. A significant minority of patients with tuberculosis (9-17%) fail to react with intermediate strength PPD; a 2d strength dose is then indicated.

5. Biopsy: Miliary tuberculosis is usually widely disseminated in the body via hematogenous spread. When routine clinical and culture methods fail, biopsy of bone marrow or liver may be useful. Liver biopsy shows a fairly good positive yield, considering that a needle biopsy specimen is such a tiny random sample of a huge organ. However, it is usually difficult to demonstrate acid-fast organisms on liver biopsy even when tubercles are found—and, without organisms, the diagnosis is not absolutely certain. Bone marrow aspiration is probably the best procedure in such cases. It yields much better results for mycobacterial culture than for demonstration of tubercles. Routine marrow (Wright-stained) smears are worthless for histologic diagnosis in tuberculosis. Aspirated material may be allowed to clot in the syringe, then Formalin-fixed

---

TABLE 5.—COMPARISON OF TUBERCULOSIS SKIN TESTS

Old Tuberculin (OT) and Purified Protein Derivative (PPD)

| Tuberculin Units (TU) | 1 | 10 | 250 |
|---|---|---|---|
| Micrograms of PPD | 0.02 | 0.2 | 5.0 |
| "Strength" of PPD | 1st | Intermediate | 2nd |
| OT equivalent | 1:10,000 | 1:1000* | 1:100 |
| Milligrams of OT | 0.01 | 0.1 | 1.0 |

*Some use the equivalent of a 1:2000 intermediate strength (5 TU or 0.1 mcg. of PPD).

and sent through as a regular biopsy specimen for histologic slides. Before clotting, some of the aspirate is inoculated into suitable tuberculosis culture media. It should be emphasized that bone marrow aspiration or liver biopsy is not indicated in pulmonary tuberculosis (since this disease is relatively localized), only in miliary tuberculosis.

Besides Mycobacterium tuberculosis, there are other mycobacteria which are pathogenic for man. These have been termed the "atypical" mycobacteria (sometimes also called "unclassified" mycobacteria). At present, the most useful classification is that of Runyon, which subdivides the atypical mycobacteria into four groups, depending on growth and colony characteristics (Table 6). These divisions have clinical value. Group III (Battey strains) cause the majority of significant "atypical" infections, followed by group I. These organisms produce a disease similar to pulmonary tuberculosis, although often milder or more indolent. They are much more frequent in adults. Group II organisms are more frequent in children, and clinically tend to cause cervical lymphadenopathy. Diagnosis of the "atypical" mycobacteria is essentially the same as for M. tuberculosis. Skin tests (OT or PPD) for M. tuberculosis will also cross-react with the atypical mycobacteria. In general, the atypical mycobacteria tend to give less reaction to standard tuberculin skin tests than does M. tuberculosis infection. In fact, several studies claim that the majority of positive intermediate strength tuberculin skin tests which are less than 10 mm. (reaction diameter) are due to atypical mycobacterial infection rather than tuberculosis. Skin test antigens are available for each of the atypical mycobacterial groups, although some reports challenge the specificity of these preparations. The main clinical importance of these "atypical" organisms is the fact that many are resistant to one or more of the standard antituberculous chemotherapeutic agents.

Other Bacterial Infections: Coverage of bacterial infections in this chapter has been limited to the common organisms in clinical practice and a few which enter the differential diagnosis of certain common situations, such as hepatitis or fever of unknown origin. Many others have been omitted, such as those which cause plague, cholera, relapsing fever, and chancroid. In general, most of these are diagnosed through culture of appropriate specimens, such as stool for cholera and blood culture for plague. In addition, common laboratory contaminants such as the diphtheroids and B. subtilis have not been mentioned. The reader is referred to standard textbooks on microbiology for consideration of these organisms and for more information on those which are discussed briefly.

General Isolation and Identification Techniques: It is useful to know certain technical information involved with isolation and identification of bacteria. These facts may be of assistance to aid communication between the physician and the microbiology laboratory, for the benefit of each. It usually takes at least 48 hours, and often

TABLE 6.—CLASSIFICATION OF THE ATYPICAL MYCOBACTERIA

| Group I | Photochromogens | (M. Kansasii) |
| Group II | Scotochromogens | (M. scrofulaceum) |
| Group III | Nonphotochromogens | (Battey) |
| Group IV | Rapid growers | (M. fortuitum and others) |

longer, for definitive diagnosis, 1 day to culture the organism, 1 to isolate it, and often 1 or more days extra to identify it. A technician uses knowledge of the site and source of culture material in deciding what media or techniques (such as anaerobic conditions) to use for isolation. Some organisms are normal inhabitants of certain body areas but pathogens in other areas, so that an experienced technician knows to some extent what to subculture from a mixture of organisms growing in a specific location and also what special media to use for the pathogens usual in that anatomic location. This knowledge can easily save a day's time. Information that a certain specific organism is suspected may save even more, by allowing original inoculation of the culture material onto special test media. Even if definitive isolation is not yet accomplished, the technicians can often provide useful information or even a presumptive diagnosis. For example, among the enteric gram-negative rods, E. coli, Aerobacter, and Klebsiella ferment lactose, while most of the other pathogens do not. Therefore, a lactose-fermenter cannot be Salmonella or Shigella. The Pseudomonas group, in addition, does not ferment glucose, while most of the other pathogens do. Some of these organisms have characteristic appearances on isolation media. Some of the gram-positive aerobic bacteria produce a fairly typical appearance on original blood agar culture plates; combining this with gram stain morphology may yield a rapid presumptive diagnosis.

When any culture is taken, three things should be done. First, the culture must be taken to the laboratory as soon as possible, since many organisms die on prolonged exposure to air or drying. This is especially true for swab preparations. Second, the source of the culture should be written on the request form. Finally, if a specific organism is suspected, this information should also be written on the request, so that if special culture methods are required for that organism, the requisite techniques will be anticipated and used.

To obtain material for blood culture, not only must proper aseptic techniques be followed, but extra precautions must be taken to avoid contamination by skin bacteria. Iodine should be used, if possible, because it has the most efficient bactericidal effect of the common solutions available. However, since iodine is irritating to the skin, it must be removed shortly after application with less-powerful antiseptics such as alcohol or benzalkonium chloride.

For urine cultures, contamination with vaginal or labial bacteria is a serious problem. Catheterization is one way to solve this, but approximately 2% of patients develop urinary tract infection following a single catheterization. Therefore, a "midstream" voided specimen is the next best procedure. The urinary opening is cleansed. The labia are held apart in the female and the foreskin pulled back in the male. The first portion of urine is allowed to pass uncollected; then the sterile container is quickly introduced into the urine stream to catch the specimen. Quantitative urine cultures have now replaced simple cultures, since it has been shown that a titer of 100,000 or more organisms per milliliter has excellent correlation to clinical infection, whereas less than 10,000 organisms per milliliter very rarely proves significant. However, in some cases of pyelonephritis, cultures may be positive at some times but not at others, depending on the fluctuations of the disease and its anatomic location. A culture containing fewer than 10,000 organisms per milliliter is considered negative, but may have to be repeated if clinically indicated. On the other hand, although this dilution procedure is supposed to compensate for small degrees of unavoidable contamination, contamination can easily be severe enough to give a positive result. Therefore, good technique in collecting the specimen is essential. Also essential is getting the specimen to the laboratory as soon as possible after collection. Urine is an excellent culture medium, and specimens which stand for over 1 hour allow bacterial incubation and proliferation to the point at which quantitative counts are not reliable. If delivery to the laboratory must be delayed, the specimen should be refrigerated. The specimen can be preserved up to 12 hours in a refrigerator ($4^{\circ}$ C).

Quantitative urine culture has two other drawbacks. Culture involves trained technical personnel and relatively expensive media, thus curtailing use for mass screening to detect urinary tract infection. Culture takes 24 hours to determine bacterial quantity and another 24-48 hours to identify the organism, thus delaying treatment in suspected infection. Therefore, several screening tests have been introduced for rapid detection of significant degrees of bacteriuria. Gram stain of uncentrifuged urine roughly indicates, if organisms are seen, a good probability of a positive quantitative culture; the same is said to be true of direct examination of unstained centrifuged urine sediment. Gram-stained centrifuged sediment apparently gives too many false positives. Gram-stained uncentrifuged urine and unstained urine sediment examination are said to give relatively few false positives. Several chemical methods have been advocated; the most successful include the triphenyl tetrazolium chloride (TTC) test, the Greiss nitrate test and the catalase test. Best results have been reported with the TTC. Nevertheless, reports vary as to its accuracy, with a range of 70-90% correlation with quantitative culture, including both false positive and false negative results. The Greiss technique gives similar results, although slightly less good. The catalase test is considerably less reliable. Positive tests by any of these methods must be confirmed with quantitative culture; negative tests do not completely rule out urinary tract infection.

Although quantitative culture is widely considered the most reliable index of urinary tract infection, there are at least five major limitations:

1) A positive culture has reduced, but has not entirely eliminated, the possibility of contamination (as noted earlier).

2) A positive culture does not localize the actual area involved.

3) Bacteremia from many causes, even if transient, is filtered by the kidney and may give a temporarily positive quantitative culture.

4) Tuberculosis of the urinary tract will give a negative result on ordinary culture media.

5) Some cases of urinary tract infection may give negative cultures at various periods. In several studies, a sizable minority of patients required repeated cultures before one became positive. This may be due to the location of the infection in the kidney and to its degree of activity.

In summary, two cautions are required when a quantitative urine culture report is received. If the report is positive, the physician must be sure the specimen was properly collected, especially in the female; if the report is negative, this does not rule out chronic pyelonephritis. The problem of pyelonephritis and bacteriuria was discussed in Chapter 12.

Febrile agglutinins are serologic tests for a group of unrelated infectious diseases which are sometimes responsible for so-called fever of unknown origin (FUO). They include typhoid and enteric (Salmonella) fever, certain rickettsial diseases, brucellosis, and tularemia. Since these organisms are the ones most frequently considered in FUO situations, and since relatively simple slide agglutination serologic techniques are available for each, most laboratories automatically include the same selection of tests when "febrile agglutinins" are ordered. Typhoid or enteric ("paratyphoid") fever may be caused by several organisms of the Salmonella gram-negative rod family (p. 159). The more common Salmonella organisms are separated into groups on the basis of antigens prepared from these organisms; these antigens are used to detect antibodies in the patient's serum (Widal test). The groups are given a letter designation; for example, S. typhi (S. typhosa) is included in Salmonella D (p. 444). The Widal agglutination test involves antibodies produced to the somatic (O) and flagellar (H) antigens of Salmonella organisms. These antibodies appear approximately 7-10 days after onset of illness. In nonvaccinated individuals or most of those vaccinated over 1 year previously, a titer of 1:40 for the H antigen and 1:80 for the O antigen are suspicious; 1:80 for the H antigen and 1:160 for the O antigen are definitely significant. However, recent (less than 1 year) vaccination may cause greatly increased titer of either or both the O and the H antigen. The O antigen is more significant for diagnosis than the H antigen.

Antibody-antigen agglutination tests for brucellosis and tularemia are also included.  Again, titers of 1:80 are suspicious and
1:160 are definitely indicative.  Antibodies appear 2-3 weeks after
onset of the illness.  Similar slide agglutination tests for rickettsia
(Weil-Felix reaction) complete the febrile agglutinin battery.  Interpretation of Weil-Felix results is given on page 196.

General Concepts in Bacterial Infection:  The main systemic
signs and symptoms of severe bacterial infection in general are fever and weakness; the most characteristic laboratory finding is a
leukocytosis with an increase in number and immaturity of the neutrophils.  However, in overwhelming infection, sometimes leukocytosis may be minimal or even absent; and occasionally fever may
be minimal or may not be present.  This is not frequent, but happens
more often in infants and the elderly.  It is also more frequent in
debilitated persons, especially those with other severe diseases
which may impair the ability of the body to respond normally to infection.  Overwhelming infection may be focal, such as massive
pneumonia; or generalized, such as septicemia.

The concept of septicemia should probably be separated from
that of bacteremia.  In many focal infections, a few bacteria escape
from time to time into the peripheral blood.  However, the main
focus remains localized, and symptoms are primarily those which
are secondary to the particular organ or tissues involved.  In septicemia there is widespread and relatively continuous peripheral blood
involvement; characteristically, the symptoms are systemic, such
as marked weakness, shock, or near shock.  This is usually accompanied by high fever and leukocytosis, although, as mentioned earlier, sometimes leukocytosis may be absent and occasionally even
fever may be slight.  Any bacteria may cause septicemia.  The most
common types are gram-negative rod organisms, with Staphylococcus aureus probably next most frequent.  Of the gram negatives,
E. coli and Aerobacter are the most numerous.  The portal of entry
of the gram negatives is usually from previous urinary tract infection.  Many cases follow surgery or instrumentation.  The source
of Staphylococcus is often very difficult to trace, even at autopsy.
However, pneumonia and skin infections (sometimes very small) are
the most frequent findings.  Blood cultures are the mainstay of septicemia diagnosis.  They should be drawn before antibiotic therapy is
begun, although they may often be positive  despite antibiotics.  If
penicillin has previously been given, this should be noted on the request slip, so that the antipenicillin enzyme penicillinase may be
added to the culture media (there is, however, some controversy
over this technique; some authorities believe that penicillinase is of
little value and might actually be a source of contamination).  Strict
aseptic techniques should be used in obtaining cultures, since contamination from skin bacteria may give false or confusing results.
In cases of bacteremia or in septicemia with spiking types of fever,
the best time to draw blood cultures is just before or at the rise in

temperature.  Three cultures, drawn once every 3 hours, are a
reasonable compromise among the widely diverging recommendations in the literature.

Subacute bacterial endocarditis is a disease about halfway between the concepts of bacteremia and septicemia.  Bacteria grow in
localized areas on damaged heart valves and seed the peripheral
blood; this may be infrequent, intermittent, or relatively continuous,
with gradations between the two extremes.  Classic signs and symptoms include fever, heart murmurs, petechial hemorrhages in the
conjunctivas, small "splinter hemorrhages" in the fingernail beds,
and splenomegaly.  Hematuria is very frequent, and red cell casts
are a common and very suggestive finding.  There often, but not always, is a normocytic and normochromic anemia.  Leukocytosis is
often present, but it too may be absent.  Signs and symptoms are
fairly variable in many individual patients, and the diagnostic problem is often that of a fever of unknown origin.  The most frequent
organisms responsible are alpha streptococci (strep viridans) and
enterococci ("heat-resistant" streptococci).  Some areas report that
staphylococci are almost as common.  However, almost any pathogenic bacteria may be the cause, and, under certain special conditions (such as severe debilitation), even some ordinarily nonpathogenic organisms.  For specific diagnosis, blood cultures must be
obtained; the methods used are the same as those described under
septicemia.  Repeated cultures are much more necessary, because
of the often intermittent nature of the blood involvement, and avoid-
ance of culture contamination becomes even more important.  It is
said that up to 20% of cases will not produce a positive blood culture.

Among other bacterial syndromes, gastrointestinal infection
has been covered earlier, and meningitis is discussed in Chapter 18.
Pneumonia, however, has not been examined as a separate entity.
Although the term "pneumonia" denotes only inflammation of the lung,
which could result from noninfectious sources such as a chemical
inflammation secondary to aspiration, the great majority of cases
are due to bacterial or nonbacterial infectious agents.  Except for
the newborn, in the early pediatric age group viruses are the most
common etiology, followed by Staphylococcus.  In older children and
young adults, viruses still markedly predominate, but Pneumococcus
becomes more prevalent.  In middle-aged and older adults, Pneumococcus assumes considerable importance, although viruses still are
more frequent numerically.  In debilitated persons, alcoholics, those
persons with depressed immunologic defenses, and in the elderly,
Pneumococcus is still very important, but other bacteria become
much more common, especially Staphylococcus and Klebsiella.
Staphylococcic pneumonia is particularly likely to occur following a
viral pneumonia such as influenza.  The most important nonbacterial
agents are respiratory syncytial virus, influenza virus, and Mycoplasma pneumoniae (Eaton agent).  Diseases caused by viruses and
mycoplasma are discussed in Chapter 16.

Finally, a word should be said about antibiotic sensitivity procedures. Two techniques are employed; tube-dilution and agar diffusion. Of these, agar diffusion is by far the more common, and the Kirby-Bauer modification of this technique is becoming standard. Kirby-Bauer involves isolating a bacterial colony from original growth media, allowing the bacteria to grow in broth medium to a certain predetermined visual density, covering the entirety of a Mueller-Hinton agar plate with the bacterial isolate, placing antibiotic sensitivity discs at intervals on the surface, incubating 18-20 hours, examining for clear areas around individual discs representing bacterial growth inhibition by the antibiotic-impregnated disc, and measuring the diameter of these inhibition zones. Results are reported as resistant, sensitive, or intermediate, depending on previously established values for zone size based on tube-dilution studies most often furnished by the disc manufacturer. Consistent results will depend on strict adherence to good technique at each step, as well as the quality of the antibiotic discs and agar used. Variation in potency of antibiotic discs from different shipments and disc or agar deterioration during storage necessitate a good quality control program. The Kirby-Bauer technique has limitations. To be accurate, it can only be used when the bacterium to be tested is aerobic and grows rapidly (produces colonies within 24 hours) on the agar growth medium.

Most organisms, fortunately, may be classified as sensitive or resistant. Intermediate sensitivity is a controversial area. In general, many feel that "intermediate" zones should be considered resistant although certain organisms such as enterococcus may be exceptions. The test should be repeated to rule out technical variation or error. Interpretation may be influenced by location of the infection source if the antibiotic in question can reach this area readily. Antibiotic treatment dose may occasionally be increased, especially in subacute bacterial endocarditis. Another subject of dispute is the need for sensitivity testing in those bacteria which almost always are sensitive to certain antibiotics. These organisms include Group A aerobic streptococci, pneumococci, Neisseria, and Diphtheria.

An occasional laboratory problem is requests by physicians to include additional sensitivity discs in sensitivity panels. Laboratories frequently include only one representative of an antibiotic family in sensitivity test panels because sensitivity differences between antibiotic family members (e. g., the various tetracycline derivatives) are usually very minor.

## REFERENCES

Alston, J. M. , and Broom, J. C. : Leptospirosis in Man and Animals (Edinburgh: E. & S. Livingstone, Ltd. , 1958).

Barnett, R. N. , et al. : Conference on the medical usefulness of microbiology, Am. J. Clin. Path. 54:521, 1970.

Bornstein, D. L. , et al. : Anaerobic infections: Review of current experience, Medicine 43:207, 1964.

Chapman, J. S. : Present status of the unclassified mycobacteria, Am. J. Med. 33:471, 1962.

Dearing, W. H. : Micrococcic enteritis and pseudomembranous enterocolitis as complications of antibiotic therapy, Ann. New York Acad. Sc. 65:235, 1956.

Dubos, R. J. , and Hirsch, J. G. (eds.): Bacterial and Mycotic Infections of Man (4th ed. ; Philadelphia: J. B. Lippincott Company, 1965).

Duma, R. J. , et al. : Septicemia from intravenous infusions, New England J. Med. 284:257, 1971.

Felner, J. M. , and Dowell, V. R. : "Bacteroides" bacteremia, Am. J. Med. 50:787, 1971.

Fields, B. N. , et al. : The so-called "paracolon" bacteria—a bacteriologic and clinical reappraisal, Am. J. Med. 42:89, 1967.

Finegold, S. M. : Intestinal bacteria—the role they play in normal physiology, pathologic physiology, and infections, California Med. 110:455, 1969.

Forkner, C. E. : Pseudomonas Aeruginosa Infections, Modern Medical Monograph, no. 22 (New York: Grune & Stratton, Inc. , 1960).

Galton, M. M. : Methods in the laboratory diagnosis of leptospirosis, Ann. New York Acad. Sc. 98:675, 1962.

Gardner, P. , et al. : Nonfermentative gram-negative bacilli of nosocomial interest, Am. J. Med. 48:735, 1970.

Goodman, J. S. : Bacteroides sepsis; diagnosis and therapy, Hosp. Practice 6:121, 1971.

Gray, M. L. : Listeria monocytogenes and listeric infection in the diagnostic laboratory, Ann. New York Acad. Sc. 98:686, 1962.

Guckian, J. C. , et al. : Arizona infection of man, Arch. Int. Med. 119:170, 1967.

Hable, K. A. , et al. : Bacterial and viral throat flora, Clin. Pediat. 10:199, 1971.

Haggerty, R. J. , and Ziai, M. : Acute Bacterial Meningitis, in Levine, S. Z. (ed.): Advances in Pediatrics (Chicago: Year Book Medical Publishers, Inc. , 1964), Vol. XIII, p. 129.

Huckstep, R. L. : Typhoid Fever and Other Salmonella Infections (Edinburgh: E. & S. Livingstone, Ltd. , 1962).

Jones, F. L. , Jr. : The relative efficacy of spontaneous sputa, aerosol-induced sputa, and gastric aspirates in the bacteriologic diagnosis of pulmonary tuberculosis, Dis. Chest 50:403, 1966.

Kent, D. C., and Schwartz, R. : Active pulmonary tuberculosis with negative tuberculin skin reactions, Am. Rev. Resp. Dis. 95:411, 1967.

Kestle, D. G., and Kubica, G. P. : Sputum collection for cultivation of mycobacteria. An early morning specimen or the 24-to-72 hour pool? Am. J. Clin. Path. 48:347, 1967.

Koenig, M. G. : Diagnosis of bacterial endocarditis, Hosp. Med. 5:80, 1969.

Lang, G. R., and Levin, S. : Diagnosis and treatment of urinary tract infections, M. Clin. North America 55:1439, 1971.

Lester, W. : Unclassified Myobacterial Diseases, in DeGraff, A. C., and Creger, W. P. (eds.): Annual Review of Medicine (Palo Alto, Calif. : Annual Reviews, Inc., 1966), Vol. 17, p. 351.

Martin, W. J., et al. : Epidemiologic significance of Klebsiella pneumoniae, Mayo Clin. Proc. 46:785, 1971.

Mascher, W. : Tuberculin-negative tuberculosis, Am. Rev. Tuberc. 63:501, 1951.

McDermott, W. : The problem of staphylococcal infections, Ann. New York Acad. Sc. 65:58, 1956.

O'Neil, F. S. : Salmonellosis: Review of 124 cases, Postgrad. Med. 38:269, 1965.

Parker, R. L., et al. : Brucellosis in the United States, J. Infect. Dis. 125:289, 1972.

Pryles, C. V., and Lustik, B. : Laboratory diagnosis of urinary tract infection, Pediat. Clin. North America 18:233, 1971.

Schmale, J. D., et al. : Observations on the culture diagnosis of gonorrhea in women, J. A. M. A. 210:312, 1969.

Schroeter, A. L., and Lucas, J. B. : Gonorrhea—Diagnosis and treatment, Obst. and Gynec. 39:274, 1972.

Segura, J. W., et al. : Anaerobic bacteria in the urinary tract, Mayo Clin. Proc. 47:30, 1972.

Smith, D. T., and Johnston, W. W. : New aspects of mycobacterial skin tests. II., Arch. Environ. Health 10:704, 1965.

Spink, W. W. : The Nature of Brucellosis (Minneapolis: University of Minnesota Press, 1956).

Taylor, A., et al. : Outbreaks of waterborne diseases in the United States 1961-1970, J. Infect. Dis. 125:329, 1972.

Taylor, W. I., and Schelhart, D. : Isolation of Shigella. IV. Comparison of plating media with stools, Am. J. Clin. Path. 48:356, 1967.

Thoburn, R., et al. : Infections acquired by hospitalized patients, Arch. Int. Med. 121:1, 1968.

Tillotson, J. R., and Lerner, A. M. : Pneumonias caused by gram-negative bacilli, Medicine 45:65, 1966.

Von Graevenitz, A., and Kontnick, C. : Bacteriologic laboratory reports, Postgrad. Med. 49:49, 1970.

Wallace, C. K. : Enteric infections, Hosp. Med. 6:72, 1970.

# CHAPTER 15

# Mycotic Infections

Certain fungi, known as the "deep" or "systemic" fungi, are characterized by involvement of visceral organs or penetrating types of infection. Actinomycosis is a gram-positive non-acid-fast anaerobic organism which often produces deep-seated abscesses. A gram-stained smear of aspirated material from the lesion will often show typical organism colonies (sometimes called "sulfur granules" from their gross appearance). Biopsy material gives similar information. Culture on special media provides definitive diagnosis. Nocardia organisms may produce a somewhat similar clinical picture. These fungi are also gram positive and may resemble actinomycosis in histologic appearance. Nocardia, however, is aerobic and is partially acid-fast.

Blastomycosis may primarily involve either the skin or visceral organs. It forms granulomatous lesions somewhat similar histologically to those of tuberculosis. There are three helpful means of diagnosis: (1) a skin test, which shows infection by the organism, either past or present, (2) demonstration of typical organisms by direct wet-mount examination of material aspirated from a lesion or histologic examination of a biopsy specimen and (3) culture of a lesion for definitive organism isolation.

Coccidioidomycosis is most often contracted in the San Joaquin Valley of California, but occasionally appears elsewhere in the Southwest. It has a predilection for the lungs and hilar lymph nodes, but occasionally may become systemic to varying degrees. Clinical symptoms are most often pulmonary, manifested usually by mild or moderate respiratory symptoms and sometimes by fever of unknown origin. Rarely, overwhelming infection much like miliary tuberculosis develops. Diagnosis is made by the same combination of methods that were outlined under Blastomycosis.

Cryptococcosis (torulosis) is a fungal disease with a marked predilection for the brain. Diagnosis is made by spinal fluid culture and by direct microscopic examination of spinal fluid for organisms, using an India ink preparation, or by serologic tests.

Histoplasmosis is the most common of the systemic fungal infections. It is most often encountered in the Mississippi and Ohio Valley areas, but may appear elsewhere. In endemic areas, 60% or more of those infected are asymptomatic. The remainder manifest a variety of illness patterns, ranging from mild or severe acute or chronic pulmonary forms to disseminated infection. Histoplasmosis begins with a small primary focus of lung infection much like the early lesion of pulmonary tuberculosis. Thereafter, the lesion may heal or progress, or reinfection may occur. Mild acute pulmonary infection with influenza-like symptoms may develop. The illness lasts only a few days, and skin tests, cultures, and chest x-rays are usually negative. More severe acute pulmonary involvement produces a syndrome resembling primary atypical pneumonia. Chest x-rays may show hilar adenopathy and single or multiple pulmonary infiltrates. Histoplasmin skin tests and complement fixation tests eventually convert to positive, but remain negative until after the first 3-4 weeks of illness. Sputum culture may be positive, but not often. Chronic pulmonary histoplasmosis resembles chronic pulmonary tuberculosis clinically. Cavitation sometimes develops. Skin tests and complement-fixation tests usually are positive by the time the disease is chronic. Sputum is the most accessible material for culture, although reportedly negative in 50-60% of cases. Histoplasmosis is a localized pulmonary disease in the great majority of patients, so there is usually little help from cultures obtained outside the pulmonary area. In the small group which does have disseminated histoplasmosis, either acute or chronic, there is a range of symptoms from a febrile disease with lymphadenopathy and hepatosplenomegaly to a rapidly fatal illness closely resembling miliary tuberculosis. Bone marrow aspiration is the diagnostic method of choice; it is useful both for cultures and for histologic diagnosis of the organisms within macrophages on Wright-stained smear or clot section. Occasionally lymph node biopsy may be helpful; if performed, a culture should also be taken from the node before it is placed in fixative.

Skin test and serologic test results in histoplasmosis depend on the duration of illness. They may especially be negative in the acute disseminated form, just as tuberculin skin test anergy may develop in miliary tuberculosis. A skin test may itself convert the serologic tests from negative to positive. In histoplasmosis endemic areas, many persons have positive skin or serologic tests from past infection. Therefore, a (fourfold) rising titer is much more significant than a single positive result.

Complement fixation tests are available for all of the "systemic" fungi except actinomycosis and nocardia. If no local or state

health laboratory can do these tests, serum specimens may be sent
to the USPHS National Communicable Disease Center, Atlanta,
Georgia 30333. As was mentioned, skin tests are available. These
have the same general application and limitations as the tuberculin
skin test; i. e. , they do not separate past or recent infection, and
take several weeks after initial infection to become positive. Also,
conversion of a negative to a positive reaction is highly significant.
There is a good deal of cross-reaction between skin tests of these
fungal diseases. The histoplasmin skin test reacts with about 30%
of patients who actually have blastomycosis and about 40% of those
with coccidioidomycosis. However, only about 2% of patients with
histoplasmosis give a positive coccidioidomycosis skin test; since
blastomycosis infection is relatively rare, performing the different
skin tests simultaneously helps to overcome this drawback.

In serious localized infection or widespread dissemination of
these fungi, there is often a normocytic normochromic or slightly
hypochromic anemia. The anemia is usually mild or moderate in
localized infection.

"Opportunistic" Fungi: Other fungi may, under certain circumstances, produce visceral or systemic infection. The most
common of these conditions are candidiasis, aspergillosis, and
mucormycosis. Situations predisposing to infection include aged
persons, cachetic or debilitated patients, diseases such as leukemia
which affect the body's immunologic mechanisms, and, most commonly, treatment by certain drugs which impair the same immunologic mechanisms. Such drugs include many types of antileukemic
or anticancer chemotherapy, and sometimes heavy or prolonged use
of adrenocortical steroids. Occasionally, overgrowth of Candida
may be caused by prolonged oral antibiotic therapy which destroys
normal gastrointestinal bacterial flora. Candida fungemia may be
associated with indwelling intravenous catheters. Mucormycosis is
characteristically but not exclusively associated with diabetics.
Diagnosis in many of these patients is difficult, since the original
underlying disease usually overshadows advent of the fungal infection. If the patient has a condition which predisposes to infection by
fungi, culture of a fungus from an area where it is normally absent
should not be disregarded as mere contamination, but should be investigated further.

When fungal culture is indicated, the laboratory must be notified, because bacterial culture media are not generally suitable for
fungi. All-purpose fungal culture media such as Sabouraud's, under
aerobic conditions, is satisfactory for most of the "systemic" fungi,
except for Actinomyces and Nocardia.

The dermatophytes include a number of fungi which attack the
nails and skin. A presumptive etiologic diagnosis may be made by
scrapings of the affected area examined microscopically in a wet
mount of 10% potassium hydroxide. Definitive diagnosis is by culture, usually on all-purpose media such as Sabouraud's. Skin, mu-

cous membrane, or female vaginal infection by Candida (Monilia) is a fairly common fungus problem. This is more frequent in diabetics. Diagnosis is by essentially the same methods as the dermatophytes.

## REFERENCES

Buechner, H. A.: Clinical Aspects of Fungus Disease of the Lungs Including Laboratory Diagnosis and Treatment, in Banyai, A. L., and Gordon, B. L. (eds.): Advances in Cardiopulmonary Disease (Chicago: Year Book Medical Publishers, Inc., 1966), Vol. 3, p. 123.

Butler, W. T., et al.: Diagnostic and prognostic value of clinical and laboratory findings in cryptococcal meningitis, New England J. Med. 270:60, 1964.

Conn, H. F. (ed.): Symposium on efficacy of antibiotic and antifungal agents, M. Clin. North America 54:1077, 1970.

Friese, M. J.: Coccidioidomycosis (Springfield, Ill.: Charles C Thomas, Publisher, 1958).

Furcolow, M. L.: Tests of immunity in histoplasmosis, New England J. Med. 268:357, 1963.

Goldstein, E., and Hoeprich, P. D.: Problems in the diagnosis and treatment of systemic candidiasis, J. Infect. Dis. 125:190, 1972.

Hendry, W. S., and Patrick, R. L.: Observations on thirteen cases of pneumocystis carinii pneumonia, Am. J. Clin. Path. 38:401, 1962.

Littman, M. L., and Zimmerman, L. E.: Cryptococcus (New York: Grune & Stratton, Inc., 1956).

Louria, D. B., et al.: Disseminated moniliasis in the adult, Medicine 41:307, 1962.

Louria, D. B., et al.: Fungemia caused by "nonpathogenic" yeasts, Arch. Int. Med. 119:247, 1967.

Negroni, P.: Histoplasmosis (Springfield, Ill.: Charles C Thomas, Publisher, 1965).

Quie, P. G., and Chilgren, R. A.: Acute disseminated and chronic mucocutaneous candidiasis, Seminars Hemat. 8:227, 1971.

Reeves, D. L., et al.: Phycomycosis (mucormycosis) of the central nervous system, J. Neurosurg. 23:82, 1965.

Sweany, H. C.: Histoplasmosis (Springfield, Ill.: Charles C Thomas, Publisher, 1960).

Symposium on Diseases Caused by Fungi, Am. J. Clin. Path. 25:2, 1955.

Utz, J. P.: Pulmonary Infection Due to Opportunistic Fungi, in Stollerman, G. H., et al. (eds.): Advances in Internal Medicine (Chicago: Year Book Medical Publishers, Inc., 1970), Vol. 16, p. 427.

Winslow, D. J., and Steen, F. G.: Considerations in the histologic diagnosis of mycetoma, Am. J. Clin. Path. 42:164, 1964.

Young, R. C., et al.: Aspergillosis—The spectrum of the disease in 98 patients, Medicine 49:147, 1970.

# CHAPTER 16

# Viral, Rickettsial, and Miscellaneous Infectious Diseases

This chapter will deal with the laboratory procedures available for diagnosis of viral and rickettsial infection, and will also include certain other organisms which are not bacterial but are not truly viral or rickettsial. In some cases the etiologic agent is unknown or in dispute.

Viral diseases form a large heterogeneous group. A general classification (including only the most important viruses) is presented in Table 7. In general, diagnostic methods depend on the type of illness produced. In the great majority of situations, including infection by enterovirus, respiratory viruses, and arboviruses, the only available laboratory methods are culture and serologic tests. Culture techniques have made significant advances in the past few years but, unfortunately, still must be described as difficult and expensive. Culture is done in living cell preparations or in living tissues. This fact in itself rules out "mass production" testing. Partly because of this, facilities for work of this kind are limited, and are available mainly at sizable medical centers or large Public Health laboratories. Recent application of fluorescent antibody techniques may simplify some of the procedures and possibly provide rapid screening tests in some situations; at present, these techniques are not routine. In addition to culture, serologic tests are available for most viruses. There are several different techniques; although they are considerably less exacting than culture, most are still rather tedious and time-consuming, with the result that here again, these tests are not immediately available except at reference laboratories. Serologic tests have the additional disadvantage that antibodies usually take 1-2 weeks to develop after onset of illness, and, unless a significantly (fourfold) rising titer is demonstrated, do not prove

TABLE 7.—CLASSIFICATION OF VIRUSES

A.  Taxonomic Classification

RNA Viruses

| | |
|---|---|
| Picornovirus | enterovirus (polio, Coxsackie, ECHO) and rhinovirus |
| Reovirus | |
| Arbovirus | (equine encephalitis, St. Louis encephalitis, yellow fever) |
| Myxovirus | (influenza, parainfluenza, respiratory syncytial virus, measles, mumps) |
| Rabies | |

DNA Viruses

| | |
|---|---|
| Adenovirus | |
| Herpesvirus | (herpes simplex, herpes zoster-varicella, cytomegalic inclusion virus) |
| Poxvirus | (smallpox, vaccinia, molluscum contagiosum) |

B.  Clinical Classification (characteristic organ systems involved clinically)

Central Nervous System

| | |
|---|---|
| Arbovirus | (arthropod-borne virus) |
| Enterovirus | |
| Rabies | |

Gastrointestinal

| | |
|---|---|
| Enterovirus | (ECHO) |

Respiratory

Rhinovirus
Myxovirus
Adenovirus
Reovirus

Liver

| | |
|---|---|
| Hepatitis viruses | (short-incubation and long-incubation hepatitis virus) |

Yellow fever

Skin

Poxvirus

Salivary Glands

Cytomegalic inclusion virus
Mumps

current activity of the viral agent in question.  Nevertheless, it is considered good practice to attempt specific etiologic diagnosis of viral diseases in order to provide the community with information that may alert it to an epidemic, as well as to confirm the clinical

impression and perhaps rule out other etiologies which would call
for different therapy.

## VIRAL RESPIRATORY DISEASE

Respiratory disease may take several forms, and the predominant etiologies are different in different age groups. Statistics also
vary depending on the geographic area and the population selected.
Of the known viruses, rhinoviruses seem to be predominantly associated with acute upper respiratory disease (including the common
cold) in adults, while in children, rhinovirus, adenovirus, parainfluenza, and the enteroviruses all are important. Acute bronchitis
in children is most often due to parainfluenza and respiratory syncytial virus. In croup, parainfluenza is said to be the most important
virus. Respiratory syncytial virus is the predominating etiology of
pediatric pneumonia, followed by adenovirus or parainfluenza. In
adults, nonbacterial pneumonia is most often associated with Mycoplasma pneumoniae (Eaton agent); among viral agents known to cause
pneumonia, the most common cause is probably influenza. In
any study, a large minority of cases did not yield a specific etiologic
agent.

## VIRAL MENINGITIS

Viruses are an important cause of meningitis, especially in
children. They produce the laboratory picture of aseptic meningitis,
with cerebrospinal fluid findings of variable but often mildly increased protein, increased cell counts with mononuclears predominating, and normal sugar. It should be remembered, however, that
tuberculous meningitis gives similar findings, except for decreased
cerebrospinal fluid sugar, and also will show a sterile culture on
ordinary bacterial culture media. Enteroviruses form the largest
etiologic group causing aseptic meningitis. Among the enteric viruses, poliomyelitis used to be the most common organism, but
since the advent of widespread vaccination programs, ECHO and
Coxsackie have replaced polio in terms of frequency.

After the enterovirus group, mumps is most important. A
small but significant number of patients with mumps develop clinical
signs of meningitis, and a large number will show spinal fluid
changes without demonstrating enough clinical symptoms to warrant a diagnosis and work-up for meningitis. Cerebrospinal fluid
changes or the clinical picture of meningitis may occur in patients
without parotid swelling or other evidence of mumps. Lymphocytic
choriomeningitis and leptospirosis are uncommon etiologies for
aseptic meningitis.

Encephalitis is a syndrome which presents spinal fluid alterations similar to those of meningitis. The two cannot always be separated, but the main difference is clinical; encephalitis features de-

pression of consciousness (lethargy, coma) over a prolonged period, whereas meningitis usually is a more acute episode including fever, headaches, physical signs of central nervous system irritation, and possibly convulsions. In severe bacterial infection, encephalitis may be the sequel of meningitis. Encephalitis is most frequently caused by mumps and measles. The next largest group are those of unknown etiology. Arbovirus is third in frequency. Sometimes encephalitis appears as a complication of vaccination.

## VIRAL GASTROENTERITIS

Viruses are likely to be blamed for diarrhea which cannot be explained otherwise. In most cases, definitive evidence is lacking, because enteric virus is present in a significant number of apparently healthy children. In those studies where strong evidence of a viral etiology is presented, ECHO virus is by far the most frequent organism. Bacterial infection should always be carefully ruled out.

## VIRAL INFECTIONS IN PREGNANCY

By far the most dangerous viral disease during pregnancy is rubella. Statistics are variable, but they suggest about a 15-25% risk of fetal malformation when rubella infection occurs in the 1st trimester. The true incidence is not certain; estimates and studies generally fall within 10-15%, although some report as high as 80%. Besides this, 5-15% of fetuses probably die in utero. Risk in the 2d trimester is about 5%. After the 4th month of pregnancy, there is no longer any danger to the fetus. Most viral diseases other than rubella exert ill effects in the 3d trimester, like cytomegalic inclusion virus. Many viruses are thought to have potential to cause neonatal disease or malformation, but evidence is somewhat inconclusive as to exact incidence and effects. Herpes simplex and infectious hepatitis have some documentation.

## DIAGNOSIS OF VIRAL DISEASES

These are investigated by two main types of laboratory procedures—direct isolation by culture, and demonstration of antibodies in the patient's blood to specific organisms. Serologic test results without isolation of an organism by culture allow only a presumptive diagnosis, and cultural isolation of certain viruses without serologic confirmation does not absolutely prove that the virus is causing current disease, since many viruses are quite prevalent in the general population. If possible, both techniques should be done together, since they supplement each other. Since culture methods are still rather difficult and expensive, serologic tests are probably more widely used. One serum specimen is obtained as early in the disease as possible ("acute" stage) and a second sample is obtained

2-3 weeks later ("convalescent" stage). Blood should be collected into sterile tubes or vacutainer tubes and serum processed aseptically to avoid bacterial contamination. Hemolyzed serum is not acceptable; to help prevent hemolysis, serum should be separated from blood clot as soon as possible. The serum should be frozen as soon as possible after collection (to minimize bacterial growth) and sent still frozen (packed in dry ice) to the virus laboratory. Here a variety of serologic tests can be done to demonstrate specific antibodies to the various organisms. A fourfold rise in titer from acute to convalescent stage of the disease is considered diagnostic. If only a single specimen is taken, an elevated titer could be due to previous infection rather than currently active disease. A single negative test is likewise difficult to interpret, since the specimen might have been obtained too early, before antibody rise occurred.

In any kind of meningitis with negative spinal fluid cultures or severe respiratory infection of unknown etiology, it is a good idea to freeze a specimen of serum as early in the disease as possible. Later on, if desired, another specimen can be drawn and the two sent off for virus studies. As noted, serum specimens are generally drawn 2 weeks apart.

There is one notable exception to the rule of acute and convalescent serologic specimens. In some circumstances, it is desirable to learn whether a person has an antibody titer to a particular virus sufficient to prevent onset of the disease. This is especially true for a woman in early pregnancy exposed to rubella. A significant antibody titer to rubella would suggest immunity to the virus.

When obtaining specimens for viral culture, the type of specimen depends on the type of illness. In aseptic meningitis, cerebrospinal fluid should be obtained. In addition, stool culture for virus should be done, since enteroviruses are frequent etiologies of meningitis. In enterovirus meningitis, stool culture is 2-3 times more effective than spinal fluid culture.

In suspected cases of (nonbacterial) encephalitis, whole blood should be collected for virus culture during the first 2 days of illness. During this short time there is a chance of demonstrating arbovirus viremia. This procedure is not useful in aseptic meningitis. Spinal fluid should also be sent for virus culture; even though the yield is relatively small in arbovirus infections, the specimen sometimes is positive, and also helps to rule out other organisms such as enterovirus. In upper respiratory illness, throat or nasopharyngeal swabs are preferred. These should be placed in trypticase broth (a standard bacterial medium). Swabs without some type of media such as trypticase or Hank's solution are usually not satisfactory, since they dry out quickly and most viruses are killed by drying. Throat washings or gargle material can be used, but are difficult to obtain properly. In viral pneumonia, sputum or throat swabs are needed. If throat swabs are used they should be placed in acceptable collection solutions. Whether throat swabs or sputum, the specimen must be frozen immediately, and sent to the virus laboratory packed in dry ice. In addition, a sputum specimen (or throat swab) should be obtained for mycoplasma culture (p. 194). In possible viral gastroenteritis, stool culture is the logical procedure. In any situation where a stool culture for virus is needed, actual stool specimens are preferred rather than rectal swabs, since there is a better chance of isolating an organism from the larger sample. The stool specimen should be frozen in the same manner as the serum samples. It is better to mail any virus specimens early in the week, so as to avoid arrival on weekends. An insulated container helps to prolong effects of the dry ice.

In any case, an adequate clinical history with pertinent physical and laboratory findings should accompany any virus specimen, whether for culture or serologic studies. As a minimum, the date of clinical illness onset, collection date of each specimen, and clinical diagnosis must be included. The most likely organism should be indicated. This information helps the virus laboratory in determining what initial procedures or techniques to use. For example, certain tissue culture cell types are better adapted than others for certain viruses. Considerable time and effort can be saved and a meaningful interpretation of results can be provided.

## SPECIFIC VIRAL DISEASES

Certain specific viruses deserve individual discussion. The method of diagnosis or type of specimen required for some of these organisms is different from the usual procedure. In others, it is desirable to emphasize certain aspects of the clinical illness which suggest the diagnosis.

German measles (rubella) is especially important in pregnancy. The "rubella syndrome" includes one or more of the following: congenital heart disease, cataract, deafness, and cerebral damage. Diagnosis is made by documenting active rubella infection in the mother during early pregnancy, or by proving infection of the infant after birth. A significant (fourfold) rise in antibody titer using one of several varieties of serologic tests is the easiest way to demonstrate maternal infection. At present, the hemagglutination inhibition (HI or HAI) and complement fixation (CF) serologic tests form the backbone of diagnosis. HI antibodies appear during the first week after onset of rash; they are often detectable after only 2-3 days. Peak levels are reached during the second week. An elevated titer persists for many years or for life. CF antibodies develop in the more conventional time of 7-14 days after onset of rash and generally disappear in a few years. Absence of HAI antibody indicates susceptibility to rubella, since it usually persists whereas CF antibody titer returns to normal. Presence of HI antibody means either past or recent infection. In a person who is clinically well, this means immunity to subsequent infection. In a person with suspected clinical rubella, an immediate serum specimen and a second one drawn at least 7 days later must be obtained, the standard procedure with all serologic tests. A fourfold rise in titer confirms very recent (active) infection. However, if the first serum specimen was not obtained until several days after onset of rash, the HI peak may already have been reached. In some of these cases, a significant (fourfold titer or two-tube dilution) rise in CF antibody may be demonstrated, since these antibodies develop later than HI. If both antibodies are at peak, there is no way to distinguish recent infection from one occurring months or even years previously.

In the neonatal period, congenital rubella can best be established by virus culture of nasopharyngeal swab material. Infant serum antibodies come from the mother. By 6-8 months, maternal antibody in the child has disappeared, so that persistence of antibody past this time indicates congenital or neonatal infection. For some reason, however, at least 20% of children with congenital rubella lose their HI titer by age 5.

The HI test at the present time takes considerable experience to produce reliable results. Therefore, since false positive results may occur, it is probably wise to obtain the CF test at the same time. If the patient is pregnant and the diagnosis may lead to some action, it may be advisable to split each sample, keeping part of each frozen, in case a recheck is desired.

Measles (rubeola) is still quite important, since widespread vaccination has just begun. The two main complications of this disease are encephalitis and pneumonia. Encephalitis is fortunately rare, the incidence being 0.01-0.2%; due to the great frequency of the disease, however, the total number of cases is appreciable. About a third of those with encephalitis die, about a third recover completely, and the remainder survive but show moderate-to-severe residua. This encephalitis is considered postinfectious, because it develops 4-21 days after onset of rash. Measles involves lymphoid tissue and respiratory epithelium early in the illness. Therefore, pneumonia is fairly frequent. The majority of cases are due to superimposed bacterial infection (staphylococcus, pneumococcus, streptococcus), but some occur from primarily viral effects. For diagnosis, culture and serologic tests are available. Culture depends on the stage of disease. For a period of 1 week ending with the first appearance of the rash, blood, nasopharyngeal swabs, or urine provide adequate specimens. After appearance of the rash, urine culture is possible up to 4 days. Beyond this, culture is not useful, and serologic tests must be employed.

Mumps is a disseminated virus infection, although the main clinical feature is salivary gland enlargement. Evidence of nonsalivary gland involvement is most commonly seen in adults. In adult males, orchitis (usually unilateral) is reported in about 20% of cases. Adult females occasionally develop oophoritis. Any age group may be affected by meningoencephalitis, the most serious

complication of mumps.  This is reported in 0.5-10% of patients.
Many persons with spinal fluid changes are asymptomatic.  Females
are affected five times more frequently than males.  Complications
of mumps may appear before, during, or after parotitis, sometimes
even without clinical parotitis.  Diagnosis is made by culture or
serologic tests.  Saliva is probably best for culture; mouth swabs
or spinal fluid can be used.

Viral hepatitis is one of the major unsolved problems in diagnostic virology.  Two types of hepatitis viruses seem evident: short-
incubation hepatitis (hepatitis A), with an incubation period of 10-40
days, and long-incubation hepatitis (hepatitis B), whose incubation
period is 60-120 days.  Both types may be transmitted via the oral
route from fecal contamination or by parenteral infection from a
contaminated needle or injection of contaminated blood or blood
products.  Until recently, hepatitis B was thought to be transmitted
only by blood transfusion, and was called "serum hepatitis"; hepatitis
A was known as "infectious hepatitis."  This concept changed when a
geneticist discovered an antigen in the blood of an Australian native
("Australia antigen"); eventually it was found that many persons
carry the Australia antigen and that it occurs in a high proportion
of patients with hepatitis.  Some have felt that it is actually a hepatitis virus; however, at present, it is considered only a hepatitis-
associated antigen (HAA).  Studies have linked HAA to hepatitis B
but not to hepatitis A, and have shown that HAA can be transmitted
via the oral route.  HAA is found in a significant percentage (over
5%) of persons with diseases other than hepatitis (hemophilia,
mongolism, Hodgkin's disease, leukemia, lepromatous leprosy,
chronic active hepatitis), in hemodialysis patients, and in natives of
various South Pacific and Asia regions.  Some of these instances
could be due to blood transfusions and some to close-contact trans-
mittal; many are unexplained.

In hepatitis B, HAA can often be detected 30-40 days after exposure and 2-4 weeks before a rise in serum glutamic oxaloacetic
transaminase (SGOT).  After onset of hepatitis symptoms, HAA may
disappear in 1-2 days, but more often persists for 1-6 weeks.  About
10% of patients are still positive after a year.  Various test systems
have been devised to detect HAA.  Sensitivity in hepatitis B patients
is variable: immunodiffusion, about 30%; counterimmunoelectro-
phoresis, about 40%; complement fixation, about 50%; radioimmunoassay, over 60%.  Interpretation of HAA results thus must take into
account (1) the knowledge that only about half of the cases of hepatitis-
virus hepatitis are hepatitis B and, therefore, potentially detectable
by HAA; (2) the type of test used; and (3) how early in the clinical
course the specimen was obtained.

Both hepatitis A and hepatitis B can produce asymptomatic infection; in fact, such a situation is probably more common than
clinical illness.  It is estimated that up to 10% of those who receive
a blood transfusion will develop hepatitis, although the incidence of

jaundice is only about 1%.

Cytomegalic inclusion virus may cause localized infection of the salivary glands without any clinical symptoms. If it becomes disseminated, a variety of manifestations may be produced, depending on the age of the patient, the presence of underlying diseases which might alter the patient's immunologic response to the virus, or the visceral organs affected.

In the newborn, the disseminated disease may appear in two forms:

1. A subacute form with predominantly cerebral symptoms, manifested by the picture of cerebral palsy or mental retardation.

2. An acute form with various combinations of hepatosplenomegaly, thrombocytopenia, hepatitis with jaundice, and cerebral symptoms such as convulsions. There usually is anemia, and there may be nucleated RBC and a shift to the left on peripheral blood smear.

In young children, the most common manifestation is probably mild fever or a febrile illness; one report indicates that hepatitis (usually mild, often nearly asymptomatic) is frequent.

In older children and adults, clinical disease is very uncommon. It is most often superimposed on pre-existing malignancy such as leukemia or malignant lymphoma, and has predominantly pulmonary or hepatic involvement which usually is overshadowed by the pre-existing nonviral disease.

In the newborn, periventricular cerebral calcification is demonstrable by x-ray in about 25%; this is highly suggestive, although the same pattern may be found in congenital toxoplasmosis. Characteristic inclusion bodies may be demonstrated within renal epithelial cells in stained smears of the urinary sediment in about 60% of cases; this may be an intermittent finding which may require specimens on several days. A fresh specimen is preferable to a 24-hour collection, since the cells tend to disintegrate on standing. Probably the best procedure, when available, is virus culture of a urine specimen. For best results, this must reach the virus culture laboratory within 1-2 days. The specimen should not be frozen, as freezing progressively inactivates the virus; this is in contrast to most other viruses, where quick freezing is the procedure of choice for preserving specimens. The specimen should be refrigerated without actual freezing where it may be preserved up to a week. It should be sent to the virus laboratory packed in ordinary ice (not dry ice); if possible, in an insulated container. Isolation of the cytomegalic virus may take several weeks.

In older children and adults, the kidney is not often severely affected, so that urine specimens for cytomegalic inclusion bodies usually are not helpful. Urine, sputum, or mouth swab culture for the virus is the method of choice. Fresh specimens are essential.

Infectious mononucleosis: A virus named Barr-Epstein is now considered responsible; the same virus is also thought to be associated with a peculiar type of malignant lymphoma called Burkitt's lymphoma.  Infectious mononucleosis patients are most often young adults, but a good percentage are children and some are older adults.  The most common features are fever, pharyngitis and adenopathy, with lymph node enlargement being the most frequent.  It may be localized or generalized.  The posterior cervical nodes are the most commonly enlarged.  Soft-palate petechiae are found in 10-30% of the cases.  Jaundice due to mild hepatitis is found in approximately 5% of the large patient series.  Uncommon symptoms are skin rashes and supraorbital edema.  The spleen is enlarged in about 40%.  Laboratory data show normal hemoglobin and platelets, although rare cases of thrombocytopenia are reported.  Incidentally, normal hemoglobin values help in differentiation from lymphoma and leukemia which the clinical symptoms may resemble, but which usually have anemia.  There is a leukocytosis, usually by the second week or by the time lymphadenopathy is well established.  However, during the first week there may be leukopenia.  The differential white count is characteristic and includes two of the three criteria for diagnosis (serologic tests being the third).  There is usually lymphocytosis with lymphocytes comprising over 50% of the total WBC; of these lymphocytes, a significant number (amounting to over 20%) must be atypical.  These so-called atypical lymphs are of three main types: type I has vacuolated or foamy blue cytoplasm and rounded nucleus, type II has an elongated flattened nucleus and large amounts of pale cytoplasm with sharply defined irregular borders, and type III has an immature irregular nucleus which may have a nucleolus or show folding.  All three types are larger than normal mature lymphocytes, and their nuclei are somewhat less dense.  These atypical lymphocytes are not specific for infectious mononucleosis, but may be found in small-to-moderate numbers in a variety of viral diseases including infectious hepatitis.  Many choose to call them all virocytes.  In addition, some of the type II variety may be created artificially by crushing and flattening normal lymphocytes near the edge of the blood smear.  Infectious mononucleosis cells are sometimes confused with those of acute leukemia or lymphosarcoma, although in the majority of cases there is no problem.

The serologic test for infectious mononucleosis known as the Paul-Bunnell test is based on the discovery that the antibody produced in infectious mononucleosis will agglutinate sheep RBC.  Dilutions are set up for 1:7, 1:14, 1:28, 1:64, 1:112, and so on serially, and the last tube dilution to show agglutination is reported as the titer.  Normally, the titer is less than 1:112 and most often is almost or completely negative.  The Paul-Bunnell test is also known as the "presumptive test," because later it was found that certain antibodies different from those of infectious mononucleosis will also attack sheep RBC.  This is true of antibodies produced to the so-called Forssman antigen found naturally in man and certain other animals.  Thus, if the Paul-Bunnell test is elevated, one does not

know if this means infectious mononucleosis antibody or a nonspecific Forssman antibody.  Fortunately, Forssman antibodies are
usually not produced in high titers, so this fact may help in many
cases.  Eventually, the so-called differential absorption test (Davidsohn differential test) was developed.

It seems that guinea pig kidney is a good source of Forssman
antigen.  Therefore, if a serum containing Forssman antibody is allowed to come in contact with guinea pig kidney material, the
Forssman antibody will combine with the kidney antigen and be removed from the serum when the serum is taken off.  The serum will
then show either a very low or negative titer, whereas before it had
been strongly positive.  The infectious mononucleosis antibody will
not be significantly absorbed by guinea pig kidney, but will be nearly
completely absorbed by beef RBC, which do not significantly affect
the Forssman antibody.  The only other antigen which may be involved is that produced in serum sickness, and this will absorb both
with beef RBC and guinea pig kidney.  In the absorption test, there
must be at least a three-tube decrease in titer to be considered significant absorption.  In other words, true infectious mononucleosis
antibody will not drop more than three tubes dilution when treated
with guinea pig kidney, whereas Forssman antibody will.  The height
of the titer after absorption has no diagnostic value.  However, the
original presumptive test must have at least a 1:28 titer in order to
allow the differential to be done at all.  The Paul-Bunnell test remains elevated for several weeks or months after clinical symptoms have disappeared.  The level of Paul-Bunnell titer does not
correlate well with the clinical course of infectious mononucleosis.
Titer is useful only in making a diagnosis, and should not be relied
on to follow the clinical course of the disease or to assess results
of therapy.

In suspected mononucleosis, the presumptive test should be
done first; if necessary, it can be followed by a differential absorption procedure.  The Paul-Bunnell and differential tests are usually
positive by 3 weeks after onset of symptoms.  Most cases are positive during the second week, although the Paul-Bunnell titer may
not yet have risen to its full height.  Many cases have such high
presumptive titers that a differential is not necessary.  Some never
reach 1:112, and it is in these patients and those with only moderate titer elevation that the differential absorption is most helpful.

False positive differential results have been reported but are
extremely rare.  Elevated titer from infectious mononucleosis may
persist for months, and it is possible that even the few reported
false positive cases had subclinical mononucleosis sometime earlier.  On the other hand, there are reports describing outbreaks of
a disease which clinically was identical to infectious mononucleosis
with typical blood changes, but with the Paul-Bunnell test negative
in many or even all cases.  A similar situation has been reported
following blood transfusions; some of these post-transfusion patients

prove to have cytomegalic inclusion virus on culture.  This raises a question as to what criteria to use in differentiating infectious mononucleosis.  When all three criteria are satisfied, there is no problem.  When the Paul-Bunnell test and/or differential absorption are positive, most authors believe that the diagnosis can be made, although there are reports that viral infections occurring after infectious mononucleosis can cause anamnestic "false positive" heterophil re-elevations.  When the blood picture is characteristic both regarding number and type of lymphocytes, but the Paul-Bunnell test is negative as late as 3 weeks after onset, most believe that the diagnosis can be considered probable but not established.  Parenthetically, many articles in the literature give only the results of the presumptive test; as mentioned, one can have a presumptive test within normal range (which is less than 1:112) and still have a positive differential absorption (if the titer is at least 1:28).

A technique ("Monospot") has recently been devised in which the Paul-Bunnell and differential absorption tests are converted to a rapid slide procedure without titration.  Citrate-preserved horse red blood cells are used instead of sheep RBC.  The antigen-antibody reactions and absorptions are carried out visually by adding drops of reagents to areas on a slide or piece of paper, rather than by titration in test tubes.  If properly done, preliminary reports indicate that the method is as sensitive and nearly as specific as the classic procedure.  However, at least one report indicates that false positives may occur in malignant lymphoma using this particular technique.

A rapid modification of the heterophil procedure called Mono-Test uses formalin-fixed RBC without differential absorption.  The Mono-Test has been reported to have almost the same specificity as the differential absorption technique.  There is some question whether Formalinized horse RBC are as sensitive as citrate-preserved horse RBC or sheep RBC.

In summary, the three criteria for the diagnosis of infectious mononucleosis are:

1) Lymphocytosis over 50% of total WBC count.

2) Atypical lymphocytes over 20% of the total lymphocytes.

3) Significantly elevated Paul-Bunnell test or differential absorption test.  A positive Mono-Test or spot test, from current reports, satisfies this criterion.

Work has been done using antibodies to Barr-Epstein virus for diagnosis, but this has not proved very useful clinically.

## NONVIRAL, NONBACTERIAL INFECTIOUS AGENTS

Several unrelated groups of organisms will be discussed.

Primary atypical pneumonia: This is a name describing pulmonary infection by a variety of viruses and virus-like organisms which nevertheless produce a fairly characteristic syndrome.  It consists of cough, fever, headache, and malaise lasting about 10 days. Chest x-ray shows mottled infiltrates which are most pronounced in the hilar areas of the lower lobes and are more often unilateral. Despite the symptoms and x-ray findings there is characteristically very little abnormal on physical examination. The blood count is either normal or close to it. About half the cases have been found due to Mycoplasma pneumoniae, the so-called Eaton agent, a pleuropneumonia-like (PPLO) organism. The PPLO group is intermediate in size and other characteristics between viruses and bacteria. In the primary atypical pneumonia cases due to M. pneumoniae, cold agglutinins can be found in 50-60%.

Cold agglutinins are antibodies which are able to agglutinate type O red blood cells at icebox temperatures but not at room temperature. They are found in other diseases, and thus are nonspecific, but usually in adults with an acute respiratory syndrome, their presence in significant titer is associated with Eaton agent pneumonia. Cold agglutinins elevated over 1:32 are abnormal and can be found during the second week of illness, reaching a peak in the third or fourth week. A rising titer is more significant than a single determination. The PPLO organisms can be cultured on special media, but this takes about a week. Sputum or pharyngeal swabs may be used. If preservation is necessary, specimens should be frozen and transported with dry ice.

The bedsoniae are organisms which are intermediate between viruses and rickettsiae in size, but which resemble bacteria more than viruses. They cause psittacosis, lymphogranuloma venereum, and trachoma. Psittacosis organisms are contracted from birds, most commonly parakeets. Two syndromes may be produced: a typhoid-like picture or a respiratory illness. Pulmonary involvement is the more frequent, resembling a viral bronchopneumonia or influenza syndrome. White blood counts are usually normal or subnormal. Diagnosis is usually made through serologic (antibody) tests and a history of contact with birds. The antibodies of psittacosis cross-react with those of lymphogranuloma venereum.

Lymphogranuloma venereum (LGV) is transmitted by sexual contact. After an incubation period, the inguinal lymph nodes become swollen and tender in males; in females, the lymphatic drainage is usually to the intra-abdominal, perirectal and pelvic lymph nodes. In a considerable number of cases, the perirectal nodes develop abscesses and the nearby wall of the rectum is involved, eventually leading to scar tissue and constriction of the rectum. In either male or female, in the acute stage of lymphatic involvement, there may be fever, malaise, and headache with sometimes joint aching—but all these may be absent. In the majority of cases the main findings are acute inguinal node enlargement in the male and chronic rectal stricture in the female. Laboratory findings in active disease include mild anemia, moderate leukocytosis, and serum protein disturbances with considerable hyperglobulinemia and hypoalbuminemia.

The elevated globulin gives a high diffuse gamma elevation on serum protein electrophoresis, similar to that seen with far-advanced tuberculosis. Laboratory diagnosis includes a skin test called the Frei test, and serologic complement fixation studies. The complement fixation reaction becomes positive about a month after infection and will remain elevated for years. Acute and convalescent serum should be obtained to demonstrate a rising titer. The Frei test is an intradermal skin injection of lymphogranuloma antigen giving a papule after 48-72 hours. This becomes positive about 2-3 weeks after the lymph node inflammation and remains positive for years. Either the serologic tests or the Frei test cross-react with psittacosis, although this usually is not a problem. Lymph node biopsy shows a characteristic histologic pattern which, however, is also seen with tularemia and cat-scratch fever. At present, the Frei test is the most convenient method for diagnosis. One drawback is the fact that the Frei test will itself produce a positive LGV complement fixation test. There is a relatively high incidence of syphilis serology biologic false positive reactions (p. 374) in lymphogranuloma venereum. This may cause confusion because, due to the venereal nature of transmission, syphilis may also be present, and early syphilis can give inguinal lymph node enlargement similar to lymphogranuloma venereum.

The bedsoniae and PPLO groups were included among the viruses for a long time. In the older literature there is frequent reference to them as "large viruses."

The rickettsiae to some extent resemble small bacteria, but are not stained with gram stain and cannot be cultured on artificial media. These organisms are spread only by insect vectors which have fed on blood from a patient with the disease—not from personal contact with a patient. Blood culture is the method of definitive identification for rickettsiae, especially in Rocky Mountain spotted fever. The blood specimen should be frozen and sent to the virus laboratory packed in dry ice. However, chick embryo or live animal inoculation must be done, since artificial culture medium is not available, and thus serologic tests by far overshadow culture as diagnostic aids. The most commonly used procedure is the Weil-Felix reaction. This test takes advantage of the fact that certain rickettsial diseases produce antibodies which also react (or cross-react) with antigen contained in certain strains of Proteus bacteria. These Proteus groups are called OX-19 and OX-K. Titers of 1:80 are suspicious and 1:160 are definitely significant. Antibodies appear 7-10 days after onset of illness. Rickettsial diseases which may be diagnosed by means of the Weil-Felix reaction are the following:

| Disease | Proteus Strain | Vector | Organism |
|---------|---------------|--------|----------|
| Epidemic typhus | OX-19 | body louse | R. prowazekii |
| Endemic (murine) typhus | OX-19 | rat flea | R. mooseri |
| Scrub typhus | OX-K | mite | R. tsutsugamushi |
| Rocky Mountain spotted fever | OX-19 | tick | R. akeri |

Unfortunately, there are certain limitations to the Weil-Felix test. First, there are a fairly large number of borderline false positive results as well as occasional outright false positives. Since the Weil-Felix reaction depends on Proteus antigen, urinary tract infection by Proteus should be ruled out if the Weil-Felix test is positive. Second, about two-thirds of patients with Rocky Mountain spotted fever and Brill's disease (recrudescent typhus) give false negative reactions. In these two diseases, serologic complement fixation tests are preferred to the Weil-Felix. The serum specimens should be frozen and sent to the laboratory packed in dry ice.

## REFERENCES

Blattner, R. J., and Heys, F. M.: Viral Encephalitis, in Levine, S. Z. (ed.): Advances in Pediatrics (Chicago: Year Book Medical Publishers, Inc., 1962), Vol. XII, p. 11.

Blumberg, B.: Australia antigen and hepatitis: a comprehensive review, CRC Critical Reviews in Clin. Lab. Sc. 2:473, 1971.

Chanock, R. M., and Purcell, R. H.: Role of mycoplasmas in human respiratory disease, M. Clin. North America 51:791, 1967.

Cheever, F. S.: Viral agents in gastrointestinal disease, M. Clin. North America 51:637, 1967.

Clyde, W. A., Jr., and Denny, F. W., Jr.: The etiology and therapy of atypical pneumonia, M. Clin. North America 47:1201, 1963.

Coriell, L. L.: Clinical syndromes in children caused by respiratory infection, M. Clin. North America 51:819, 1967.

Curnen, E. C.: The Coxsackie viruses, Pediat. Clin. North America 7:903, 1960.

Davidsohn, I., and Lee, C. L.: The laboratory in the diagnosis of infectious mononucleosis, M. Clin. North America 46:225, 1962.

Davidson, R. J. L.: New slide test for infectious mononucleosis, J. Clin. Path. 20:643, 1967.

Davis, D. C., and Melnick, J. L.: Poliomyelitis and aseptic meningitis, J. Lab. & Clin. Med. 51:97, 1958.

Dupont, J. R., and Earle, K. M.: Human rabies encephalitis, Neurology 15:1023, 1965.

Evans, A. S.: Clinical syndromes in adults caused by respiratory infection, M. Clin. North America 51:803, 1967.

Gifford, H.: Cat scratch disease, Pediat. Clin. North America 2:33, 1955.

Gwaltney, J. M. , Jr. , and Jordon, W. S. , Jr. : The present status of respiratory viruses, M. Clin. North America 47:1155, 1963.

Hardy, J. B. : Viruses and the fetus, Postgrad. Med. 43:156, 1968.

Horsfall, F. L. , Jr. , and Tamm, I. (eds.): Viral and Rickettsial Diseases of Man (4th ed. ; Philadelphia: J. B. Lippincott Company, 1965).

Horstman, D. M. : Rubella and the rubella syndrome: Problems and progress, M. Clin. North America 51:587, 1967.

Kennedy, C. , and Wangle, P. : Encephalitis: A variable syndrome in response to viral infection, Pediat. Clin. North America 14:809, 1967.

Krugman, S. : Varicella and Herpes virus infections, Pediat. Clin. North America 7:881, 1960.

Langmuir, A. : Medical importance of measles, Am. J. Dis. Child. 103:224, 1962.

McAllister, R. M. : ECHO virus infections, Pediat. Clin. North America 7:927, 1960.

Rifkind, D. : Cytomegalovirus mononucleosis, Ann. Int. Med. 69:842, 1968.

Sadoff, L. , and Goldsmith, O. : False-positive infectious mono-nucleosis spot test in pancreatic carcinoma, J. A. M. A. 218:1297, 1971.

Saylor, L. F. : Laboratory diagnostic services for rubella in public health laboratories in California, California Med. 111:62, 1969.

Scott, T. F. M. : Postinfectious and vaccinal encephalitis, M. Clin. North America 51:701, 1967.

Seitanides, B. : A comparison of the Monospot with the Paul-Bunnell test in infectious mononucleosis and other diseases, J. Clin. Path. 22:321, 1969.

Sever, J. L. : Viral teratogens; a status report, Hosp. Practice 5:75, 1970.

Stevens, D. P. , et al. : Asymptomatic cytomegalovirus infection following blood transfusion in tumor surgery, J. A. M. A. 221:1341, 1970.

Texter, E. C. , and Laureta, H. C. : The problem of anicteric hepatitis, Am. J. Digest. Dis. 10:968, 1965.

Weller, T. H. : The cytomegaloviruses: Ubiquitous agents with protean clinical manifestations, New England J. Med. 285:203, 267, 1971.

Ziring, P. R. , et al. : The diagnosis of rubella, Pediat. Clin. North America 18:87, 1971.

# CHAPTER 17

# Medical Parasitology

Toxoplasmosis is caused by a protozoan organism, Toxoplasma gondii. There may be a congenital form transmitted to the fetus through the placenta from maternal infection acquired just before or during the early stages of pregnancy, or an acquired form. The congenital form is manifested most often by brain damage shown by convulsions, by intracerebral calcification on x-ray, and by eye damage caused by chorioretinitis. There may also be a disseminated type which gives a clinical picture similar to bacterial septicemia. The acquired form is usually seen in adults, where the most common manifestations are lymphadenopathy and low-grade fever. Diagnosis includes isolation of the organisms and serologic tests for antibody formation. Culture has proved to be very difficult, and most laboratories are not equipped to do this. Lymph node biopsy often shows a histologic pattern which is nonspecific but still characteristic enough to be suggestive, although not diagnostic, of the disease. Serologic tests form the backbone of diagnosis. There are two main types, the Sabin-Feldman dye test and a complement fixation (CF) test. The dye test demonstrates specific antibody to Toxoplasma. Usually it begins to become positive as early as the tenth day after infection, although some cases may take considerably longer. The titer climbs rapidly and remains elevated for months, eventually falling to a stable low level of less than 1:256 which persists for years or life. To make a diagnosis of acute infection requires a change from negative to positive, a rapid fourfold or greater rise in titer, preferably from a low level, or a very high stable titer. The dye test has the disadvantage just mentioned that antibody levels tend to persist. Therefore, it is often difficult to be certain whether an elevated titer from a single specimen represents recent or old infection. This is made worse by the fact that exposure to Toxoplasma is very common. Surveys have shown posi-

198

tive dye studies in 20-70% of the various populations studied.  Also, the antibody crosses the placenta and will appear in the fetus if the mother has an elevated titer either from old or recent infection. Therefore, to make a diagnosis of congenital toxoplasmosis, it is necessary to have either very high titer in both mother and infant, or to demonstrate a rising titer in the infant from specimens taken in the 1st and 6th weeks of life.  If no active infection was present and antibody was only passively acquired from the mother, instead of rising, the titer should fall during this time.  In acute acquired toxoplasmosis the diagnosis is made as described earlier.  If the infection is chronic, titer levels may be relatively low, as mentioned previously, so clinical findings may be more important than the laboratory results.  A CF test has been described which reacts with a different but still specific antibody.  This test becomes positive a few weeks after the dye test in a dilution greater than 1:2, rapidly rises and then gradually falls to negative, usually within 5-7 years.  An indirect hemagglutination (IHA) test is now being used.  Although quite sensitive, it is not as specific, with false positives reported in persons with rheumatoid-collagen diseases and antinuclear antibodies.  Both the CF and the IHA test may sometimes be negative in congenital toxoplasmosis.

Malaria is a widespread cause of serious infection in Asia and Africa, and may be acquired by travelers or military personnel. Diagnostic procedures were discussed under Anemia (p. 48).

Gastrointestinal parasites: Ascaris, hookworm, Strongyloides, Trichinella, the tapeworms, and the amebas form the majority of gastrointestinal parasites which have clinical significance in the United States.  Diagnosis usually depends on examination of the feces for larvae or eggs.  In most situations (except for amebiasis), three routine stool specimens, collected one every other day, and sent for "ova and parasites," is adequate.

Entamoeba histolytica, however, is more difficult to isolate and requires special precautions.  If the specimen for amebas is soft or liquid, it should be sent to the laboratory immediately with the time of collection noted, because fresh specimens are essential to demonstrate the trophozoite stage.  Well-formed stools usually contain only cysts, and may be refrigerated temporarily.  For collection routine, three specimens, one specimen collected every other day, are more reliable than a single specimen.  Multiple specimens collected the same day are not much better than a single specimen. If the stools on three alternate days are all negative, and if strong clinical suspicion is still present, a saline purge should be used. After a saline purge (such as Fleet Phosphosoda), the patient should be passing liquid stools within a few hours.  Oily laxatives (such as mineral oil or magnesia) make the stools useless for examination. Enema specimens are not advisable, because they are too dilute to be of much value and, in addition, may destroy the trophozoites. Barium, if present, also makes the preparation unfit to read.  If

stool specimens for ameba must be sent by mail, they should be
placed in a preservative (1 part specimen to 3 parts of 10% Formalin). If possible, a second portion using a special polyvinyl alcohol
fixative (PVA) as a preservative (in the same proportions) should be
included along with the Formalin-fixed portion of the specimens (Formalin preserves ameba cysts, and also eggs and larvae of other
parasites; PVA preserves ameba trophozoites, although ameba cysts
are often distorted).

The preceding discussion was concerned with the usual type of
amebiasis—amebiasis localized to the colon. Visceral amebiasis is
not common. Liver involvement with abscess formation constitutes
a majority of these cases. Clinical hepatic amebiasis is always associated with chronic ameba infection rather than acute. Stools for
ameba are usually negative. Liver function tests most often give
results compatible with a space-occupying lesion (p. 224). Liver
scan is often very helpful, both for detection and localization of a
lesion.

Serologic tests for amebiasis are now becoming available in
reference laboratories. The most commonly used are gel diffusion
and latex slide agglutination. Both detect over 95% of hepatic
amebiasis. Latex is more sensitive for intestinal amebas; more
likely positive in severe cases. Antibody levels persist for some
time, so that a positive test does not necessarily mean active infection.

Schistosoma mansoni is sometimes encountered in the United
States, because it is endemic in Puerto Rico. Routine stools for
parasite ova are often not sufficient, because the adult lays its eggs
in the venous system, and the ova must penetrate the intestinal mucosa in order to appear in the stool. In difficult cases, proctoscopic
rectal biopsy with a fresh unstained crush preparation of the biopsy
specimen has been advocated.

Pinworm (Enterobius vermicularis or Oxyuris) infection is
fairly common in children. The female worm lays her eggs at night
around the anal region. The best diagnostic procedure, therefore,
is some method to swab the anal region thoroughly with an adhesive
substance such as transparent celluloid tape ("Scotch tape"). The
sticky surface with the eggs can then be directly applied to a microscope glass slide and later examined for the characteristic pinworm
ova. Such slides can also be sent through the mail, if necessary.
The best time for obtaining specimens is early in the morning, before the child gets up. Stool samples are not satisfactory for diagnosis of enterobiasis. Since the worms do not lay eggs every night,
repeated specimens may be necessary.

Hookworm is a problem in some areas of the southern United
States, and occasionally may be the etiology of an iron-deficiency
anemia in children. Routine stool examinations for ova and parasites are usually adequate for diagnosis.

The fish tapeworm (Diphyllobothrium, or Dibothriocephalus
latum) is only rarely a problem in the United States. Infection is

caused by eating raw pike fish from the Great Lakes area. Usually very few symptoms are produced, but occasionally the syndrome of megaloblastic anemia may result from ingestion of dietary vitamin B12 by the parasite. Diagnosis consists of stool examinations for ova.

Trichinella spiralis infection is caused chiefly by eating raw or insufficiently cooked pork, or insufficiently cooked meat products contaminated by infected pork. During the first week after ingestion, symptoms consist of nausea and diarrhea; this may be minimal or absent. Seven to 8 days after ingestion, there is onset of severe muscle pain, which sometimes begins in the face. Bilateral periorbital edema often develops. Eosinophilia may begin as early as 10 days after ingestion, and, with muscle pain and periorbital edema, forms a very suggestive triad. The eosinophilia reaches its peak during the third week. The most helpful laboratory test is a skin test; this becomes positive near the end of the third week after ingestion. A positive result consists of a wheal and erythema reaction within 15 minutes. A delayed reaction after 24 hours has been described, but this is apparently less specific. A negative result does not rule out the diagnosis. A positive result does not guarantee that symptoms are due to trichinosis, because a skin test remains positive for many years. Muscle biopsy is occasionally useful; it is considered best to wait until at least 3 weeks after ingestion to do this procedure, in order to allow the larvae time to encyst. A painful area of a skeletal muscle has been recommended as the preferred site for biopsy.

A latex agglutination slide test is now available; 20-30% of cases are positive by 7 days after onset of symptoms and 80-90% in 4-5 weeks. False positive results have been recorded in polyarteritis nodosa (also in tuberculosis, typhoid, and infectious mononucleosis, but these would ordinarily not be considered in differential diagnosis).

Trichomonas vaginalis is a protozoan parasite which infects the vagina and labial area in the female and occasionally produces a urethritis in the male. The diagnosis is accidentally made in many cases by a microscopic examination of a fresh urine centrifuged sediment. The living organism has a typical appearance and motility. However, on dying, the parasite rounds up and resembles a large white blood cell or small epithelial cell; therefore, a fresh specimen is essential. The urine specimen must be taken without cleansing the genitalia, since the organism is actually a contaminant. A more reliable method consists of a cervical and a vaginal swab, which are then placed into a small amount of 0.9% saline. A wet preparation is then made from this material and examined microscopically. The organism may sometimes be diagnosed from a PAP smear.

## REFERENCES

Barrett-Connor, E.: Amebiasis, today, in the United States, California Med. 114:1, 1971.

Faust, E. C., and Russell, P. F.: Clinical Parasitology (7th ed.; Philadelphia: Lea & Febiger, 1964).

Feldman, H. A.: Toxoplasmosis, New England J. Med. 279:1370, 1431, 1968.

Feldman, H. A.: Toxoplasma and toxoplasmosis, Hosp. Practice 4:64, 1969.

Harrison, E. G., et al.: Human and canine dirofilariasis in the United States, Mayo Clin. Proc. 40:906, 1965.

Healy, G. R.: Laboratory diagnosis of amebiasis, Bull. New York Acad. Med. 47:478, 1971.

Jacobs, L., et al.: A comparison of the toxoplasma skin tests, the Sabin-Feldman dye tests, and complement fixation tests in various forms of uveitis, Bull. Johns Hopkins Hosp. 99:1, 1956.

Jones, T. C., et al.: Acquired toxoplasmosis, New York J. Med. 69:2237, 1969.

Kagan, I. G.: Evaluation of routine serologic testing for parasitic diseases, Am. J. Pub. Health 55:1820, 1965.

Markell, E. K., and Voge, M.: Diagnostic Medical Parasitology (2d ed.; Philadelphia: W. B. Saunders Company, 1965).

Maynard, J. E., and Kagan, I. G.: Intradermal test in the detection of trichinosis, New England J. Med. 270:1, 1964.

Salfelder, K., and Schwarz, J.: Pneumocystosis, Am. J. Dis. Child. 114:693, 1967.

Smith, M. H. D., and Beaver, P. C.: Visceral larva migrans due to infection with dog and cat ascarids, Pediat. Clin. North America 2:163, 1955.

Sterman, M. M.: Amebae of man: Classification and practical laboratory diagnosis, Ann. New York Acad. Sc. 98:725, 1962.

Stoll, N. R.: For hookworm diagnosis, is finding an egg enough? Ann. New York Acad. Sc. 98:712, 1962.

Turner, J. A., et al.: Amebiasis—A symposium, California Med. 114:44, 1971.

# CHAPTER 18

# Cerebrospinal Fluid Examination

Pressure: Normal values for cerebrospinal fluid (CSF) are 100 to 200 mm. of water. Elevations are due to increased intracranial pressure. The two most common causes are meningitis and subarachnoid hemorrhage. Brain tumors and brain abscess will, in most cases, develop increased intracranial pressure but only after a varying period—days or even weeks. An increase is present in many cases of lead encephalopathy. CSF pressure varies directly with the venous pressure, but has no constant relationship to arterial pressure. The Queckenstedt sign makes clinical use of this information; increased venous pressure via jugular vein compression increases CSF pressure at the lumbar region, whereas a subarachnoid obstruction above the lumbar will prevent this.

Appearance: CSF normally is clear. It may be pink or red with many RBC present, or white and cloudy if there are many WBC or especially high protein content. There usually have to be more than 500 WBC per cu. mm. before cloudiness can begin to appear. When blood has been present in the CSF for more than 4 hours, xanthochromia (yellow color) may occur, although the RBC may eventually disappear due to lysis. Severe jaundice may give false xanthochromic appearance.

Sugar: Normal values are 50 mg./100 ml. or over (Somogyi or "true glucose" methods). Values of 40-50 mg./100 ml. are equivocal, although it is rare to get below 45 mg./100 ml. normally. The CSF level depends on the blood glucose values and is usually about half the blood level. The main pathologic significance of CSF sugar occurs when it is decreased. This is seen classically in bacterial and tuberculous meningitis. It is important to know, however, that when seen very early these patients may still have normal cerebrospinal glucose, although later it begins to decrease. Other conditions which may cause decrease are occasional cases of metastatic carcinoma to the meninges and also, sometimes, subarachnoid hemorrhage, probably due to release of glycolytic enzymes from the red cells and dying tissue. Most other central nervous system diseases, including viral meningitis, encephalitis, brain abscess, and syphilis, classically have normal cerebrospinal fluid sugar when the meninges are not infected bacterially.

Protein: CSF protein is normally 15-40 mg./100 ml. Generally speaking, but not always, increased protein is roughly proportional to the degree of leukocytosis in the CSF; protein concentration is also increased by the presence of blood. There are, however, certain diseases which may have mild-to-moderate protein increase with relatively slight leukocytosis; these include brain tumors, multiple sclerosis, chronic infections such as syphilis, and similar conditions. Diabetics with peripheral neuropathy frequently have elevated CSF protein, of unknown cause. A marked protein elevation without corresponding cell increase is known as albuminocytologic dissociation; this is found classically in the Guillain-Barre syndrome. Protein may be measured in the laboratory quantitatively by any of several methods. A popular semiquantitative bedside method is Pandy's test, which consists of a few drops of saturated phenol agent into the spinal fluid. This test reacts with all protein but apparently much more with globulin. Chronic infections or similar conditions such as (tertiary) syphilis or multiple sclerosis tend to accentuate globulin elevation, and thus may give positive Pandy's test results, although the total CSF protein may not be tremendously high. Contamination by blood will often give false positive test results.

Cell Count: Generally speaking, any conditions which affect the meninges will cause cerebrospinal fluid leukocytosis whose degree will depend on the type of irritation, its duration, and its intensity. Usually, the highest white cell counts are found in severe acute infections. The classic variety is the acute bacterial infection. One important thing to keep in mind is that if the patient is seen very early, leukocytosis may be minimal or possibly even absent, just as mentioned previously with the CSF sugar. However, in a few hours a repeat lumbar puncture usually finds steadily increasing white cell counts. This does not happen too often, but does occur and should be remembered. Another general rule is that bacterial infections usually have polymorphonuclear neutrophils as the predominating cell type, whereas viral infections, chronic nervous system diseases of varying types, and tertiary syphilis ordinarily have a predominance of lymphocytes or mononuclears. The main exception is tuberculous meningitis, which combines a bacterial with a chronic type of infection; in this case, the cells are predominantly lymphocytes. On the other hand, Coxsackie and ECHO virus infections may have a predominance of neutrophils in the early stages; in most of these patients, the CSF subsequently shifts to lymphocytosis.

In cases of subarachnoid hemorrhage or traumatic spinal fluid taps, approximately 1 WBC is added for every 500 RBC, and approximately 1 mg./100 ml. of protein for every 1,000 RBC. Also, the presence of blood may sometimes cause moderate meningeal irritation with subsequent increase in polymorphonuclear leukocytes. Another exception is so-called aseptic meningeal reaction which is secondary to either a nearby infection or sometimes to acute localized brain destruction. In these cases, which actually are not too common, there may be a wide range of WBC values with neutrophils often predominating. When this occurs, however, there should be normal CSF sugar, since the meninges are not directly infected. Aseptic meningitis is not the same as aseptic meningeal reaction. Aseptic meningitis is due to direct involvement of the meninges by nonbacterial organisms. Viruses cause most cases, but organisms such as Leptospira sometimes do also. Bacterial CSF cultures are negative. Sugar is usually normal; protein is usually, but not always, increased. The WBC count is elevated to varying degree, the predominant type of cell depending on the etiology.

Serology: This subject is discussed in Chapter 31. Nevertheless, some of that discussion will be repeated here, for the sake of continuity. The standard serologic tests for syphilis (STS), such as the VDRL, are usually, but not always, positive in the blood when they are positive in the CSF. A lack of relationship is most often found in the tertiary stage, when the blood VDRL sometimes reverts to normal. Conversely, the CSF is very often negative when the peripheral blood STS is positive, since central nervous system syphilis is usually a tertiary form developing symptoms only after years of infection, and, in many cases of syphilis, the central nervous system is not clinically involved at all. The more specific tests such as the TPI or FTA-ABS are usually positive in the blood if CNS syphilis exists. Increased CSF white cell counts and protein are better guides to actual syphilitic activity than the CSF serology, and may be present as early as the secondary stage. A positive serology alone, either in the blood or the CSF, does not indicate if the disease is currently active. The CSF serology is usually negative in those patients with so-called biologic false positive blood reactions. The three most important forms of central nervous system syphilis are: general paresis, tabes dorsalis, and vascular neurosyphilis. In general paresis, the serology (STS) in the spinal fluid is almost always positive in untreated cases. In tabes, the CSF serology is said to be usually positive in early untreated cases, but up to 50% of late or so-called burnt-out cases may be negative. In vascular neurosyphilis approximately 50% are positive.

Colloidal Gold Reaction: This is based on the fact that in certain pathologic CNS conditions, a suspension of colloidal gold in sodium chloride will be precipitated, giving characteristic color changes in standard dilutions. The color normally is wine-red, but may change to a blue and even to a clear color, depending on the degree of precipitation.  Each dilution tube is given a number 0 to 5, depending on the degree of color change.  There are 10 tubes, each with a different dilution, so the results are reported as a series of 10 numbers.

A reading of 1 in all tubes is within normal limits.  A reading of 2 is of doubtful significance and, to be significant, at least one of the 10 tubes must be 3 or over.  According to classic theories, globulin tends to precipitate the gold particles in the solution, while albumin tends to "protect" the finely dispersed colloidal state.  More recent work indicates that the gamma globulins have the strongest precipitating action, while most but not all of the protective function seems to be in the albumin and alpha globulins.  When gamma globulin is increased without significant albumin or alpha globulin increase, color changes are mostly in the lower dilution tubes, producing a "first zone" curve (for example, 5553211111).  This is characteristically found in syphilitic general paresis and in multiple sclerosis, but not all cases of either.  When both the albumin and the globulin are increased in the same general proportions, but only moderately, or when the gamma globulin is only very slightly increased, a "second zone" curve is produced in which the middle dilution tubes show precipitation and thus have color change (for example, 1113321111).  Theoretically, the albumin or alpha globulin was present in sufficient quantities to prevent precipitation in the first zone, but was diluted out after the first few tubes.  Due to the relatively mild gamma globulin increase, this globulin also is supposed to be diluted out, but not until the last tubes.  A second zone curve is classically found in tabes dorsalis; again, many other conditions can occasionally produce a similar effect.  In cases with high total protein, the precipitating action of the gamma globulin may not appear until the last dilution tubes, by which time the albumin and alpha globulin are diluted enough to unmask the gamma globulin effect.  This is called a "third zone" or "end zone" curve and classically is found in acute bacterial meningitis.  The colloidal gold curve, however, is not nearly as specific as one would gather from this simplified account, since, for example, acute bacterial meningitis can give any of the three types of curves as well as no curve at all, and many other diseases can occasionally give one or the other type of curve.  Again, for example, although multiple sclerosis classically gives a first zone curve, a considerable number show a midzone or no curve.  The main clinical use of the colloidal gold curve is in the diagnosis of multiple sclerosis, general paresis, and tabes dorsalis.  It is not a routine test and its use should be confined mainly to situations in which these three diseases are possibilities.

CSF electrophoresis can substitute for colloidal gold; chronic infections or diseases produce elevated gamma globulin.

Bacteriology:  The diagnosis of acute bacterial meningitis will often depend on the isolation of the organisms in the spinal fluid.  In children, there is some regularity of the types of infection most commonly found. In infants under the age of 6 months, gram-negative coliform organisms are most frequent. In children from 1 to 5 years, Haemophilus influenzae and meningococcus are the two most common organisms. In young adults, meningococcus is by far the most usual. In middle age, the meningococcus is first and pneumococcus probably second. In old age, there may be practically any type of organism, including an increasing number of fungi. Also, in patients who are debilitated or have underlying serious diseases such as leukemia or carcinoma, fungi are not uncommon. In many cases, a centrifuged spinal fluid sediment can be smeared and gram stained with the organisms seen easily. A (bacterial) culture should be done in all cases suspicious for bacterial meningitis or in any cases where bacterial meningitis could be even a remote possibility. Special provision should be made for spinal fluid reaching the laboratory as quickly as possible; and, if any particular organism is suspected, the laboratory should be informed so that special media may be used if necessary. For example, the meningococcus grows best in a high $CO_2$ atmosphere, and Haemophilus influenzae should be planted on media provided with a staph. streak.

When meningitis or brain abscess due to Cryptococcus is suspected, an India ink spinal fluid preparation should be requested. Cryptococcus is a yeast-like (fungus) organism (also known as Torula) whose peculiarity is a thick gelatinous capsule. This capsule shows up well in the dark background of black India ink. Sometimes this organism is demonstrated only after repeated spinal fluid examinations. A culture should also be done. Fungi require different culture media from bacteria, so the laboratory must be notified that fungi are suspected. Meningitis due to Cryptococcus produces a CSF pleocytosis consisting predominantly of mononuclears. The protein is elevated and the sugar usually is decreased. As noted above, cultures on ordinary bacterial (or tuberculosis) culture media will be negative. Serologic tests are now available and may replace India ink.

Brain Abscess: Apparently the CSF findings in brain abscess are not significantly influenced by the causative organism or the location of the lesion. The spinal fluid is most often clear, and about 70% are said to have increased pressure. Protein levels are normal in nearly 25% of patients, with about 55% of the values between 45 and 100 mg./100 ml. and the remaining 20% over 100 mg./100 ml. Spinal fluid sugar is normal. The cell count is variable; about 30% are between 5 and 25, about 25% between 25 and 100, and about 25% between 100 and 500 per cu. mm. Lymphocytes generally predominate, but a significant percentage (5-25%) of polymorphonuclear neutrophils are said to be nearly always present. In occasional cases, an abscess breaks through to the subarachnoid space and results in purulent meningitis.

Brain Tumor: In primary cortical brain tumor, the CSF usually is clear and colorless, although xanthochromia may be present.

Spinal fluid pressure is elevated in 70%. Seventy per cent show increased protein, with about half of these over 100 mg./100 ml. CSF sugar is normal. The majority (70%) of brain tumor patients have normal cell counts; of the remainder, about two-thirds have counts less than 25 per cu. mm., mostly lymphocytes. In the few cases with high cell counts there may be appreciable numbers of neutrophils, and the spinal fluid pattern would then resemble brain abscess. Other methods for diagnosis are discussed in Chapter 32. Most metastatic tumors behave like primary neoplasms. In occasional instances, metastatic carcinoma may spread widely over the meninges; in such cases, the findings are similar to those of tuberculous meningitis (high cell count, lymphocytes predominating, elevated protein, and decreased sugar). Cell blocks and cytologic smears of spinal fluid sediment are helpful for diagnosis; these would not be useful in the ordinary case of metastatic carcinoma or in primary intracranial neoplasms, where the meninges are not directly involved.

One or two other subjects should be mentioned. Too often, unfortunately, when doing a lumbar puncture, the question is brought up whether blood has been introduced into the spinal fluid by the spinal needle, resulting in a so-called traumatic tap. There are several useful differential points. Xanthochromia, if present, suggests previous bleeding. However, a nonxanthochromic supernatant fluid does not rule out the diagnosis, since xanthochromia may be absent even when subarachnoid bleeding has occurred many hours before. A second point utilizes the fact that the standard method for collecting CSF involves catching the specimen in three consecutively numbered tubes. If blood was introduced by a traumatic tap, more blood should appear in the first tube, less in the second, and least in the third, as the bleeding decreases. Previous CSF bleeding should distribute the RBC equally throughout the spinal fluid and characteristically show approximately equal numbers of RBC in each of the three tubes. Therefore, RBC counts can, if necessary, be requested for all three tubes. However, sometimes traumatic taps, if severe, can have roughly equal numbers of RBC in each tube. As noted previously, blood in the CSF may falsely alter the various chemical tests.

## RADIOISOTOPE SCANNING IN BRAIN DISEASES

Brain scanning is similar to scanning any other organ. An appropriate compound labeled with a radioactive isotope is injected; later, a radioactivity counting device surveys ("scans") various areas of the brain, producing an over-all pattern of radioactivity in those areas. A special device translates focal variations in cerebral radioactivity into a visual picture of light and dark areas.

The brain scan has become an important screening technique in certain brain disorders. Brain scanning originated from the observation that certain radioactive isotopes seemed to localize in brain tumors. It is not certain whether this phenomenon is due to focal alterations of cerebral vascular permeability ("blood-brain barrier"), to the increased vascularity which most tumors possess, or to both. In subsequent experience, it was shown that subdural hematomas and cerebral infarctions also displayed increased isotope pickup over normal brain tissue, so that brain scanning was useful for diagnosis of these conditions. Unfortunately, brain scan cannot differentiate with certainty between tumor and cerebral infarct. Brain scan is also helpful in diagnosis of brain abscess.

In brain tumors, best results are obtained with meningiomas and the higher-grade astrocytomas. Grade I astrocytomas, histologically very similar to normal cerebral tissue, often do not concentrate the isotopes enough to stand out from normal surrounding brain. In addition, scanning with present equipment will miss the great majority of tumors under 2 cm. in size, regardless of type. Posterior fossa tumors are difficult to detect and require special techniques. Pituitary tumors are frequently not detected because of high vascularity in surrounding structures. Scanning is less useful for spinal cord tumors. Despite these limitations, brain scanning is the best screening test for either primary or metastatic brain tumors, since it can be done with negligible risk on an outpatient basis. Accuracy in diagnosis is quoted as 80-90%. Cerebral arteriography can have a similar success rate, but requires a neuroradiologist for best results and is more complicated and dangerous to perform. If both cerebral arteriography and brain scan are to be done, the brain scan should be performed first. Angiography causes cerebral vessel dilatation, and may produce a false positive brain scan. It is necessary to wait at least 48 hours after cerebral arteriography to do a brain scan.

In cerebral infarction, less than half the patients have a positive brain scan if the scan is done before the end of the second week after cerebral damage occurs. During the second to fourth week postinfarction, 75% or more patients have abnormal scans. After 6 weeks, the abnormal findings often disappear. The optimal time for scanning to detect cerebral infarction is during the third week after onset of symptoms. Cerebral arteriography can detect lesions soon after damage occurs, but carries a definite risk.

A helpful alternative to angiography is available to those institutions that possess a stationary radioactive imaging device such as the Anger scintillation camera. Certain isotopes can be injected intravenously and followed through major arteries by means of rapid-sequence photography. Results do not have the same degree of detail as x-ray angiography, but complete or nearly complete large-vessel occlusion can be visualized.

Cerebral isotope angiography ("flow study") of the carotid and major cerebral vessels is frequently abnormal in the early stage of a cerebral vascular accident or subdural hematoma when brain scan is normal. Both these lesions very often give a similar pattern; occasionally a subdural does have characteristic features. Arteriovenous malformations are frequently diagnosable.

Subdural hematoma is frequently a diagnostic problem. According to one study, 20% of patients did not have any history of head trauma and 30% had no localizing neurologic signs. Textbook CSF findings of protein increase and xanthochromia were present in only 50% of subacute and chronic cases. In subdural hematoma, cerebral isotope "dynamic flow study" is a good screening procedure, and cerebral arteriography is the procedure of choice for diagnosis during the first 2 weeks after onset. Brain scans most often do not become positive until after 2 weeks. It is thought that increased isotope pickup is not due to the hematoma itself but to the "membrane" which develops around the hematoma, consisting of highly vascular granulation tissue. Therefore, brain scanning is not very accurate for diagnosis of acute subdural hematoma, but is very useful in detecting chronic subdurals.

An abnormal scan must be interpreted with the aid of skull x-rays, since lesions of bone (such as hyperostosis or Paget's) or scalp (hematoma or laceration) may concentrate the isotope.

Brain scan technique can aid the diagnosis and management of hydrocephalus. A small amount of special isotope-tagged albumin (RISA) can be injected into the lumbar spinal fluid, and sequential scans can follow the distribution of this material throughout the CSF ("cisternogram"). This is especially valuable in patients with normal-pressure hydrocephalus (Hakim's syndrome); these are predominantly older persons with progressive dementia. When cisternography displays classic findings of lateral ventricle filling plus inability of CSF to reach the superior sagittal sinus by 48 hours, ventricular shunting frequently produces dramatic improvement.

## REFERENCES

Blahd, W. H. (ed.): Nuclear Medicine (2d ed.; New York: McGraw-Hill Book Company, Inc., 1971).

Bloomfield, N.: Behavior of isolated plasma proteins in the colloidal gold test, Am. J. Clin. Path. 41:15, 1964.

Bossak, H. N., et al.: A quantitative turbidimetric method for the determination of spinal fluid protein, J. Ven. Dis. Inform. 30:100, 1949

Brain, R. W.: Diseases of the Nervous System (6th ed.; London: Oxford University Press, 1962).

Butler, W. T., et al.: Diagnostic and prognostic value of clinical and laboratory findings in cryptococcal meningitis, New England J. Med. 270:59, 1964.

Dattner, B.: Significance of spinal fluid findings in neurosyphilis, Am. J. Med. 5:709, 1948.

Dawson, D. M., and Taghavy, A.: A test for spinal-fluid alcohol in Torula meningitis, New England J. Med. 269:1424, 1963.

DeJesus, P. V. , Jr. , and Poser, C. M. : Subdural hematomas, a clinicopathologic study of 100 cases, Postgrad. Med. 44:172, 1968.

Deland, F. H. : Nuclear medicine in diseases of the central nervous system, Hosp. Practice 6:57, 1971.

Fiumara, N. J. : Diagnosis of neurosyphilis (Questions and Answers), J. A. M. A. 192:1111, 1965.

Glasgow, J. L. , et al. : Brain scans at varied intervals following cerebrovascular accidents, J. Nuclear Med. 6:902, 1965.

Hooshmand, H. , et al. : Neurosyphilis: A study of 241 patients, J. A. M. A. 219:726, 1972.

Ivers, R. R. , et al. : Spinal fluid gamma globulin in multiple sclerosis and other neurologic disease, J. A. M. A. 176:137, 1961.

Madonick, M. J. , and Margolis, J. : Protein content of spinal fluid in diabetes mellitus, A. M. A. Arch. Neurol. & Psychiat. 68:641, 1952.

Merritt, H. H. , and Fremont-Smith, F. : The Cerebrospinal Fluid (Philadelphia: W. B. Saunders Company, 1937).

Miller, J. L. , et al. : Significance of the treponema pallidum immobilization test on spinal fluid, J. A. M. A. 160:1394, 1956.

Papadopoulos, N. M. , et al. : Spinal fluid protein determination for the differentiation of neurologic disorders, Clin. Chem. 9:97, 1963.

Schumacher, G. A. : Multiple sclerosis, J. A. M. A. 143:1146, 1950.

Wehrle, P. F. , et al. : Seminar on infectious diseases: Infections of the central nervous system, J. Florida M. A. 57:15, 1970.

# CHAPTER 19

# Liver and Biliary Tract Tests

## LIVER FUNCTION

Liver function tests form a very important segment of laboratory medicine, since both primary and secondary liver diseases are common. Most liver diseases can be diagnosed by means of these tests if they are understood and intelligently selected.

Bromsulphalein Test (BSP): The liver excretes bilirubin by conjugating it with glucuronide molecules and then releasing it into the bile. It was found that certain synthetic substances such as BSP dye are handled by the liver in a similar manner. On injection into the blood stream, the dye is mostly bound to serum albumin. As it passes through the intrahepatic sinusoidal circulation, BSP is somehow absorbed into the hepatic cells. Once there, some of the dye is conjugated with glucuronide molecules, and all the absorbed BSP, whether conjugated or still free, is excreted into the bile. About 1% is excreted in urine without liver involvement, and a small percentage seems to be removed by other tissues. The rate of hepatic uptake is proportional to the amount of BSP in the plasma, meaning that a fairly constant percentage is removed by the liver on each passage through it. Therefore, the great bulk of the dye is removed from plasma relatively early, with the remaining amount getting progressively less as time passes. The four variables concerned in the test may be summarized as follows: the amount of dye injected, the plasma volume in which it is diluted, the ability of the hepatic parenchymal cell mass to remove the BSP, and the patency of the bile ducts through which the excreted final products must pass to the duodenum.

The standard dose of BSP has been empirically set at 5 mg./kg. of body weight, after experimentation with other concentrations. The reason this particular value is used comes from studies that showed the ability of the liver in normal persons to remove practically all of the dye in the test period of 45 minutes. While normal persons al-

most always had less than 5% remaining in the serum at 45 minutes
and less than 2% serum retention at 60 minutes, a large majority of
patients with damaged liver due to various causes showed elevated
serum values, allowing good separation of normal from abnormal.
Furthermore, plasma volume is normally not a significant factor
due to the extremely efficient ability of the liver to take up and excrete BSP. In order to report values as percentage of test dose retained, it was assumed that body weight is related to plasma volume in a proportion of 1 kg. to 50 ml., meaning that 5 mg. is injected for each 50 ml. of plasma, giving a theoretical initial concentration of 10 mg. per 100 ml. plasma. The amount of BSP remaining in the plasma in mg. per 100 ml. is measured at the end of
the test period, and the percentage of the initial dose then calculated.

Since normal liver removal and excretion of the dye depends
on normal hepatic blood flow, normal liver cells and normal bile
duct excretory channels, it follows that a variety of diseases affecting one or more of these components will lead to impaired BSP
excretion. In posthepatic bile obstruction such as may be caused by
common duct stone or carcinoma of the head of the pancreas, there
will be BSP retention if the obstruction is complete, sometimes even
if obstruction is incomplete. Gallbladder disease will not affect BSP
values unless infection spreads to the biliary duct system or stones
reach the common bile duct. Severe acute liver damage will cause
BSP serum elevation due to lack of ability to extract the dye. Small
degrees of acute damage may not show values above the normal
range, even if there is an increase in serum retention over what the
same patient would show with his normal liver. Therefore, in hepatitis, BSP results are variable; if jaundice is present, however, BSP
is almost invariably elevated. The jaundice of acute viral hepatitis
is an intrahepatic type due to cell edema and destruction with collapse of bile sinusoids and thus temporary obstruction. BSP is the
best single test for detection of cirrhosis, and may be the only one
with elevated values when the cirrhosis is inactive. The same is
true for fatty liver. The reason for this behavior in cirrhosis is
the presence of fibrosis and irregularly regenerating liver cell
nodules which cause distortion and rearrangement of intrahepatic
blood flow as well as actual loss of liver cells by fibrous tissue replacement. Nevertheless, despite reasonably good sensitivity, BSP
may occasionally be normal in moderate degrees of cirrhosis or in
severe fatty liver. Passive congestion of the liver secondary to congestive heart failure may cause temporary BSP elevation due to
intrahepatic blood stasis and hepatic cell anoxia. Shock or hypotension from various causes will cut down hepatic blood flow and
give elevated values. BSP is normal in hemolytic anemias unless
some different cause of liver damage is present. BSP elevation is
the most frequent abnormality in metastatic carcinoma to the liver,
although the mechanism involved is often obscure. The same is

true for granulomas and other space-occupying lesions. Transient degrees of BSP elevation have been reported in some cases of acute pancreatitis, high fever, recent abdominal surgery, severe stress situations such as trauma, and acute severe upper gastrointestinal hemorrhage. In summary, BSP elevation by itself means that something abnormal is taking place in the liver, but more information from history, physical examination, laboratory studies, or the clinical situation is needed to show the etiology.

Certain substances will interfere with the test. These include PSP, iodine, morphine and other opium derivatives, and sometimes barbiturates. Some of the x-ray contrast media for gallbladder studies will produce false results, so that doing a BSP should wait until 3 days afterward if gallbladder x-rays have been done. Otherwise, the x-ray department should be asked whether the particular substance they use is one which will affect the BSP.

False negatives may result from incorrect estimation of the dose or losing some of the dye outside the vein when it is injected. The dose is estimated according to the formula: weight in pounds divided by 22 equals ml. of BSP to be used. Regarding dosage, the problem of obesity sometimes arises. The weight-volume correlation obviously does not hold true in a markedly obese patient, whose adipose tissue will cause a significant overdose of dye when calculated on the same basis as a normally built person. There is no formula to correct for obesity. Since adipose tissue has about two-thirds of the blood flow found in muscle, it may be possible to find the ideal weight for the patient from published tables and add two-thirds of the weight he possesses over that value in order to calculate the BSP dose more accurately. However, this is just a rough approximation and is no guarantee that true compensation is achieved.

Another important question is the usefulness of the BSP test when jaundice is present. When jaundice is over 5 mg./100 ml. bilirubin level, the BSP will almost always be elevated unless the elevated bilirubin is due to pure hemolysis. In milder degrees of jaundice, the test still may be worth while, since a normal or near normal result can be of considerable help, especially in differentiating cirrhosis from other causes of bilirubinemia or indicating only slight degrees of parenchymal liver damage. The test is most helpful in patients with normal or only minimally elevated bilirubin. As mentioned earlier, elevated values may be caused by upper GI bleeding, but normal values in such a case would be helpful in ruling out cirrhosis as a cause for the bleeding. BSP may be given by syringe injection or intravenous tubing. Care should be taken to avoid extravasation of dye out of the vein, since the dye is very irritating to tissue and also the test results may be affected. A few patients get hypersensitivity reactions to BSP; these are usually mild and treatable with antihistamines. Rarely, they are severe.

Indocyanine green (Cardio-Green) is a dye which is metabolized by liver cells in a manner similar to BSP. Evaluations suggest results equivalent to BSP, although the dye is slightly less sensitive for inactive cirrhosis. Cardio-Green has one advantage: no tissue toxicity or hypersensitivity reactions have been reported. The dye is 5 times more expensive than BSP and has not had the same degree of clinical evaluation and publicity.

Serum Bilirubin: Bilirubin is formed from breakdown of hemoglobin molecules by the reticuloendothelial system. Bilirubin is carried in plasma to the liver, where it is extracted by hepatic parenchymal cells, conjugated with two glucuronide molecules to form bilirubin diglucuronide, and then excreted in the bile. It has been well documented that the addition of a certain diazo compound, discovered by van den Bergh, in the presence of conjugated bilirubin would result in the development of color maximal within 1 minute. If alcohol is then added, additional color development takes place up to 30 minutes. This second component, which precipitates with alcohol, corresponds to unconjugated bilirubin. Actually it is true that color continues to develop slowly up to 15 minutes after the simple van den Bergh reaction maximal at 1 minute, and this extra fraction used to be known as the delayed or biphasic reaction. It has since been shown that a considerable proportion of the substance involved is actually unconjugated bilirubin. Since this is measured more completely in the 30-minute alcohol precipitation technique, most laboratories do not report the biphasic reaction. The 1-minute van den Bergh is also called the "direct reaction," and the conjugated bilirubin it measures is known as "direct-acting bilirubin," whereas the 30-minute alcohol measurement of unconjugated bilirubin is called the "indirect reaction" and its substrate "indirect bilirubin." Normal values for total bilirubin are less than 1.5 mg./100 ml. and for 1-minute bilirubin less than 0.5 mg./100 ml.

Visible bile staining of tissue is called jaundice. Three major causes predominate—hemolysis, biliary obstruction, and liver cell damage.

Hemolysis causes increased breakdown of RBC and thus increased formation of unconjugated bilirubin. If hemolysis is severe enough, more unconjugated bilirubin may be present in the plasma than the liver can handle. Therefore, the level of total bilirubin will rise, most of this due to the indirect-acting fraction. The direct-acting fraction stays normal or is only slightly elevated. Certain congenital diseases of the bilirubin conjugation system show similar values without hemolysis, since ability to conjugate bilirubin is decreased. Elevated serum indirect (nonconjugated) bilirubin is a classic finding in hemolytic anemia, but may occur in many other conditions. The reason is often obscure. In one study, the most common associated diseases (collectively 60% of total cases) included cholecystitis, cardiac disease (only 50% having overt congestive failure), acute or chronic infection, GI tract disease (mostly ulcerative or inflammatory), and cancer.

Obstructive jaundice may be extrahepatic or intrahepatic in location.  The classic example is extrahepatic common bile duct obstruction from stone or carcinoma.  Here, one expects increased
serum bilirubin mostly due to the direct-acting fractions, since conjugated bilirubin cannot escape into the small intestine and backs up,
regurgitating into the blood stream.  After a time, however, some
of the conjugated bilirubin breaks down in the plasma to the unconjugated form, so that there may be a sort of false increase of the indirect fraction producing a less clear-cut direct-to-indirect ratio.
Also, after a prolonged period of cholestasis there often is some
degree of secondary liver damage, which may tend to obscure results.  In jaundice due to liver cell damage, such as is found in
hepatitis and often in decompensated (considerably active) cirrhosis,
both direct and indirect bilirubin are elevated in varying proportions.  Indirect may be increased due to inability of the damaged
cells to conjugate normal amounts of unconjugated serum bilirubin,
while the direct fraction is usually increased due to intrahepatic
cholestasis secondary to bile sinusoid blockage by damaged hepatic
cells.  Jaundice due to carcinoma may be caused by extrahepatic
direct biliary obstruction or secondary to intrahepatic blockage of
small biliary ducts by expanding tumor masses.  Drug toxicity jaundice is due to hypersensitivity reactions to certain drugs, notably
Thorazine, causing intrahepatic jaundice of a type which simulates
extrahepatic obstruction.

In patients with considerable jaundice in whom liver function
tests or other evidence do not delineate a clear-cut pattern, a steroid
test may be of value in differentiating hepatocellular damage (due to
viral hepatitis, cholangitis, or active cirrhosis) from extrahepatic
obstruction.  Prednisone (10 mg. every 6 hours) is given for 5 days,
after baseline bilirubin values are obtained.  The anti-inflammatory
effect of adrenocorticosteroids will usually demonstrate acute hepatocellular damage by a decrease in total bilirubin values of more than
50% before 5 days.  In extrahepatic obstruction due to a tumor, or
intrahepatic obstruction due to drugs, no significant decrease (or
less than 50% decrease) occurs in total bilirubin.  The behavior of
obstructing common bile duct stones is variable, because in some
cases the obstruction may be due to edema around a stone and will
be relieved by steroids.  As in similar nonspecific tests, occasional
false positives and negatives occur.

Urine Bilirubin and Urobilinogen follow much the same pattern
as direct and indirect bilirubin.  After bile reaches the duodenum,
intestinal bacteria convert most of the bilirubin to urobilinogen.
Much urobilinogen is lost in the feces but part is absorbed into the
blood stream.  Once in the blood, most of the urobilinogen goes
through the liver and is extracted by hepatic cells.  Thence, it is
excreted in the bile and once again reaches the duodenum.  Not all
the blood-borne urobilinogen reaches the liver; some is lost through

kidney removal into the urine.  A positive 1:20 dilution is the maximum normal quantity (see p. 124 ).  Direct-acting (conjugated) bilirubin will also be partially excreted by the kidney if the serum level
of conjugated bilirubin is elevated.  Indirect (unconjugated) bilirubin
apparently cannot pass the glomerular filter, so it does not appear
in urine.  However, when serum indirect bilirubin is high, more
conjugated bilirubin is produced and excreted into the bile, so more
urobilinogen is produced in the intestine.  A fraction of this gets
back into the blood stream and thence into the urine, so that increased urine urobilinogen is found when increased indirect bilirubin is present.  When increased serum indirect bilirubin is due
only to increased red blood cell destruction, the serum direct-acting
(conjugated) bilirubin is close to normal, because the liver excretes
most of what it produces into the bile ducts.  Since the serum direct-
acting bilirubin is normal, the urine does not contain increased
direct-acting bilirubin in jaundice due to hemolytic anemia.  When
complete biliary obstruction occurs, no bile can reach the duodenum
and no urobilinogen can be formed.  The stool normally gets its color
from bilirubin breakdown pigments, so that in complete obstruction
the stools lose their color and become gray-white (so-called clay-
color).  The conjugated bilirubin backs up ("regurgitates") into the
blood stream, and tests for urine direct-acting bilirubin are positive.  In cases of severe hepatocellular damage, urobilinogen is
formed and absorbed into the blood stream, but the damaged liver
cells cannot extract it adequately, and thus increased amounts get
into the urine.  In addition, there may be direct-acting bilirubin in
the urine secondary to leakage back into the blood from damaged
liver cells as described earlier.  Incidentally, urine bilirubin is often called bile, which is technically incorrect, since direct-acting
bilirubin is only one component of bile.  However, custom and convenience make the term widely used.

        Alkaline Phosphatase is an enzyme produced mainly in liver
and bone.  Much is still unknown regarding mechanisms of formation and excretion.  Apparently formation is relatively small in the
normal liver, and the compound is excreted into the bile by a different mechanism from that of bilirubin.  The great usefulness of
alkaline phosphatase in liver disease is its unusual sensitivity to
partial or mild degrees of biliary obstruction, either extrahepatic
or intrahepatic.  Under such circumstances, the alkaline phosphatase may be elevated with a normal serum bilirubin.  In mild cases
of acute liver cell damage there may be little if any alkaline phosphatase elevation.  When a phase of temporary intrahepatic obstruction exists in acute liver cell damage, the alkaline phosphatase is
usually elevated, but promptly decreases once the acute episode is
finished, whereas the serum bilirubin is often still climbing.  In
cirrhosis, the alkaline phosphatase is variable, depending on degree of decompensation and obstruction.  Inactive mild or moderate
cirrhosis and uncomplicated fatty liver usually do not show elevation.

Active cirrhosis may or may not have increased values. Alkaline phosphatase is one of the best indications of liver space-occupying lesions, whether carcinoma or infection. It may be elevated in these cases when all other tests are negative, even the BSP. The reason is not always clear.

Since osteoblasts in bone produce large amounts of alkaline phosphatase, greatly increased osteoblastic activity destroys its usefulness as a liver function test. Paget's disease, hyperparathyroidism, rickets and osteomalacia, and osteoblastic metastatic carcinoma to bone all give consistently elevated values.

Leucine Amino Peptidase (LAP) is an enzyme produced exclusively by the liver. In general, it tends to parallel the alkaline phosphatase although it is not as sensitive. Bone lesions do not affect this test. When originally reported, LAP was thought to indicate pancreatic carcinoma, but all agree now that this theory was wrong and that the only association occurs when pancreatic carcinoma causes biliary obstruction, just as alkaline phosphatase is elevated in the same situation.

Prothrombin Time (PT): In certain situations, this can be a useful liver test. Prothrombin is synthesized in the liver but apparently needs vitamin K to do so. Vitamin K is a fat-soluble vitamin, present in most adequate diets, which is also synthesized by intestinal bacteria; in either case, it is absorbed from the small bowel in combination with dietary fat molecules. This means that interference with vitamin K metabolism can take place either from deficiency due to diet or destruction of intestinal bacteria, defective intestinal absorption due to lack of bile salts or through primary small bowel malabsorption, or inadequate utilization secondary to destruction of liver parenchyma. Normally, the body has considerable tissue stores of vitamin K, so that it usually takes several weeks to get significant prothrombin deficiency on the basis of inadequate vitamin K alone. The usual cause of prothrombin difficulties is liver disease. The main point to remember is that it takes very severe liver disease, more often chronic but sometimes acute, before prothrombin levels become significantly abnormal. In the usual case of viral hepatitis, the PT is either normal or only slightly increased. In massive hepatocellular necrosis the PT may be significantly elevated, but it seems to take a few days to occur. In mild or moderate degrees of cirrhosis there is usually little change. In severe end-stage cirrhosis the PT is often elevated and usually does not give much response to vitamin K therapy. In metastatic carcinoma, PT is usually normal except with biliary tract obstruction.

SGOT—SGPT—LDH: Serum glutamic oxaloacetic transaminase (SGOT) is an enzyme found in several tissues, but especially in heart and liver. In cases of acute cellular destruction in either organ, the enzyme is released into the blood stream from damaged cells. Elevated values may be found by 8 hours after injury. If the original episode is not continued or repeated, serum levels reach a peak in 24-36 hours and fall to normal (usually by 4-6 days). In mild injury, serum levels may be only transiently and minimally elevated, or may even remain within normal limits. In acute hepatitis, the SGOT usually is elevated according to the severity and extent of hepatocellular damage and the particular time the test was drawn. In the acute phase, values are often over 10 times normal. However, later the values fall toward normal, so that a test drawn in the subsiding phase may show moderate or possibly only mild abnormality. In extrahepatic obstruction there is no elevation unless secondary parenchymal acute damage is present; when elevations occur, they are usually only mild to moderate (less than 10 times normal values). In cirrhosis, SGOT may or may not be abnormal, depending on the degree of hepatic decompensation or cell necrosis taking place. SGOT elevation is generally mild to moderate in these cases (less than 10 times normal). Usually, but not always, only active cirrhosis shows significant abnormalities. The same is true in fatty liver. In alcoholic patients in delirium tremens, the SGOT is usually elevated even without demonstrable liver damage. In liver passive congestion there may be variable degrees of SGOT elevation if the episode is severe and acute; since congestive heart failure with secondary liver passive congestion is common in heart disease, this makes it difficult to interpret whether SGOT elevation is due only to liver congestion or to a possible myocardial infarct. In metastatic carcinoma, up to half the cases show abnormality, but generally only if metastases are extensive, and usually with only mild or moderate elevation.

Serum glutamic pyruvic transaminase (SGPT) is an enzyme found mostly, although not exclusively, in liver. In liver disease, it is elevated under roughly the same circumstances as the SGOT, but seems less sensitive, apparently requiring somewhat more extensive or severe acute parenchymal damage to give abnormal values. It has the advantage that it is relatively specific for liver cell damage, although occasionally slight elevations in myocardial infarct have been reported. It usually returns to normal ranges before the SGOT.

Lactic dehydrogenase (LDH) is found in most of the same tissues as SGOT and is elevated in many of the same conditions. For some reason, acute liver damage does not ordinarily release much LDH, so that LDH is a relatively insensitive indicator of acute hepatocellular destruction, usually not rising over twice normal even in hepatitis. One exception is infectious mononucleosis, which frequently does cause both SGOT and LDH elevation. Nevertheless, in some cases of passive congestion from heart failure or in an occasional case of viral hepatitis, LDH can rise to levels several times normal, so that LDH values have not been very reliable in differentiating cardiac from hepatic damage. LDH enzyme fractionation (p. 232) may help solve this problem. LDH can often rise to levels higher than twice normal in metastatic carcinoma to the liver, and is thus valuable as an addition to the usual tests for metastasis, especially when jaundice is present. It is interesting that LDH becomes elevated in a significant number of patients with various malignancies even without liver metastases.

Serum Proteins: Albumin is chiefly synthesized in the liver, so that most acute or chronic destructive liver diseases of at least moderate severity show decreased serum albumin on electrophoresis. In addition, there may be other changes. In cirrhosis of moderate to severe degree, there is a decreased albumin and usually a diffuse gamma globulin elevation, sometimes fairly marked. Far-advanced cirrhosis sometimes has a characteristic pattern with a gamma globulin configuration which even includes the beta range (so-called "slurring into the beta"). However, a considerable number show only the gamma range elevation, and a few have normal gamma levels. Hepatitis may also have moderate elevation of the gamma globulins. Biliary obstruction eventually causes elevated beta globulins, since beta globulins carry cholesterol.

Blood Ammonia: One function of the liver is the synthesis of urea from various sources of ammonia, most of which comes from protein-splitting bacteria in the GI tract. In cirrhosis, there is extensive liver cell destruction and fibrous tissue replacement of areas between nodules or irregularly regenerating liver cells. This architectural distortion also distorts the hepatic venous blood supply, leading to shunting into the systemic venous system often manifested by esophageal varices. Thus, two conditions should exist for normal liver breakdown of ammonia: enough functioning liver cells must be present, and enough ammonia must reach these liver cells. With normal hepatic blood flow, blood ammonia elevation occurs only in extremely severe liver decompensation. With altered blood flow in cirrhosis, less severe decompensation is needed to produce elevated blood ammonia. Nevertheless, the blood ammonia is not directly dependent on the severity of cirrhosis, only on the presence of hepatic failure.

Hepatic failure produces a syndrome known as prehepatic coma (hepatic encephalopathy), which progresses to actual hepatic coma. Clinical symptoms of prehepatic coma include mental disturbances of various types, characteristic changes in the electroencephalogram, and a peculiar flapping intention type tremor of the distal extremities. However, each element of this triad may be produced by other causes, and one or more may be lacking in some patients. The ensuing coma of liver disease may also be simulated by the hyponatremia or hypokalemia that cirrhotic patients often manifest, or by gastrointestinal bleeding, among other causes. Blood ammonia shows the best correlation with hepatic encephalopathy or coma of any current laboratory test. However, blood ammonia is not elevated in all of these patients, so that a normal blood ammonia does not rule out the diagnosis. Arterial ammonia levels are slightly more reliable than venous ones. The blood ammonia has been proposed as an aid in the differential diagnosis of massive upper gastrointestinal bleeding, since elevated values would mean severe liver disease and thus suggest esophageal varices as the cause of the bleeding. However, since cirrhotics may also have acute gastritis or peptic ulcer, this use of the blood ammonia has not been widely accepted. At present, the blood ammonia is mainly utilized as an aid in diagnosis of hepatic encephalopathy or coma, since elevated values would suggest liver failure as the cause of the symptoms. Otherwise, ammonia is not a useful liver function test, since elevations usually do not occur until hepatic failure.

Liver Scan: If radioactive colloidal preparation is injected intravenously, it is picked up by the reticuloendothelial system. The Kupffer cells of the liver take up the great majority in normal circumstances, with a small amount in spleen and bone marrow. If a sensitive radioactive counting device is placed over the liver, a sort of photograph can be obtained of the distribution of radioactivity. A similar procedure can be done with thyroid and kidney, using radioactive material that these organs normally take up, such as iodine in the case of the thyroid. Certain diseases may be suggested on liver scan if the proper circumstances are present.

1. Space-occupying lesions, either tumorous or inflammatory, often show as discrete filling defects if they are over 2 cm. in size.

2. Cirrhosis has a characteristic although nonspecific appearance, but has to be well established, and best results are obtained in far-advanced cases.

3. Fatty liver may sometimes be diagnosable, but only if severe, and may be confused easily with the cirrhosis pattern.

4. Liver scanning may be useful to differentiate abdominal masses from an enlarged liver.

Undoubtedly, more sensitive equipment will become available and perhaps also better radioactive isotopes. At present, useful as the liver scan may be, it is often difficult to distinguish between cirrhosis, fatty liver, and disseminated metastatic carcinoma with nodules less than 2 cm. in diameter. Also, liver scan is reported to miss about 15% of cases with metastatic carcinoma, and to suggest a false positive diagnosis in about 10% without cancer. The majority of these false positive studies are in patients with cirrhosis.

Liver Biopsy: This procedure has been greatly simplified, and its morbidity and mortality markedly reduced, by the introduction of small-caliber biopsy needles such as the Menghini. Nevertheless, there is a small but definite risk. Contraindications to biopsy include a prothrombin time near the anticoagulant range or a platelet count under 50,000 per cu. mm. Liver biopsy is especially useful in the following circumstances:

1. To differentiate between cirrhosis, subsiding hepatitis, and extrahepatic obstruction, when the clinical picture or laboratory values are confusing or atypical. In classic cases, there usually is

no need for biopsy, although some believe that a tissue diagnosis is worth the risk.

2.  To prove the diagnosis of metastatic or primary hepatic carcinoma in a patient who would otherwise be operable or who does not have a known primary lesion (in a patient with an inoperable known primary lesion, such a procedure would be academic).

3.  In hepatomegaly of unknown origin whose etiology cannot be determined otherwise.

4.  In a relatively few selected patients who have systemic diseases affecting the liver, such as miliary tuberculosis, in whom the diagnosis cannot be established by other means.

A discussion of liver biopsy should be concluded with a few words of caution. Two disadvantages are soon recognized by anyone who deals with a large number of liver specimens. First, the procedure is a needle biopsy, and this means a very small fragment of tissue, often partially destroyed, taken in a random sample manner from a large organ. Localized disease is easily missed. Second, many diseases produce nonspecific changes which may be spotty, may be healing, or may be minimal. Even with an autopsy specimen it may be difficult to put a definite label on many situations, including the etiology of many cases of cirrhosis. The pathologist should be furnished with the pertinent history, physical findings, and laboratory data; sometimes these have as much value for interpretation of the microscopic findings as the histologic changes themselves. In summary, liver biopsy is often indicated in difficult cases, but do not expect it to be infallible or even invariably helpful.

Fetoprotein Test: Fetal liver produces a serum alpha-1 globulin called fetoglobulin which disappears shortly after birth. It was found that hepatomas produce a similar protein; therefore a test for hepatoma could be devised using antibodies against the "fetoprotein" antigen. Extensive studies have shown that approximately 30% of hepatoma patients who are white have positive tests, while the rate among Chinese and blacks is 60-75%. Men seem to have a higher positive rate than women. Besides hepatoma, embryonal carcinoma of the testis has an appreciable positivity rate. Scattered reports of false positives in other conditions include gastric carcinoma with liver metastases (six cases), pregnancy in the second trimester (a few cases), viral hepatitis, cirrhosis, and pancreatic carcinoma with hepatic metastases (one case). In summary: thus far the fetoprotein test seems moderately sensitive and reasonably—although not completely—specific for hepatoma.

Having discussed various individual liver function tests, it may be useful to summarize the typical laboratory abnormalities associated with certain common liver diseases.

Acute viral hepatitis, after an incubation period, most often begins with some combination of gastrointestinal symptoms, fever, chills, and malaise, lasting 4-7 days. During this phase there is no clinical jaundice. Leukopenia with a relative lymphocytosis is

common, and there may be a few atypical lymphocytes. Hemoglobin
and platelet counts usually are normal. Liver function tests reflect
acute hepatocellular damage, with marked elevation of SGOT and abnormal SGPT levels. The alkaline phosphatase usually is elevated.
In the last 1-2 days of this period, urine tests often are positive for
bile, even without icterus, and sometimes even with the serum bilirubin within normal range. Serum bilirubin values begin climbing
toward the end of this initial phase. The next development is visible
jaundice; during this period, clinical symptoms tend to subside. The
serum bilirubin continues to rise for a time, then slowly falls. Both
direct and indirect fractions are increased. Alkaline phosphatase
often begins to fall shortly after clinical icterus begins. A convalescent phase eventually ensues, with return of all tests to normal,
beginning with the alkaline phosphatase and ending with the ceph.
floc. (p. 415) and BSP. Some patients continue to manifest a low-
grade or intermittent hepatitis (called subacute hepatitis), which is
reflected by variable and intermittent SGOT abnormalities with or
without alkaline phosphatase or BSP elevations. Some patients never
develop jaundice during viral hepatitis; this is known as anicteric
hepatitis. In such situations, function tests reveal mild-to-moderate
acute hepatocellular damage, with minimal obstructive indications.

Biliary obstruction may be complete or incomplete, extrahepatic or intrahepatic. Extrahepatic obstruction is most often produced by gallstones in the common bile duct or by carcinoma of the
head of the pancreas. Intrahepatic obstruction is most often found
in the obstructive phase of acute hepatocellular damage, as seen in
"active" cirrhosis or infectious hepatitis, or by liver reaction to
certain drugs such as Thorazine. Serum bilirubin becomes markedly elevated, with the direct-acting fraction predominating. Usually, but not always, complete extrahepatic obstruction has a more
marked total bilirubin elevation with a greater proportion of the
direct-acting fraction than does acute hepatocellular necrosis, in
which the direct and indirect fractions are often nearly equal. As
time goes on, the serum bilirubin in extrahepatic obstruction may
not have a marked direct-indirect fraction disproportion. Drug-
induced jaundice mimics extrahepatic obstruction closely in all respects. Alkaline phosphatase tends to parallel serum bilirubin in
biliary obstruction. SGOT is normal in the early phase of complete
extrahepatic obstruction, but later may become abnormal when prolonged obstruction creates liver cell damage. This contrasts to the
marked elevations in viral hepatitis. The most common diagnostic
problems involve differentiating extrahepatic obstruction from drug
jaundice, some cases of severe active cirrhosis, and occasional
cases of subsiding hepatitis. If the PT time is markedly prolonged,
a good response to parenteral vitamin K would suggest extrahepatic
obstruction. The steroid test may be of help. It usually is not possible to differentiate extrahepatic obstruction from drug jaundice
except by history and elimination of the drug. Liver biopsy often

cannot demonstrate the etiology of obstruction, and is mainly useful to rule out certain of the intrahepatic etiologies, such as cirrhosis or hepatitis.

Fatty liver is a common cause for hepatomegaly of unknown etiology. In uncomplicated fatty liver, function tests are variable. There may be no abnormality at all. However, 75% reportedly have an abnormal BSP, the degree of abnormality being variable. Alkaline phosphatase may be elevated in nearly 48%, usually less than twice normal. Forty per cent of patients have elevated SGOT, usually less than 5 times normal, and more often with severe degrees of fatty metamorphosis. Serum bilirubin may be raised in 35% of patients, but most have minimal abnormality, usually less than twice normal and without jaundice. Very uncommonly, however, severe fatty liver may present clinically with jaundice.

Cirrhosis exhibits a wide spectrum of test results, depending on whether the disease is active or inactive and on degree of hepatocellular destruction. With inactive cirrhosis, the most frequent abnormality is found in the BSP. Early cases may not show any abnormal tests, or may have an elevated BSP. In more advanced cases, the BSP usually is abnormal to a varying degree. In moderate degrees of inactive cirrhosis there may, in addition, be minimal or mild abnormalities in the SGOT, alkaline phosphatase, and serum bilirubin, although no definite pattern can be stated. In advanced cases, the PT time begins to become elevated, and mild abnormalities in other liver function tests become more frequent.

In "active" cirrhosis ("florid cirrhosis" or "alcoholic hepatitis"), liver function tests show evidence of mild-to-moderate acute hepatocellular damage. Serum bilirubin may be normal or elevated; if elevated, usually only to mild extent, but occasionally to severe degree. Alkaline phosphatase is most often less than 3 times normal, although occasionally it may be higher, and SGOT usually is less than 10 times normal. Active cirrhosis may have a clinical and chemical pattern simulating either the minimal changes of advanced fatty liver, the moderate abnormalities of subacute hepatitis, or the picture of obstruction with secondary liver damage. A history of chronic alcoholism and physical findings of spider angiomata and splenomegaly would help point toward cirrhosis. Liver biopsy is the best diagnostic test.

Metastatic carcinoma may produce a clinical picture compatible with obstructive jaundice, active cirrhosis, or hepatomegaly of unknown origin, or it may be completely occult. The liver is a frequent target for metastases, some of the most common primary sites being lung, breast, prostate, and both the upper and lower gastrointestinal tract. Earlier reports frequently stated that metastases to a cirrhotic liver were rare, but later studies dispute this. Depending on the number, size, and location of tumor deposits, the patient may or may not develop jaundice; some may do so even without much involvement. In carcinoma of the head of the pancreas, obstruction of the common bile duct may occur relatively early, with onset of a typical picture of posthepatic obstruction. About 25% of patients with metastatic carcinoma to the liver become clinically jaundiced, and about the same number have elevated bilirubin (most often, the direct-acting fraction) without evident jaundice. By far the most frequently noted abnormality is hepatic enlargement. A significant minority may have physical findings compatible with portal hypertension or cirrhosis.

In many cases of metastatic carcinoma to the liver the patient is not jaundiced. Alkaline phosphatase and BSP are very often elevated in these circumstances; and this may be true, although not always, even when only a relatively few nodules are present. Therefore, the typical pattern for metastatic carcinoma to the liver is a normal bilirubin with elevated alkaline phosphatase. Since cirrhosis often is confused with metastatic carcinoma, and since BSP usually is elevated in cirrhosis (whereas the alkaline phosphatase with inactive cirrhosis often is normal), BSP is less useful than alkaline phosphatase to suggest hepatic metastases. If the serum bilirubin is elevated, the "typical" metastatic pattern becomes much less frequent, or is obscured, and a significant minority develop abnormal enzyme tests indicative of acute hepatocellular damage. Diagnosis, therefore, is much more difficult in the presence of jaundice, since these tests are often elevated (at least temporarily or at some time) from any of a great variety of etiologies. As mentioned previously, a liver scan is very useful, and LDH may be of some further help. Liver biopsy may be indicated, depending on the circumstances.

To conclude liver function tests, perhaps some comments are indicated on the use of these procedures. Some doctors order every test available and keep repeating them all, even those which give essentially the same information. For example, the SGPT is ordered along with the SGOT because of its relative specificity for liver disease. If either test is normal, it usually is not necessary to keep repeating the one which is normal, because it ordinarily will stay normal except in special circumstances. It is usually sufficient to follow a few selected abnormal enzyme tests. The same is true of alkaline phosphatase and LAP. If the LAP is abnormal, that gives all the information needed from it; namely, that an alkaline phosphatase elevation is due to liver disease rather than bone disease. Since the presence of significant liver disease is often obvious, most of the time the LAP is not needed, and the alkaline phosphatase is easier to follow. Serum cholesterol is not a very helpful liver function test, since the PT time gives essentially the same information and is technically more easy and reliable. Urine bile is not necessary if the serum direct-acting bilirubin value is known. Electrophoresis is valuable mainly in helping pick up some cases of cirrhosis. Liver scan is most helpful in showing metastatic carcinoma. Liver biopsy can frequently provide a definitive answer, thereby shortening the patient's stay in the hospital and making lengthy repetition of lab tests unnecessary. The earlier a biopsy is obtained, the more chance one has to see clear-cut diagnostic changes. If, for some reason, a liver biopsy is thought to be contraindicated, and if the serum bilirubin is more than twice normal limits, the steroid test may be helpful in differentiating intrahepatic from extrahepatic obstruction.

Liver function tests should be selected to fit the clinical situation. Therefore, one suggestion for a good initial liver test "battery" might include bilirubin (total and direct); SGOT, alkaline phosphatase, and PT time. The SGOT should demonstrate the presence of acute hepatocellular injury; the alkaline phosphatase, obstruction and also many cases of space-occupying lesions; and the PT time, if abnormal, would suggest a serious degree of hepatic damage. Of course, to interpret these tests, one must know what conditions (such as cardiac failure with liver congestion) could affect each of these tests, have other clinical information, and perhaps may have to repeat certain of the procedures in 3-4 days to establish a pattern. The clinical circumstances dictate to some extent the choice of tests in any situation. If hepatitis is suspected, an SGOT level contributes the most toward establishing the diagnosis. In possible cirrhosis, the BSP, SGOT, and PT time are useful (the LDH and liver scan also may be helpful, since metastatic carcinoma may closely mimic cirrhosis). In possible metastatic carcinoma, the BSP, alkaline phosphatase, LDH, and liver scan are the best tests. If the patient has considerable jaundice, the BSP would not be helpful in any of these situations. Other hepatic tests may be indicated in special circumstances. Liver biopsy may be necessary in any difficult case; biopsy is the only way to prove a diagnosis. There are too many exceptions to any of the so-called diagnostic or typical liver function test patterns.

## EXTRAHEPATIC BILIARY TRACT

The major subdivisions of the biliary tract are the intrahepatic bile ducts, the common bile duct, and the gallbladder. The major diseases of the biliary system are gallbladder infection (cholecystitis, acute or chronic), gallbladder stones, and obstruction to the common bile duct by stones or tumor. Obstruction to intrahepatic bile channels can occur due to acute hepatocellular damage, but this aspect was noted in the discussion of liver function tests and will not be included here.

Acute cholecystitis usually presents with upper abdominal pain, most often accompanied by fever and a leukocytosis. Occasionally, difficulty in diagnosis may be produced by a right lower lobe pneumonia or peptic ulcer; and cholecystitis occasionally results in ST and T-wave electrocardiographic changes which might point toward myocardial disease. Acute cholecystitis is very frequently associated with gallbladder calculi, usually in the cystic duct. Some degree of increased bilirubin is found in 25-30% of patients, and some report as high as 50%. Bilirubinemia may occur even in patients without stones. Acute cholecystitis without stones is said to be most common in elderly persons. SGOT is said to be elevated in nearly 75% of cholecystitis patients; this is more likely if jaundice is present. In one study, about 20% had SGOT levels over 6 times normal, and 6% over 10 times normal. Of these, some had jaundice and some did not. About 20% of cholelithiasis patients are reported to have common duct stones. About 40% with common duct stones do not become jaundiced. Common duct stones usually occur in association with gallbladder calculi, but occasionally may be present alone. Cholecystitis patients sometimes develop elevated serum amylase, usually less than twice normal limits. About 15% of patients are said to have some degree of concurrent acute pancreatitis.

In uncomplicated obstructive jaundice due to common duct stones or tumor, SGOT and LDH are usually normal. Nevertheless, in some instances SGOT may become elevated very early, sometimes over 10 times normal, in the absence of demonstrable hepatocellular damage. The striking SGOT elevation may lead to a misdiagnosis of hepatitis. Several reports indicate that LDH was also considerably elevated in these patients, usually 5 times upper limits of normal. Since LDH is usually less than twice normal in viral hepatitis (although occasional exceptions occur), higher LDH values point toward the "atypical obstruction" enzyme pattern. Both SGOT and LDH values may fall steadily after 2-3 days.

Radiologic Procedures: Diagnosis of stones in the gallbladder or common bile duct rests mainly with the radiologist. About 20-25% of gallbladder stones are said to be visible on plain films of the abdomen. Oral cholecystography consists of oral administration of a radiopaque contrast medium which is absorbed by intestinal mucosa and secreted by liver cells into the bile. When bile enters the common duct, it takes a certain amount of pressure to force open the ampulla of Vater. During the time this pressure is building up, bile enters the cystic duct into the gallbladder, where water is reabsorbed, concentrating the bile. This process allows concentration of the contrast medium as well as the bile and therefore outlines the interior of the gallbladder as well as delineates any stones which are of sufficient size. An average of 70% of those with gallbladder calculi may be identified by oral cholecystography. Repeat examination (using a double dose of contrast medium or alternative techniques) is necessary if the original study does not show any gallbladder function. In most of the remaining patients with gallbladder calculi, oral cholecystography reveals a poorly functioning or a nonfunctioning gallbladder. Less than 5% of patients with gallbladder stones are said to have a completely normal oral cholecystogram. (Over 50% of patients with cholecystitis and gallbladder tumor have abnormal oral cholecystograms.)

There are certain limitations to the oral method. Although false negative examinations (gallbladder calculi and a normal test) are relatively few, false positive results (nonfunctioning gallbladder but no gallbladder disease) have been reported in some instances in over 10% of cases. In addition, neither oral cholecystography nor plain films of the abdomen are very useful in detecting stones in the common bile duct. Visualization of the common bile duct by the oral method is frequently poor, whether stones are present or not.

Intravenous cholecystography supplements the oral procedure in some respects. Nearly 50% of common duct stones may be identified. Intravenous injection of the contrast medium is frequently able to outline the common duct and major intrahepatic bile ducts.

Limitations of the intravenous technique include poor reliability in demonstrating gallbladder calculi, since there are an appreciable number of both false positive and false negative results. There also is a considerable incidence of patient reaction to the contrast medium, although newer techniques ("drip infusion") have markedly reduced the danger of reaction.

A limitation to both the oral and the intravenous procedure is the fact that both depend on a patent intrahepatic and extrahepatic biliary system. If the serum bilirubin is over 2 mg./100 ml. (and the increase is not due to hemolytic anemia), neither oral nor intravenous cholangiography is usually satisfactory.

When jaundice is present, it is sometimes possible to do transhepatic percutaneous cholangiography. This consists of inserting a cannula into one of the intrahepatic bile ducts through a biopsy needle and injecting the contrast medium directly into the duct. This procedure outlines the biliary duct system and is therefore useful in confirming the presence of extrahepatic obstruction in a patient with jaundice. The technique is not easy, and it requires considerable experience; over 25% of attempts fail. There is a definite risk of producing bile peritonitis, which occasionally has been fatal. Preparation for surgical intervention should be made in advance in case this complication does develop.

## REFERENCES

Adams, J. T., et al.: Serum glutamic oxalacetic transaminase activity in cholecystitis, Surgery 68:492, 1970.

Bessman, S. P.: Blood Ammonia, in Sobotka, H., and Stewart, C. P. (eds.): Advances in Clinical Chemistry (New York: Academic Press, Inc., 1959), Vol. 2.

Blahd, W. H. (ed.): Nuclear Medicine (2d ed.; New York: McGraw-Hill Book Company, Inc., 1971).

Bradus, S., et al.: Hepatic function and serum enzyme levels in association with fatty metamorphosis of the liver, Am. J. M. Sc. 246:35, 1963.

Breen, K. J., and Schenker, S.: Liver function tests, CRC Crit. Rev. Clin. Lab. Sc. 2:573, 1971.

Cooley, R. N.: Diagnostic accuracy of radiologic studies of the biliary tract, small intestine, and colon, Am. J. M. Sc. 246:610, 1963.

Enquist, I. F., et al.: Validity of the bromsulphalein test in patients with acute severe upper gastrointestinal hemorrhage, Am. J. Surg. 107:306, 1964.

Fenster, F., and Klatskin, G.: Manifestations of metastatic tumors of the liver, Am. J. Med. 31:238, 1961.

Feizi, T.: Immunoglobulins in chronic liver disease, Gut 9:193, 1968.

Frank, B. B., and Raffensperger, E. C.: Hepatic granulomata, Arch. Int. Med. 115:223, 1965.

Gabuzda, G. J.: Hepatic Coma: Clinical Considerations, Pathogenesis, and Management, in Dock, W., and Snapper, I. (eds.): Advances in Internal Medicine (Chicago: Year Book Medical Publishers, Inc., 1962), Vol. XI.

Ginsberg, A. L.: Very high levels of SGOT and LDH in patients with extrahepatic biliary tract obstruction, Am. J. Digest. Dis. 15:803, 1970.

Gollin, F. F., et al.: Liver scanning and liver function tests, J. A. M. A. 187:151, 1964.

Leevy, C. M.: Fatty liver: A study of 270 patients with biopsy proven fatty liver and a review of the literature, Medicine 41:249, 1962.

Levine, R. A., and Klatskin, G.: Unconjugated hyperbilirubinemia in the absence of overt hemolysis, Am. J. Med. 36:541, 1964.

Mehlman, D. J., et al.: Serum alpha-fetoglobulin with gastric and prostatic carcinoma, New England J. Med. 285:1060, 1971.

Mujahed, A., and Evans, J. A.: Percutaneous transhepatic cholangiography, Radiol. Clin. North America 4:535, 1966.

O'Conor, G. T., et al.: A collaborative study for the evaluation of a serologic test for primary liver disease, Cancer 25:1091, 1970.

Reaves, L. E., III: Syndromes of constitutional hyperbilirubinemia, Postgrad. Med. 39:270, 1966.

Schiff, L. (ed.): Diseases of the Liver (3d ed.; Philadelphia: J. B. Lippincott Company, 1969).

Shehadi, W. H.: Radiologic examination of the biliary tract: Plain film of the abdomen; oral cholecystography, Radiol. Clin. North America 4:463, 1966.

Sherlock, S.: Chronic active hepatitis, Postgrad. Med. 50:206, 1971.

Spellberg, M. A.: Intrahepatic cholestasis vs. posthepatic jaundice: Methods of diagnosis, M. Clin. North America 48:53, 1964.

Steigmann, F., and Shah, M. N.: Fatty liver with jaundice: A diagnostic enigma with surgical implications, Am. J. Gastroenterol. 54:126, 1970.

Wise, R. E. : Current concepts of intravenous cholangiography, Radiol. Clin. North America, 4:521, 1966.

Zieve, L. , et al. : Normal and abnormal variations and clinical significance of the one-minute and total serum bilirubin determinations, J. Lab. & Clin. Med. 38:446, 1951.

Zimmerman, H. J. , and Seeff, L. B. : Enzymes in Hepatic Disease, in Coodley, E. L. (ed.): Diagnostic Enzymology (Philadelphia: Lea & Febiger, 1970), p. 1.

# CHAPTER 20

# Cardiac, Pulmonary, and Miscellaneous Diagnostic Procedures

Myocardial Infarction: Clinical signs and symptoms are extremely important in both suspicion and diagnosis. The type of pain with its distribution and response to nitroglycerin may be very characteristic. A history may show predisposing factors, previous anginal pain, or symptoms of heart failure. Even when diagnosis is virtually certain on clinical grounds alone, the physician often will want laboratory confirmation, and this becomes more important when symptoms are atypical or minimal. An electrocardiogram is the most useful direct test available. Approximately 50% of myocardial infarctions show unequivocal changes on the first ECG. Another 30% have abnormalities compatible with, but not diagnostic of, infarction, often obscured by certain major conduction irregularities such as bundle branch block or previous digitalis therapy. About 20% do not show significant changes, and this occasionally happens even in otherwise characteristic cases. Laboratory tests cannot directly show infarction, but certain ones are regularly elevated in this condition and may give a pattern which is helpful when combined with the clinical picture. In classic cases, a polymorphonuclear leukocytosis begins between 12 and 24 hours after onset of symptoms, usually in the range of 10,000-20,000 per cu. mm. This generally lasts between 1 and 2 weeks, depending on the extent of tissue necrosis. Leukocytosis is accompanied by increased temperature of moderate degree and increased erythrocyte sedimentation rate (ESR). The ESR abnormality persists longer than leukocytosis, remaining elevated sometimes as long as 3-4 weeks.

Certain enzymes are present in cardiac muscle which are released when tissue necrosis occurs. Serum glutamic oxaloacetic transaminase (SGOT) becomes elevated between 8 and 12 hours after infarction, reaches a peak between 24 and 48 hours, and falls to normal within 3-8 days. The blood levels have a very rough correlation with the extent of infarct, and may be only transiently and minimally abnormal. SGOT may be elevated due to acute damage to parenchymal cells of other organs. This is very common in liver cell necrosis (p. 218), happens often with sufficient skeletal muscle damage (including trauma or extensive surgical damage), and is found fairly frequently in acute pancreatitis. In some of these situations, myocardial infarct may have to be considered in differential diagnosis of symptoms. Chronic hypokalemia may elevate SGOT (and CPK

Other conditions may elevate SGOT besides myocardial infarction, skeletal muscle disease, liver cell damage, and acute pancreatitis. Morphine or Demerol may temporarily raise SGOT. Elevations have also been reported in occasional cases of Coumadin anticoagulant therapy and with large doses of salicylates.

Lactic dehydrogenase (LDH) becomes elevated between 24 and 48 hours postinfarction, reaches a peak between 48 and 72 hours, and slowly falls to normal between 5 and 10 days. Thus, LDH tends to parallel SGOT at about double the time interval. LDH is more sensitive than SGOT, and is reported to be elevated even in small infarcts which showed no SGOT abnormality. When LDH values are quoted, total serum LDH is meant.

In acute liver cell damage, total LDH is not as sensitive as the SGOT. In acute or chronic passive congestion of the liver, LDH is most often normal or only minimally elevated, although occasionally substantial elevations do occur. Since LDH fraction 1 is contained in RBC as well as cardiac muscle, LDH is greatly influenced by accidental hemolysis in serum, and thus must be collected and transported with care. LDH is also abnormal in many patients with megaloblastic and hemolytic anemias, including sickle cell anemia. Finally, LDH may be abnormal in some cases of malignant neoplasm, especially when widespread. Pulmonary infarction or embolism can have a similar (total) LDH pattern to myocardial infarct, although the SGOT is usually normal for the first few days.

Lactic dehydrogenase is actually a group of enzymes (Fig. 8). The individual enzymes (isoenzymes) which make up total LDH have different concentrations in different tissues. Therefore, the tissue responsible for elevated total LDH may often be identified by fractionation (separation) and measurement of individual isoenzymes. In addition, since the population normal range for total LDH is rather wide, abnormal elevation of one isoenzyme may occur without lifting total LDH out of the total LDH normal range.

Five main fractions (isoenzymes) of LDH are measured. Using the standard international nomenclature (early U. S. investigators used opposite terminology), fraction 1 is found mainly in heart, RBC, and kidney, whereas fraction 5 is found mainly in liver. Various methods of isoenzyme separation are available; the two most commonly used are heat and electrophoresis. Heating at 60° C for 30

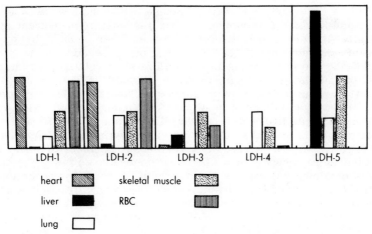

heart    skeletal muscle

liver    RBC

lung

Fig. 8.—LDH isoenzyme pattern of various tissues.

minutes destroys most activity except for fractions 1 and 2, which
are the heat-stable fractions. Using electrophoresis, the fast-
moving fractions are 1 and 2 ("heart"), while the slowest-migrating
fraction is 5 ("liver"). Electrophoresis has the advantage that one
can see the relative contributions of all five fractions.

The relative specificity of LDH isoenzymes is very useful because of the large number of diseases which affect standard "heart"
enzyme tests. For example, one study of patients in hemorrhagic
shock with no evidence of heart disease found elevated SGOT in 70%,
LDH in 52%, and SGPT in 37%. LDH enzyme fractionation offers a
way to diagnose myocardial infarction when liver damage is suspected of contributing to total LDH increase. In such situations,
fraction 1 would not be elevated proportionately as much as total
LDH, since most of the abnormality would be due to fraction 5. In
addition, the isoenzyme determination in some instances has proved
more sensitive to myocardial damage than total LDH, being definitely
abnormal with a normal or only a borderline total LDH.

There are certain pitfalls in LDH isoenzyme interpretation
which should be mentioned. Hemolysis raises the "heart" fraction
due to isoenzyme release from RBC. The same fraction is usually
elevated in megaloblastic anemia, but not invariably. Lung contains
mainly the "intermediate" fractions, especially fraction 3; although
reports in the literature have advocated this as a test for pulmonary
embolization, others have found that any of the fractions may be elevated in pulmonary embolization. Skeletal muscle contains LDH, so
that LDH or HBD values are not reliable in the first week after extensive surgery. Frozen serum specimens have rapid deterioration
of the slow ("liver") fraction. Uremia may elevate LDH.

Hydroxybutyric acid dehydrogenase (HBD) has been used as a substitute for LDH fast-moving ("heart") isoenzyme measurement. Actually, HBD is total LDH which is forced to act on an alpha-ketobutyric acid substrate instead of pyruvic or lactic acid. Under these conditions, the fast-moving LDH fractions show relatively greater activity than the slow-moving fraction, so that HBD therefore indirectly measures fast-moving fraction 1 ("heart") activity. However, if fraction 5 ("liver") is elevated sufficiently, it will also produce measurable HBD effect, so that HBD is not as specific as electrophoresis or heat fractionation in separating heart from liver isoenzymes. Nevertheless, since HBD assay is easier to perform (and therefore cheaper) than LDH isoenzymes, some follow the practice of obtaining a more specific isoenzyme method if in doubt about LDH heart vs. liver contribution. Once the "heart" fraction is proven elevated, they follow subsequent activity levels with HBD.

Creatine phosphokinase (CPK) is available as an aid in diagnosis of cardiac and skeletal muscle lesions. It is being advocated as a substitute for the SGOT in heart disease. CPK is found only in heart muscle, skeletal muscle, and brain. Use of CPK in primary diseases of skeletal muscle is discussed elsewhere (p. 404). In myocardial infarction, CPK behaves like the SGOT. However, acute liver cell damage (which frequently causes an abnormal SGOT) has no effect on CPK. This is an advantage, since the situation often arises in which an elevated SGOT (or LDH) might be due to severe hepatic passive congestion from heart failure rather than fresh myocardial infarction.

CPK is present in brain tissue as well as muscle, but reports differ to some extent as to the effect of central nervous system disease on serum CPK levels. According to one report, CPK may be elevated in a wide variety of conditions which affect the brain, including bacterial meningitis, encephalitis, cerebrovascular accident, hepatic coma, uremic coma, and grand-mal epileptic attacks. Elevation is not always present; even when present, the degree of elevation varies considerably. Elevations have been reported in some patients with the acute phase of certain psychiatric diseases, notably schizophrenia; the cause is not known.

Since CPK is frequently utilized to differentiate acute cardiac and hepatic disease, it is worth noting that hepatic coma and delirium tremens, two conditions associated with liver damage, may induce elevated CPK values due to effects on tissue other than liver. CPK is often abnormal in delirium tremens, presumably due to muscular exertion. Elevations have also been reported (for reasons unknown) in many patients with hypothyroidism and in some patients with tachyarrhythmias (mostly ventricular) and chronic hypokalemia.

CPK elevation is associated with effects of alcohol on muscle. 24-48 hours following a heavy drinking episode, CPK levels become abnormal in the majority of patients, as well in most patients with delirium tremens. CPK is said to be normal in chronic alcoholics without acute intake.

CPK is frequently elevated after intramuscular injection. Since therapeutic injections are common, this probably constitutes the most frequent cause of CPK elevation. Specimens must be drawn before injection or at least within 1 hour after injection. Trauma to muscle makes CPK unreliable for a few days postoperatively.

Pulmonary embolism is often difficult either to diagnose or to confirm. Sudden dyspnea is the most common symptom, but clinically there may be any combination of chest pain, dyspnea, and possibly hemoptysis. Diseases which must be also considered are myocardial infarction and pneumonia. Pulmonary embolism is often associated with chronic congestive heart failure, cor pulmonale, postoperative complications of major surgery, and fractures of the pelvis or lower extremities—all situations in which myocardial infarct itself is more likely. The classic x-ray findings of a wedge-shaped lung shadow are often absent or late in developing, because not all cases of embolism develop actual pulmonary infarction even when the embolus is large.

Laboratory tests in pulmonary embolism have not been very helpful. Initial reports of a characteristic test triad (elevated bilirubin and LDH with normal SGOT) proved disappointing, because only 20-25% of patients display this combination. Reports that LDH is elevated in 80% of patients are probably optimistic. In addition, LDH may be elevated in myocardial infarction or liver passive congestion, conditions which could mimic or be associated with embolism. LDH isoenzyme fractionation has not proved useful either, since a variety of patterns have been noted in pulmonary embolism. The CPK test has been advocated to differentiate myocardial infarction, but reports indicate that increased values may occur in some cases of embolism.

The most useful diagnostic procedure for pulmonary embolism is the lung scan. Serum albumin is tagged with $I^{131}$ radioisotope and the tagged albumin molecules are treated in such a way as to cause aggregation into larger molecular groups (50-100$\mu$ size). This material is injected into a vein, goes through the right side of the heart, and is sent into the pulmonary artery. The molecules then are trapped in small arterioles of the pulmonary artery circulation, so that a radiation detector scan of the lungs shows a diffuse radioactive uptake throughout both lungs from these trapped radioactive molecules. A scan is a visual chart of the radioactivity counts over a specified area received by the radiation detector. The isotope solution is too dilute to cause any difficulty from its partial occlusion of the pulmonary circulation; only a small percentage of the arterioles are affected, and the albumin is metabolized in 3-4 hours. If a part of the pulmonary artery circulation is already occluded by a thrombus, the isotope does not reach that part of the lung, and the portion of lung affected does not show any uptake on the scan ("positive" scan).

The lung scan becomes "positive" immediately after total occlusion of the pulmonary artery or any branches of the pulmonary artery which are of significant size. There does not have to be actual pulmonary infarction, since the scan results do not depend on tissue necrosis, only on mechanical vessel occlusion. However, anything which will temporarily or permanently occlude or cut down lung vascularity will show varying degrees of "positivity" on lung scan; these include cysts, abscesses, many cases of carcinoma, scars, and a considerable number of pneumonias, especially when necrotizing. However, many of these conditions may be at least tentatively ruled out by comparison of the scan results with a chest x-ray. A chest x-ray should therefore be obtained with the lung scan.

Emphysema and congestive heart failure frequently produce perfusion defects. Emphysema may do this even without x-ray changes. Asthma in the acute phase may also produce focal defects; these disappear after treatment. Emphysema can be differentiated by a follow-up lung scan after 6-8 days. Defects due to emphysema persist, whereas those from emboli tend to change configuration.

The lung scan (like the chest x-ray) is nonspecific; i.e., a variety of conditions produce abnormality. Certain findings increase the probability of embolization. Serial studies provide the best information. Pulmonary artery angiography is more definitive but is relatively complicated, entails some risk, and may miss small peripheral clots. A normal lung scan effectively rules out pulmonary embolism.

Pericardial effusion may be a consideration in differential diagnosis of an enlarged heart on chest x-ray. Two techniques are available to demonstrate increased pericardial fluid: (1) the radioisotope heart (or cardiac blood pool) scan and (2) ultrasound (echosonography). A heart scan involves placing a radioisotope compound into the blood stream, where it mixes with blood inside the heart. Scanning this region provides a picture of the interior dimensions of the heart as outlined by the intracardiac blood pool; this can be compared to the x-ray cardiac silhouette or (depending on technique) to adjacent lung and liver blood pools. Pericardial effusion separates the heart pool from the x-ray heart border or from adjacent structures. Effusion over 200 ml. can be detected with reasonable efficiency. Ultrasound is equally effective for anteriorly placed effusion, although a B-mode detector is needed.

Scanning may be helpful in demonstrating subdiaphragmatic abscess. Current technique is to scan the lung-liver junction after administering one isotope which localizes in the lungs and another which is taken up by the liver. Subphrenic abscess causes separation of the lung and liver, whereas normally they are contiguous. Ascites or right pleural effusion may produce false separation; a chest x-ray prevents misdiagnosis from effusion.

Sarcoidosis is a disease of as yet unknown etiology, manifested by noncaseating granulomatous lesions in many organ systems, most commonly in lungs and thoracic lymph nodes. The disease is much more common in Negroes. Laboratory studies may suggest or support the diagnosis. Anemia is not frequent, but appears in about 5% of cases. Splenomegaly is present in 10-30%. Leukopenia is found in approximately 30%. Eosinophilia is reported in 10-60%, averaging 25% of cases. Thrombocytopenia is very uncommon, reported in less than 2% of several large series. Serum protein abnormalities are common, with hyperglobulinemia in nearly 50% and frequently decreased albumin. Hypercalcemia is reported in about 20%, although some authors give higher figures. Alkaline phosphatase is elevated in nearly 35%, which probably reflects either liver or bone involvement. The two major diagnostic procedures available are the Kveim skin test and biopsy.

The Kveim test consists of intradermal inoculation of an antigen composed of human sarcoidal tissue. A positive reaction is given by development of a papule in 4-6 weeks which, on biopsy, yields the typical noncaseating granulomas of sarcoidosis. The test is highly reliable, with less than 3% false positives. The main difficulty is inadequate supplies of sufficiently potent antigen. For this reason, few laboratories are equipped to do the Kveim test. Between 40 and 80% of cases give positive results, depending on the particular lot of antigen and the duration of disease. In chronic sarcoidosis (more than 6 months after onset of illness), the patient is less likely to exhibit a positive Kveim test. Steroid treatment depresses the Kveim reaction, and may produce a negative test. The value of the Kveim test is especially great when no enlarged lymph nodes are available for biopsy, when granulomas obtained from biopsy are nonspecific, or when diagnosis on an outpatient basis is necessary. A recent report has challenged the specificity of the Kveim test, suggesting that a positive test is related more to chronic lymphadenopathy than to any specific disease.

Biopsy is the most widely used means for diagnosis at present. Peripheral lymph nodes are involved in 60-95% of cases, although often they are small. The liver is said to show involvement in 75% of cases, although it is palpable in 20% or less. Difficulties with biopsy come primarily from the fact that the granuloma of sarcoidosis, although characteristic, is nonspecific. Other diseases which may sometimes or often give a similar histologic pattern are early miliary tuberculosis, histoplasmosis, some fungal diseases, some pneumoconioses, and the so-called pseudosarcoid reaction sometimes found in lymph nodes draining areas of carcinoma.

Erythrocyte Sedimentation Rate (ESR): This procedure consists of filling a calibrated tube of standard diameter with anticoagulated whole blood and measuring the rate of RBC sedimentation during a specified period, usually 1 hour. When the RBC settle toward the bottom of the tube, they leave an increasingly large zone

of clear plasma, which is the area measured.  Many diseases cause
abnormally great red cell sedimentation (rate of fall in the tube system).  These include:  acute and chronic infection; tissue necrosis
and infarction; well-established malignancy; rheumatoid-collagen
diseases; abnormal serum proteins, and certain physiologic stress
situations such as pregnancy.  Most of the sedimentation effect
seems due to alterations in plasma proteins, mainly fibrinogen and
globulins.  The ESR has two main uses:  (1) as a means of following
the activity or clinical course of certain diseases (such as acute
rheumatic fever or acute glomerulonephritis) and (2) to demonstrate
or confirm the presence of occult organic disease, either when the
patient has symptoms but no definite physical or laboratory evidence
of organic disease, or in some cases when the patient is completely
asymptomatic.

The ESR has three main limitations:  (1) it is a very nonspecific test; (2) it is sometimes normal in diseases where usually it is
abnormal, and (3) technical factors may considerably influence the
results.  The tubes must be absolutely vertical; even small degrees
of tilt have great effect on degree of sedimentation.  Anemia of most
types will falsely increase the ESR as performed by the Wintrobe
method using oxalate anticoagulant; the Westergren method, using
citrate or EDTA, is not affected.  The Wintrobe method may be
"corrected" for anemia, but this is not accurate.  On the other
hand, sickle cell anemia and polycythemia falsely decrease the
ESR.  Normal values (at least for the Westergren method) usually
quoted for the ESR may be too low in persons over age 40 and definitely are too low in those over age 60.  After age 60, at least
10 mm./hour should be added to normal values.

Fat Embolization is a syndrome most often associated with
severe bone trauma, but it may also occur in fatty liver, diabetes,
and other conditions.  Symptoms may be immediate or delayed.  If
immediate, shock is frequent.  Delayed symptoms occur 2-3 days
after injury, and pulmonary or cerebral manifestations are most
prominent.  Frequent signs are fever, tachycardia, tachypnea, upper body petechiae (50% of patients), and decreased hemoglobin.
Laboratory diagnosis includes urine examination for free fat (special
technique, p. 137) which is positive in 50% of cases during the first
3 days; and serum lipase, which is elevated in nearly 50% of patients
from roughly day 3 to 7.  Fat in sputum is unreliable; it gives many
false positives and negatives.  Chest x-rays sometimes demonstrate
diffuse tiny infiltrates, sometimes coalescing, described in the
literature as having a "snowstorm" appearance.  Some patients develop a laboratory picture suggestive of disseminated intravascular
coagulation.  A recent report has indicated that diagnosis by cryostat frozen section of peripheral blood clot is sensitive and specific,
but adequate confirmation of this is not yet available.

Selected Tests of Interest in Pediatrics

(1) Neonatal IgM levels:  Maternal IgG (immunoglobulin-G,

p. 252) can cross the placenta, but not IgA or M. Chronic infections involving the fetus, such as congenital syphilis, toxoplasmosis, rubella, and cytomegalic inclusion disease, lead to IgM production by the fetus. Increased IgM levels in cord blood at birth or in neonatal blood during the first few days of life suggest chronic intrauterine infection. Infection near term or subsequent to birth results in IgM increase beginning 6-7 days post partum. Unfortunately, there are pitfalls when interpreting such data. Many cord blood samples become contaminated with maternal blood, thus falsely raising IgM values. Normal values are controversial; 20 mg./100 ml. is the most widely accepted upper limit. Various techniques have different reliabilities and sensitivities. Finally, some investigators state that fewer than 40% of rubella or cytomegalovirus infections cause elevated IgM before birth.

(2) Agammaglobulinemia: This condition may lead to frequent infections. Electrophoresis displays decreased gamma globulin, which can be confirmed by quantitative immunoglobulin technique.

(3) Chronic granulomatous disease of childhood is a rare sex-linked disorder of WBC manifested by repeated infections and death before puberty. Polymorphonuclear leukocytes are able to attack high-virulence organisms such as streptococci and staphylococci, but are unable to destroy those of lower virulence such as the gram-negative rods. The nitroblue tetrazolium test is negative. Some normal granulocytes are able to reduce this substance to a dark blue color, but those in patients with chronic granulomatous disease are unable to do so. The nitroblue tetrazolium test has also been reported to separate persons with bacterial infection from leukocytosis of other etiologies, but there is sufficient overlap to nullify much help in the individual case unless values are definitely high. It has also been advocated as a screening test for infection when the WBC count is normal; more work needs to be done to assess reliability when used thus, or in differentiating viral and bacterial disease.

Porphyria is a collection of related diseases whose main similarity is the abnormal secretion of substances which are precursors of the porphyrin compound heme (of hemoglobin). The known pathways of porphyrin synthesis begin with glycine and succinate, which are combined to eventually form a compound known as delta aminolevulinic acid (ALA). This goes on to produce a substance known as porphobilinogen, composed of a single pyrrole ring. From there, four of these rings are joined to form the tetrapyrrole compound proporphyrinogen; this is the precursor of protoporphyrin, which in turn is the precursor of heme (Fig. 9). The tetrapyrrole compounds exist in 8 isomers, depending on where certain side groups are located. The only isomeric forms which are clinically important are I and III. Normally, very small amounts of proporphyrin degradation products appear in the feces or in the urine; these are called coproporphyrins or uroporphyrins (their names refer to where they were first discovered, but both may appear in either urine or feces).

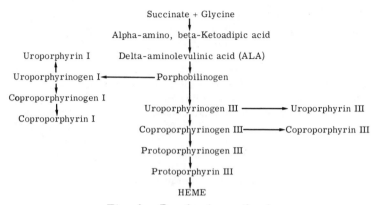

Fig. 9.—Porphyrin synthesis.

The porphyrias have been classified in several ways, none of which is entirely satisfactory. The most common system includes congenital porphyria, acute intermittent porphyria, cutanea tarda, and toxic porphyria. Congenital porphyria is a rare congenital disease characterized clinically by skin photosensitivity, pink discoloration of the teeth, and sometimes mild hemolytic anemia. Uroporphyrin and coproporphyrin I are excreted and are the only abnormal chemical findings.

Acute intermittent porphyria is manifest clinically by intermittent attacks of colicky abdominal pain. This is often accompanied by a leukocytosis, and thus can mimic a variety of diseases such as appendicitis and pancreatitis. These attacks may be precipitated by barbiturates. In addition, severe constipation and episodes of abnormal mental behavior may occur. In acute (intermittent) porphyria, an almost pathognomonic finding is the presence of porphobilinogen in the urine. Urinary porphyrins are relatively normal in many cases of acute porphyria when urine is freshly voided. Porphyrinogens may be increased; these compounds and porphobilinogen may break down to porphyrins. If this occurs, uroporphyrin type III and coproporphyrin type III are produced, but are not diagnostic, since they may be increased in other conditions. A compound called Waldenström's porphyrin—a complex of uroporphyrin type I and III—may also be present. Porphobilinogen is nearly always present during one of the clinical attacks, but the duration of excretion is highly variable. It may occasionally disappear if not searched for initially. Between attacks, some patients excrete porphobilinogen and others do not.

Porphobilinogen is usually detected by color reaction with Ehrlich's reagent and confirmed by demonstrating that the color is not removed by chloroform (Watson-Schwartz test). Since false positives may occur, it is essential to further confirm a positive test by butanol (butyl alcohol) extraction. Porphobilinogen will not be extracted by butanol, whereas butanol will remove most of the other Ehrlich-positive, chloroform-negative substances.  A positive porphobilinogen test is the key to diagnosis of symptomatic acute porphyria; analysis and quantitation of urinary porphyrins or ALA are useful only if the Watson-Schwartz test is equivocal.  Glucose administration may considerably decrease porphobilinogen excretion.

Cutanea tarda is a chronic type of porphyria.  There usually is some degree of photosensitivity, but it does not develop until after puberty.  There often is some degree of liver disease.  These patients excrete abnormal amounts of uroporphyrin and coproporphyrin III.

Toxic porphyria may be produced by a variety of chemicals, but the most common is lead.  Lead poisoning produces abnormal coproporphyrin III excretion, but not uroporphyrin III.  ALA is also excreted.

Toxicology includes a selected list of conditions which seem especially important in drug overdose and poisoning.

Lead poisoning:  The acute syndrome is uncommon; symptoms may include "lead colic" (crampy abdominal pain, constipation, occasional bloody diarrhea), and, in 50% of cases, hypertensive encephalopathy.  Chronic poisoning is more common, with varying symptoms which may include lead colic, constipation with anorexia (85% of cases), peripheral neuritis (wrist-drop) in adults, and lead encephalopathy (headache, convulsions) in children.  A "lead line" is frequently present just below the epiphyses (approximately 70% cases with clinical symptoms and 20-40% with abnormal exposure but no symptoms).  Most patients develop slight to moderate anemia, more often hypochromic but sometimes normochromic.  Basophilic stippled RBC are the most characteristic peripheral blood finding.  Some authors claim stippling is invariably present; others report stippling absent in 70-80% of cases.  Normal persons may have up to 500 stippled cells per 1 million RBC.  The reticulocyte count is usually over 4%.  Urinary coproporphyrin III excretion is usually (although not invariably) increased in clinical lead poisoning, and simple screening tests using fluorescent light are based on this fact.  Urinary delta-aminolevulinic acid (ALA) excretion is increased; this is said to provide the most sensitive screening test for significantly increased lead exposure.  In moderate degrees of exposure, urine ALA may be elevated when blood lead is within normal limits.  Light, room temperature, and alkaline pH all decrease ALA levels.  If ALA determination is not done immediately, the specimen must be refrigerated and kept in the dark (collection bottle wrapped in paper or foil) with the specimen acidified, using glacial acetic or tartaric acid.  Blood lead is still considered necessary for definitive diagnosis.  Lead-free collection containers are necessary.  The U.S. Public Health Service has recommended the following guidelines (age 1-5 years):

Blood lead: Normal up to 40 μg./100 ml. whole blood; 50-80 μg. equivocal.

Urine ALA: Normal up to 5 mg./24 hours.

Heavy metals: Mercury, arsenic, bismuth, and antimony are included. Urine is preferred over blood samples. Hair and nails are useful for arsenic examination.

Organic phosphate: Certain insecticides such as parathion and the less powerful malathion are inhibitors of the enzyme cholinesterase. This allows overproduction of acetylcholine at nerve-muscle junctions. Symptoms include muscle twitching, cramps, and weakness; parasympathetic effects such as pinpoint pupils, nausea, sweating, diarrhea, and salivation; and various central nervous system aberrations. Laboratory diagnosis is based on finding decreased cholinesterase in RBC or plasma. RBC levels reflect poisoning more accurately than plasma values, which are reduced by many conditions and drugs. Screening tests are generally based on plasma measurement; a normal result rules out anticholinesterase toxicity.

Salicylate is discussed on p. 323. The Phenistix dipstick test on plasma and the ferric chloride test on urine are useful screening procedures.

Barbiturates and glutethimide (Doriden): These are the most common vehicles of drug-overdose suicide. In testing, either anticoagulated (not heparinized) whole blood or urine can be used; blood is preferred. Thin-layer chromatography is used both for screening and to identify the individual substance involved; chemical screening tests are also available. It is preferable to secure both blood and urine specimens plus gastric contents if available.

Phenothiazine tranquilizers: Urine is tested with the Phenistix or ferric chloride procedure.

Narcotic alkaloids: Urine is most commonly used for screening purposes. A syndrome of pulmonary vasculitis in addicts caused by foreign-particle injection has been reported with lung scan findings suggestive of embolization and multiple small chest x-ray infiltrates.

Cardiac drugs: The digitalis family, procainamide, and quinidine may be toxic under certain conditions (p. 436). Radioisotope immunoassay techniques are becoming available for digitalis family serum measurement. In general, most patients with clear-cut evidence of digitalis toxicity and those who are clinically normal can be separated. In the case of borderline or questionable situations, it is very difficult to rely on any theoretical upper limit of normal, since many factors (electrolyte concentrations, medications, acid-base, thyroid status, and individual patient variation) may affect cardiac response to a given level of digitalis.

Blood alcohol: Most courts of law follow the recommendations of the National Safety Council on alcohol and drugs:

Below 0.05%: No influence by alcohol within the meaning of the law.

Between 0.05 and 0.10%: A liberal, wide zone; alcoholic influence usually is present, but courts of law are advised to consider the person's behavior and circumstances leading to the arrest in making their decision.
Above 0.10%: Definite evidence of being "under the influence," since most persons with this concentration will have lost, to a measurable extent, some of that clearness of intellect and self-control they would normally possess.

## REFERENCES

Albahary, C.: Lead and hemopoiesis, Am. J. Med. 52:367, 1972.
Aldrich, F. D.: Cholinesterase assays: Their usefulness in diagnosis of anticholinesterase intoxication, Clin. Toxicol. 2:445, 1969.
Alford, C. A.: Immunoglobulin determinations in the diagnosis of fetal infection, Pediat. Clin. North America 18:99, 1971.
Allen, J. C.: Recurrent infections in man associated with immunologic or phagocytic deficiencies, Postgrad. Med. 50:88, 1971.
Batsakis, J. G., and Briere, R. O.: Clinical enzymology and diseases of the lung—A critical reappraisal, Geriatrics 23:97, 1968.
Berger, R. L., et al.: Diagnosis and management of massive pulmonary embolism, Surg. Clin. North America 48:311, 1968.
Chisolm, J. J.: Childhood lead intoxication, M. Times 98:92, 1970.
Cohen, L.: Enzymes in Pulmonary Disease, in Coodley, E. L. (ed.): Diagnostic Enzymology (Philadelphia: Lea & Febiger, 1970), p. 113.
Coodley, E. L.: Enzymes in Cardiac Disease, in Coodley, E. L. (ed.): Diagnostic Enzymology (Philadelphia: Lea & Febiger, 1970), p. 39.
Czucs, M. M., Jr.: Diagnostic sensitivity of laboratory findings in acute pulmonary embolization, Ann. Int. Med. 74:161, 1971.
Eshchar, J., and Zimmerman, H. J.: Creatine phosphokinase in disease, Am. J. M. Sc. 253:272, 1967.
Evarts, C. M.: The fat embolization syndrome: A review, Surg. Clin. North America 50:493, 1970.
Fleigin, R. D., et al.: Nitroblue tetrazolium dye test as an aid in the differential diagnosis of febrile disorders, J. Pediat. 78:230, 1971.
Fleisher, G. A., et al.: Serum creatine kinase, lactic dehydrogenase, and glutamic-oxaloacetic transaminase in thyroid disease and pregnancy, Mayo Clin. Proc. 40:300, 1965.
Gilbertsen, V. A.: Erythrocyte sedimentation rates in older patients, Postgrad. Med. 38:A-44, 1965.
Green, M.: Immediate management of accidental poisoning in children, Hosp. Med. 3:114, 1967.
Hauman, A., et al.: Cryostat test for fat embolism, Lab. Med. 2:37, 1971.

Israel, H. L.: Diagnosis of sarcoidosis, Ann. Int. Med. 68:1323, 1968.
Israel, H. L., and Goldstein, R. A.: Relation of Kveim-antigen reaction to lymphadenopathy, New England J. Med. 284:345, 1971.
Lafair, J. S., and Myerson, R. M.: Alcoholic myopathy, Arch. Int. Med. 122:417, 1968.
Mayock, R. L., et al.: Manifestations of sarcoidosis, Am. J. Med. 35:67, 1963.
Meltzer, H. Y.: Creatine kinase and aldolase in serum: Abnormality common to acute psychoses, Science 159:1368, 1968.
Quinn, J. L., III: The lung: The challenge of nuclear medicine, Am. J. Roentgenol. 105:251, 1969.
Schrader, W. H.: Erythrocyte sedimentation rate, Postgrad. Med. 34:A-42, 1963.
Sherman, N. J., et al.: Subphrenic abscess—A continuing hazard, Am. J. Surg. 117:117, 1969.
Siltzbach, L. E.: The Kveim test in sarcoidosis, J. A. M. A. 178:476, 1961.
Smith, T. W.: Measurement of serum digitalis glycosides: Clinical implications, Circulation 43:179, 1971.
Stein, J. A., and Tschudy, D. P.: Acute intermittent porphyria, Medicine 49:1, 1970.
Taddeini, L., and Watson, C. J.: The clinical porphyrias, Seminars Hemat. 5:335, 1968.
Thurlbeck, W. M., et al.: Chronic obstructive lung disease, Medicine 49:81, 1970.
Tysinger, D. S.: Pulmonary function testing for the general hospital and physician, J. Alabama M. A. 39:658, 756, 834, 922, 1113, 1970; 40:33, 106, 1970.
Vincent, W. F., and Ullmann, W. W.: Measurement of urinary delta-aminolevulinic acid in detection of childhood lead poisoning, Am. J. Clin. Path. 53:963, 1970.
Vincent, W. F., and Ullman, W. W.: The preservation of urine specimens for delta-aminolevulinic acid determinations, Clin. Chem. 16:612, 1970.
Vorhaus, L. J., and Kark, R. M.: Serum cholinesterase in health and disease, Am. J. Med. 14:707, 1953.
Weidner, W., et al.: Roentgen techniques in the diagnosis of pulmonary thromboembolism, Am. J. Roentgenol. 100:397, 1967.
Weinsaft, P. P., and Haltaufderhyde, V.: Erythrocyte sedimentation rate in the aged, J. Am. Geriat. Soc. 13:738, 1965.
Whitaker, J. A.: Lead poisoning—A masquerade, South. M. J. 55:1184, 1962.
Windhorst, D. B.: Functional Defects of Neutrophils, in Stollerman, G. H., et al. (eds.): Advances in Internal Medicine (Chicago: Year Book Medical Publishers, Inc., 1970), Vol. 16, p. 329.

# CHAPTER 21

# Serum Proteins

Albumin and globulin, both free and combined with other substances containing lipid or carbohydrate, make up the serum proteins. Normal total protein concentration is roughly 6.5-8 Gm./100 ml. Normal globulin range is approximately 1-3 Gm. and that of albumin approximately 4-6 Gm. Plasma contains fibrinogen in addition to the ordinary serum proteins. The globulin molecule is approximately 2 1/2 times as large as that of albumin, although, quantitatively, albumin is normally 2-3 times the level of globulin. Albumin seems most concerned with maintaining the serum oncotic pressure, where its osmotic influence is about 4 times that of globulin. The globulins, on the other hand, seem to have more varied assignments and form the main transport system for many substances, as well as having an active role themselves in certain immunologic mechanisms.

There are four widely used procedures for fractionating the serum proteins. "Salting-out" by differential chemical solubility will yield rough separation into albumin and globulin. Cohn has devised a more complicated chemical fractionation method by which certain parts of the protein spectrum may be separated from one another as a large-scale industrial-type procedure. The ultracentrifuge has recently been used to study some of the subgroups of the globulins. This is possible because the sedimentation rate at high speeds depends on the molecular size and shape, the type of solvent used to suspend the protein, and the force of centrifugation. The velocity of any particular class of globulins under standard conditions is known as the Svedberg number; therefore, according to their characteristics, globulins might be designated as 7-S, 19-S, or 22-S. Electrophoresis can also be used; the three standard methods use filter paper, cellulose acetate film, or starch as a migrating field. In clinical medicine, electrophoretic techniques

are becoming routine and will form the backbone of this discussion.
The albumin to globulin (A/G) ratio is usually done by a chemical
method and should be discarded, since paper electrophoresis will
not only give the same information but also pinpoint the areas
where serum protein shifts take place, which sometimes has as
much diagnostic importance as the shifts themselves.

Different methods give slightly different values for various protein fractions. For example, serum albumin by paper electrophoresis may be about half a gram/100 ml. less than by the usual
chemical method. This is fortunately not often very important. Also,
the laboratory must rigidly standardize its electrophoretic technique,
since variations in electrical current, buffer solution, and other
technical aspects will give different results. That is why normal
values should be prepared by the individual laboratory for its own
particular procedure.

Serum protein electrophoresis on filter paper or cellulose
acetate film will show bands corresponding to albumin, alpha-1 and
alpha-2 globulins, beta globulins, and gamma globulins. According
to the quantitation or density of these bands, a special instrument
will translate this into a linear pattern which thus is a rough visual
approximation of the amount of substance present. The main problem with this method is the difficulty in separating some of the serum components. It has been found that by using potato starch in a
gel-like state, the separation of some of these fractions will be
sharper; this is especially true in some of the abnormal hemoglobins.
However, this procedure is technically somewhat more difficult
than the other techniques, and filter paper or cellulose acetate remains the routine clinical laboratory method of choice.

Most serum albumin seems produced by the liver. The origin
of various globulins is not well understood, although some, if not
all, are apparently synthesized by the reticuloendothelial system.
Both of these protein categories can be elevated and depressed in
various conditions.

Serum albumin elevation is very unusual. Most changes involve diminution, although the normal range is somewhat large, and
small decreases are thus lost without previous knowledge of the individual patient's normal levels. In pregnancy, albumin decreases
progressively until delivery and does not return to normal until
about 8 weeks post partum. In infants, adult levels are reached at
about 1 year of age. Thereafter, serum proteins are relatively
stable except for a gradual decrease after age 70. Malnutrition
leads to decreased albumin, presumably from lack of essential
amino acids, but also possibly from impaired liver manufacture and
unknown causes. Impaired synthesis may itself be a cause of decreased albumin, since it is found in most forms of clinical liver
disease. In chronic cachectic or wasting diseases such as tuberculosis or carcinoma, the albumin is often decreased, but it is not
clear whether this is due to impaired synthesis or to other factors.

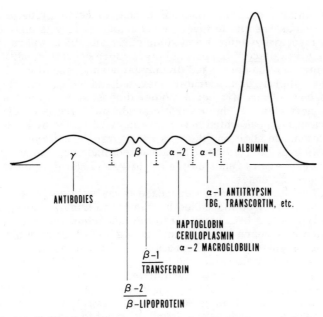

Fig. 9-A.—Some important components of serum protein fractions.

Chronic infections seem to have much the same effect as the cachectic diseases. Serum albumin may be directly lost from the
blood stream by hemorrhage, burns, exudates, or leakage into the
gastrointestinal tract in various malabsorption diseases. In many
acute illnesses or injuries, the albumin is quickly decreased. This
might be thought of as a response to stress and seems to have a different mechanism from hypoalbuminemia found in malnutrition or
simple loss of protein. This will be discussed further. Finally,
there may be a genetic cause such as familial idiopathic dysproteinemia, in which the albumin is greatly decreased while all the
globulin fractions are elevated and seem to take over most of the
functions of albumin. In nephrosis there is a marked decrease in
serum albumin secondary to direct loss in the urine.

Alpha-1 globulin is absent in alpha-1 antitrypsin deficiency, a
disease which leads to development of emphysema. Serum protein
electrophoresis detects homozygous disease, but frequently displays
a normal alpha-1 peak in those who are heterozygous. Estrogens
also tend to raise alpha-1 values. Besides alpha-1 antitrypsin deficiency, low alpha globulins are not often found, although sometimes
the alpha-1 is decreased in the nephrotic syndrome. On the other
hand, a considerable number of diseases may cause an increase.
An increase in the alpha-2 globulin is coupled with a decrease in
albumin in various stress situations. They may include acute in-

fections, injury, surgery, trauma, burns, or certain febrile illnesses such as rheumatic fever or pneumonia. This is also found
in acute myocardial infarct and some other situations where tissue
necrosis takes place. In certain other, more chronic conditions,
the albumin may be decreased or may be normal; the alpha-2 globulin may be slightly or moderately elevated and the gamma globulin
is increased. There are certain other diseases which often show
alpha-2 increases. In the nephrotic syndrome there is classically a
marked alpha-2 peak which may sometimes be joined by a beta globulin elevation. In addition, there is, of course, greatly decreased albumin. In hyperthyroidism, far-advanced diabetes, and adrenal insufficiency, there is reportedly a slightly to moderately elevated
alpha-2 in some cases.

In the beta globulins, a decrease is not very common. The
beta globulins may be increased in many conditions. In pregnancy,
there is typically a beta increase in the last trimester of varying degree which may reach twice normal levels and which may have a
homogeneous spike-like configuration. In patients in whom the serum cholesterol is elevated, the beta globulins are also likely to be
increased; this includes hypothyroidism, biliary cirrhosis, nephrosis, and some cases of diabetes. In liver disease in general, there
is some variability. It is usually, but not always, elevated in obstructive jaundice, and may be found elevated to some extent in many
cases of hepatitis, but not as often. It is often elevated in cirrhosis;
when so, it is often joined to the gamma globulin and occasionally
does not even appear as a separate peak. This will be discussed
later. Finally, beta elevations may occasionally be seen in certain
other diseases, including malignant hypertension, Cushing's disease, periarteritis nodosa, and sometimes in carcinoma. Hemolysis
may produce an artifactual needle-like spike in the beta or pregamma area. A double peak in the beta area is frequently observed when
the cellulose acetate method is used. Electrophoresis on polyacrilamide gel produces reversal of the alpha-2 and beta area positions compared to paper or cellulose acetate electrophoresis (i. e.,
the beta area on paper becomes alpha-2 on polyacrilamide gel).

Gamma globulins exhibit a wide variety of changes. They are
decreased in hypo- and agammaglobulinemia, which may be either
primary or secondary. The secondary type sometimes may be found
with long-term steroid treatment, the nephrotic syndrome, occasionally in overwhelming infection, and relatively often with chronic lymphocytic leukemia, lymphosarcoma, or multiple myeloma.

Many diseases cause increase in gamma globulin. Almost all
types of infections are followed by increased gamma globulin, although it may not be sufficient to cause abnormal changes on paper
electrophoresis, especially if mild or acute. Chronic infections
characteristically show electrophoretic gamma increase, especially
tuberculosis. Collagen diseases, including rheumatoid arthritis and
lupus erythematosus, often cause considerably elevated values, and

this may be true also in many hypersensitivity diseases.  Sarcoidosis, syphilis, and lymphogranuloma venereum are other well-known etiologies.  Gamma globulin is frequently increased in Hodgkin's disease, malignant lymphoma, and chronic lymphocytic leukemia. Multiple myeloma and certain uncommon diseases characteristically show a marked increase of a special homogeneous spike-like pattern, and this will be discussed later.  A final general category for gamma increase is the group of liver diseases.  In hepatitis, there is classically a relatively mild separate increase in both beta and gamma globulins with a decrease of albumin, but this does not always occur. In cirrhosis, there is characteristically a marked increase in gamma globulin.  The most suggestive pattern is a combination of beta and gamma without the usual separation between the two.  However, in most cases, one merely sees an ordinary gamma globulin elevation; of considerable degree in some, slight in others, and no gamma elevation in about 10%.  In obstructive jaundice, one often sees an increase in alpha-2, beta and gamma, all three, to varying degree.

By way of summary, several typical electrophoretic patterns will be presented with diseases in which they will most commonly be found (Fig. 10).  It must be strongly emphasized that these patterns are by no means pathognomonic of any one disease or groups of diseases, that they will sometimes not occur in the disease in which they should be present, and that there will be considerable variation in the shape and height of the electrophoretic peaks in individual patients which may obscure the pattern.  In other words, the patterns are simply intended as a rule of thumb.

The first of these patterns presents what is called the acute stress pattern and consists of a decreased albumin and elevated alpha-2 globulin.  This is found in acute infections in the early stages, some cases of myocardial infarct and tissue necrosis, some cases of severe burns, surgery, and other stress situations, and in some of the rheumatoid diseases with acute onset.  The second pattern consists of a slightly or moderately decreased albumin, an elevated gamma globulin, and a slightly elevated or normal alpha-2. This is the chronic inflammatory pattern and is found in chronic infections of various types, including some cases of chronic tuberculosis.  There may, of course, be various stages of transition between this chronic pattern and the previously described acute one. Next is the so-called nephrotic type in which one sees a greatly decreased albumin and a considerably increased alpha-2 with or without an increase in beta.  This differs from the acute stress pattern in that the alpha-2 elevation of the nephrotic syndrome is usually either slightly or moderately greater than that seen in acute stress, while the albumin fraction in the nephrotic syndrome has a definitely greater decrease (sometimes to extremely low levels) than the albumin values of the acute stress pattern.

Fourth is the frequently found pattern in far-advanced cirrhosis consisting of a decreased albumin with moderately or consider-

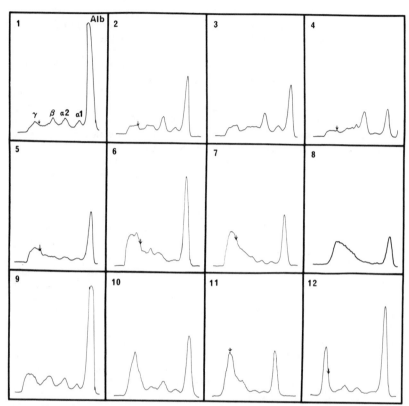

Fig. 10.—Typical serum protein electrophoretic patterns.
(1) Normal (arrow near gamma region indicates serum application
point); (2) acute stress pattern; (3) acute stress or nephrotic syndrome; (4) nephrotic syndrome; (5) chronic inflammation (mild to
moderate); cirrhosis; (6) cirrhosis; granulomatous diseases; rheumatoid-collagen group; (7) suggestive of cirrhosis, but could be found
in the granulomatous diseases or the rheumatoid-collagen group;
(8) characteristic pattern of cirrhosis; (9) slight nonspecific elevation
of gamma, possibly also beta globulin fraction (? chronic disease);
(10) same as (6); configuration of gamma peak superficially mimics
myeloma, but is more broad-based; (11) same interpretation as (10);
(12) myeloma; Waldenström's; idiopathic or secondary monoclonal
gammopathy.

ably increased gamma globulin and variable degrees of incorporation
of the beta into the gamma. The more pronounced the "slurring"
becomes, the more suggestive for cirrhosis. However, complete
incorporation of the beta into the gamma is actually uncommon, and

this is only one of several patterns that may be found in cirrhosis. The fifth pattern consists of a greatly increased, but diffuse, gamma globulin, with or without a small but independent beta increase and a moderately decreased albumin. This is most often found in some cases of cirrhosis, in granulomatous diseases such as sarcoidosis or far-advanced pulmonary tuberculosis, in subacute bacterial endocarditis, and in certain of the collagen diseases such as lupus or periarteritis.

Finally, there is a so-called monoclonal gammopathy spike (m-protein and paraprotein are synonyms). This is located in the gamma area (much less frequently in the beta and rarely in the alpha-2) and consists of a high relatively thin spike configuration which is more homogeneous and needle-shaped than the other gamma or beta elevations discussed earlier. The majority of persons with the monoclonal spike on serum paper electrophoresis have myeloma. However, a sizable minority do not, and these are divided among Waldenström's macroglobulinemia, secondary paraproteinemia, and idiopathic monoclonal gammopathy. Pregnancy often causes a peak in the beta region which occasionally may be pronounced enough to suggest a monoclonal spike. The secondary paraproteinemias may be associated with hematopoietic malignancy such as the lymphomas or leukemias, neoplasias of other types (of which colon carcinoma seems relatively frequent), and occasional cases associated with long-standing chronic urinary or biliary tract infection. The incidence of nonmyelomatous idiopathic paraproteinemias (idiopathic monoclonal gammopathy) increases with age, especially over age 60. It is not agreed whether overt myeloma will develop if followed long enough, although it is reported in some cases. In myeloma, the abnormal serum proteins are of normal (160,000 or 7-S) molecular weight. In Waldenström's, the abnormal proteins involved are macroglobulins which have high molecular weight (1,000,000 or 19-S), even though the serum spike has a configuration identical to that of the myeloma proteins. The other paraproteinemias may be either normal weight paraproteins or macroglobulins; the secondary monoclonal gammopathies tend to be more often of normal weight.

In addition to serum paraproteins, up to 50% of myeloma patients excrete an abnormal protein known as Bence Jones which is of low molecular weight (40,000 or 3.5-S) and thus is able to pass the glomerular filter into the urine. Apparently it is excreted rapidly from the plasma, and, thus, even when Bence Jones proteinuria is marked, this substance usually is not demonstrable in the serum. Bence Jones is more likely to be present when the total serum globulins are within normal range, although it must be remembered that there may be a myeloma peak on electrophoresis without the total globulins being elevated. However, Bence Jones can sometimes be found in association with hyperglobulinemia. The classic method of detecting Bence Jones is by a carefully done heat coagulability test, where it appears on heating to 60° C and disappears on boiling, only

TABLE 8.—IMMUNOGLOBULIN NOMENCLATURE

| Current Terminology | Synonyms |
|---|---|
| IgG | $\gamma$ (gamma) G |
|  | $\gamma_2$ |
|  | 7-S $\gamma$ |
| IgA | $\gamma$ A |
|  | $\gamma_1$A |
|  | $\beta_2$A |
| IgM | $\gamma$ M |
|  | $\gamma_1$M |
|  | $\beta_2$M |
|  | 19-S $\gamma$ |

to reappear if the urine is cooled. As mentioned earlier (p. 116), Bence Jones gives a positive sulfosalicylic acid test for protein. It has been found that many factors, both technical and personal, can interfere with the heat method, and that urine electrophoresis is the best method for demonstrating Bence Jones. In urine, it appears as a single homogeneous spike similar to those seen in the serum. The abnormal serum proteins of myeloma do not appear in the urine.

Gamma globulins (called immunoglobulins in current immunologic terminology) are not a homogeneous group. There are three main subdivisions: IgG (immunoglobulin-G), which migrates in the gamma region on electrophoresis; IgA, which migrates in the pregamma or the area between gamma and beta; and IgM, which migrates in the prebeta or beta (Table 8). IgA and IgG are normal weight globulins (7-S), while IgM corresponds to the macroglobulins (19-S). The serum protein abnormality of multiple myeloma may affect either IgG or IgA (although IgG is definitely the most frequent), thus explaining the variability of electrophoretic serum spike positions in myeloma patients (Fig. 11). Other abnormalities in myeloma may be better understood by considering the basic composition of the gamma globulin (immunoglobulin) molecule. This is composed of two heavy chains (each chain of 50,000 molecular weight) and two light chains (20,000 molecular weight) connected by disulfide bridges. Bence Jones protein is composed of the two light chains alone. There is a very rare disease characterized by production of abnormal immunoglobulins made up only of two heavy chains (Franklin's disease, or heavy chain disease).

In most cases of myeloma, and many with Waldenström's macroglobulinemia, standard laboratory procedures yield an adequate diagnosis. In certain problem cases, it may be necessary to resort to immunoelectrophoresis. Immunoelectrophoresis consists of three steps: First, the unknown (patient's) serum is subjected to

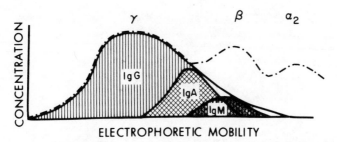

Fig. 11.—Diagrammatic relationship of the immunoglobulins to the standard filter paper serum protein electrophoretic pattern.

ordinary electrophoresis in a substance such as agar gel; this separates the immunoglobulins from one another to some extent. Second, antiserum against a specific type of human globulin (or a polyvalent antiserum against several types) is added to a trench cut near the electrophoretic bands, and the immunoglobulins and anti-immunoglobulin antibodies diffuse toward each other. Third, the areas of reaction between the patient's immunoglobulin fractions and their corresponding antibodies form visual precipitin lines (Fig. 12). The combination of electrophoresis and agar diffusion antigen-antibody reaction produces better separation of the immunoglobulin components and demonstrates abnormal quantities of any type present. Immunoelectrophoresis is currently most useful in differentiating macroglobulinemia from other types of monoclonal gammopathy. If the monoclonal peak is demonstrated to be IgM, this rules out myeloma. On the other hand, if the peak is not IgM, this rules out Waldenström's macroglobulinemia. The secondary paraproteinemias can be either IgG, IgA, or IgM (p. 251).

Other immunoglobulins exist: IgD myeloma has been reported, but is very uncommon; and IgE has been linked to certain allergic disorders.

Immunoelectrophoresis for light chains is also useful. Normally, two types of light chains (known as kappa and lambda) are present in serum. Malignant monoclonal gammopathies such as myeloma usually have an abnormal predominance either of kappa or of lambda, with the other markedly decreased or absent. Commercial companies have had problems in producing consistently good antisera to kappa and lambda light chains. Controls must be run with every lot of antiserum to guard against false results.

Occasionally, there may be other types of abnormal serum proteins in myeloma, Waldenström's macroglobulinemia, malignancy, and some of the other diseases such as lupus. Among these are cryoglobulins. These are abnormal globulins which have the interesting property of coagulating when cooled to certain temperatures. They are not generally demonstrable as distinct peaks on paper electrophoresis, but are incorporated into areas occupied by other globulins.

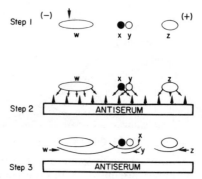

Fig. 12.—Procedure for immunoelectrophoresis (modified from Terry and Fahey). Step 1: electrophoresis of human serum globulins on agar gel. Step 2: addition of antihuman globulin antibody mixture to a nearby trough, and diffusion of the separated globulin fractions and the antibody mixture components toward each other. Step 3: formation of precipitin lines at interaction of globulin fractions and specific antibodies to these fractions from the antiglobulin antibody mixture. The globulin fractions have different rates of diffusion, and thus produce precipitin lines in different areas.

There are screening tests for both cryoglobulins and macroglobulins. The cryocrit is essentially a cold precipitation test for cryoglobulins adapted to yield a rough quantitative result. Serum of the patient is placed in the icebox overnight, then centrifuged in a Wintrobe hematocrit tube. Normally, less than 2% of precipitate will be found. To test for cryofibrinogen, heparinized plasma is used for the same procedure. Macroglobulins are screened by the Sia test, which is actually a test for euglobulin. The procedure consists very simply of adding a drop of the patient's serum to distilled water. Most of the macroglobulins are insoluble in water, so that the formation of a precipitate suggests the presence of macroglobulins. The test is not very reliable.

Thus far, discussion has concerned the serum proteins in general. There is a special category known as lipoproteins which are combinations of various lipids with the plasma proteins. Lipids, in general, are insoluble in water and most biologic fluids, and depend for transport on binding to various plasma proteins. Nonesterified fatty acids comprise about 5% of the blood lipid, are mostly carried by serum albumin, and seem to provide a readily available and excellent source of energy when carbohydrate is deficient. The other blood lipids are bound to globulin in various proportions and are known as lipoproteins. The lowest-density lipoproteins are also those of the largest molecular size and are known as chylomicrons. These are composed mainly of triglycerides with a thin covering of protein and are the particles which are initially formed after intestinal fat absorption and which give the plasma at that time its char-

TABLE 9.—MAJOR LIPOPROTEIN SUBGROUPS

| Lipid-Protein Fractions | Ultracentrifuge $S_f$ | Ultracentrifuge Specific Gravity | Electrophoresis | Composition |
|---|---|---|---|---|
| Chylomicrons | 400-40,000 | - | Neutral fat zone (point of application) | About 80% triglycerides |
| Very low-density (beta) lipoproteins | 20-400 | Less than 1.006 | Pre-beta | About half triglycerides, half cholesterol and phospholipid |
| Low-density (beta) lipoproteins | 10-20<br>0-10 | 1.006-1.019<br>1.019-1.063 | Beta<br>Beta | About half cholesterol, remainder predominantly phospholipid and protein |
| High-density (alpha) lipoproteins | - | Over 1.063 | Alpha | About half protein, remainder predominantly cholesterol and phospholipid |
| Albumin-unesterified fatty acids | - | - | - | - |

acteristic milky appearance. The chylomicrons are eventually broken down enzymatically into unesterified fatty acids and other lipid fractions. There is a class of intermediate although still relatively low-density lipoproteins which are bound to beta globulins and which are composed predominantly of cholesterol with smaller amounts of phospholipids and triglycerides. These are known as low-density beta lipoproteins. The highest-density molecules are also the smallest. These are bound to the alpha-1 globulin and are composed predominantly of protein with smaller amounts of cholesterol, phospholipids, and triglycerides. They are alpha or high-density lipoproteins. Serum lipids may be determined chemically or by paper electrophoresis. On electrophoresis, the results usually are reported in terms of immobile lipid, beta lipoprotein, and alpha lipoprotein. This corresponds to low-density, medium-density, and high-density lipoproteins respectively (Table 9).

There has been much recent interest in the significance of the lipoproteins in atherosclerosis and, indirectly, in myocardial infarction. Large numbers of studies have been carried out, various populations have been examined, various diets have been tried, and endless pages of statistics have been published. Summarizing this material, there is general but not unanimous agreement that when the beta lipoproteins are elevated there seems to be an increased tendency toward atherosclerosis, and therefore of myocardial infarct. In addition, many believe that serum triglyceride elevation has an equal significance. Since the beta lipoproteins are the main carriers of serum cholesterol, again without unanimous agreement the majority of investigators believe that the serum cholesterol can be used as an indirect measure of the beta lipoprotein and, therefore, as one parameter of increased atherogenic risk. However, certain factors have to be kept in mind. First, it has been shown that cholesterol levels may deviate 10% from mean values during any 24-hour period and show differences of 5-50 mg. /100 ml. in day-to-day variation. Some individuals display even greater changes. It has also been found that there is a well-documented tendency by the serum lipids, especially cholesterol, to fluctuate considerably for as much as 2 months after myocardial infarct. Therefore, values taken soon after a myocardial infarct may not be representative of the patient's usual levels. Third, the normal values which are quoted vary considerably from one population to the next depending on diet, heredity, age, sex, and even types of occupation where stress is a factor. For example, normal values for an average American population (Table 9a) are considerably higher than those for an average Japanese group. Normal values for total cholesterol which are probably near the true normal range are 150-250 mg. /100 ml.; those for average American populations are 150-300 mg. /100 ml. Finally, the technical aspects of lipid and cholesterol determination are very important. Many methods for cholesterol determination are in use, and surveys have shown disturbingly great fluctuation among values of different laboratories using either these different methods or even the same method. Accuracy for serum cholesterol has been relatively poor except under rigid quality control

### TABLE 9a.—LIPID NORMAL VALUES

| Age | Total Cholesterol (mg./100 ml.) | Triglycerides (mg./100 ml.) |
|---|---|---|
| 1-19 | 120-230 | 10-140 |
| 20-29 | 120-240 | 10-140 |
| 30-39 | 140-270 | 10-150 |
| 40-49 | 150-310 | 10-160 |
| 50-59 | 160-330 | 10-190 |

programs and with certain standard methods, and sometimes not even then. If one is to rely on cholesterol values, he should know the laboratory to which he sends patients and find out how they run their controls and what variation they expect from duplicate samples. Triglyceride values have been shown in laboratory surveys to be generally even less reproducible than those for cholesterol. It becomes even more necessary to send triglycerides to a reliable laboratory. Therefore, diet or other treatment may be given credit for moderate decreases in cholesterol, whereas in reality it may be due to physiologic or laboratory variability. Other diseases which characteristically cause high cholesterol are idiopathic hypercholesterolemia, biliary cirrhosis, hypothyroidism, and the nephrotic syndrome.

The lipoprotein disease classification (Fig. 12a) proposed by Frederickson's group is now becoming standard.

Tests useful in establishing and categorizing lipoprotein disease include inspection of serum (after it has been kept overnight at ice-box temperature), cholesterol, triglyceride, lipoprotein electrophoresis, and ultracentrifugation. Visual inspection, cholesterol, and triglyceride are the most important; they serve as screening procedures and in many cases as diagnostic tests. Normal values for all three are reasonable evidence (although not completely so) against serious lipoprotein disease (Table 9b).

### TABLE 9b.—PROBABILITY OF DETECTING HYPERLIPOPROTEINEMIA BY LIPID ANALYSIS ALONE

| Type | Percentage Detectable by Lipid Concentration | | |
|---|---|---|---|
| | Abnormal Cholesterol | Abnormal Triglyceride | Abnormal Cholesterol or Triglyceride |
| I | 80 | 100 | 100 |
| II | 89 | 24 | 92 |
| III | 82 | 91 | 91 |
| IV | 22 | 100 | 100 |
| V | 61 | 100 | 100 |

From Frederickson, D. S., et al.: The Typing of Hyperlipoproteinemia: A Progress Report (1968), in Holmes, W. L., et al. (eds.): Drugs Affecting Lipid Metabolism (New York: Plenum Press, 1969).

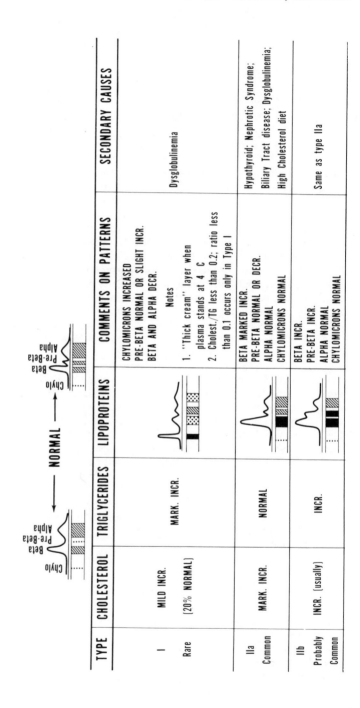

| TYPE | CHOLESTEROL | TRIGLYCERIDES | LIPOPROTEINS | COMMENTS ON PATTERNS | SECONDARY CAUSES |
|---|---|---|---|---|---|
| I<br>Rare | MILD INCR.<br>(20% NORMAL) | MARK. INCR. | | CHYLOMICRONS INCREASED<br>PRE-BETA NORMAL OR SLIGHT INCR.<br>BETA AND ALPHA DECR.<br>Notes<br>1. "Thick cream" layer when plasma stands at 4 C<br>2. Cholest./TG less than 0.2; ratio less than 0.1 occurs only in Type I | Dysglobulinemia |
| IIa<br>Common | MARK. INCR. | NORMAL | | BETA MARKED INCR.<br>PRE-BETA NORMAL OR DECR.<br>ALPHA NORMAL<br>CHYLOMICRONS NORMAL | Hypothyroid; Nephrotic Syndrome;<br>Biliary Tract disease; Dysglobulinemia;<br>High Cholesterol diet |
| IIb<br>Probably<br>Common | INCR. (usually) | INCR. | | BETA INCR.<br>PRE-BETA INCR.<br>ALPHA NORMAL<br>CHYLOMICRONS NORMAL | Same as type IIa |

| | | | Pattern | Description / Notes | Diseases |
|---|---|---|---|---|---|
| III Uncommon | INCR. (20% NORMAL) | INCR. (10% NORMAL) | 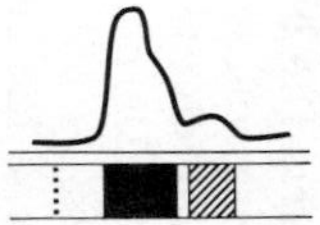 | BETA INCR. ("BROAD BETA" IN 2/3 CASES) PRE-BETA NORMAL OR MILD INCR. ALPHA NORMAL CHYLOMICRONS NORMAL — Notes: Need ultracentrifugation for diagnosis (Demonstration of "floating beta") | Diabetes Mellitus; Hepatic Disease |
| IV Most Common | NORMAL (20% INCR.) | INCR. | 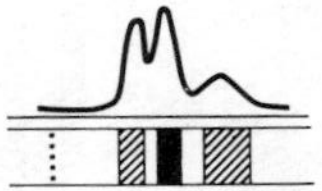 | PRE-BETA MOD. OR MARK. INCR. BETA AND ALPHA NORMAL OR MILD DECR. CHYLOMICRONS NORMAL — Notes: Sometimes called "Carbohydrate-induced hyperlipemia" | Hypothyroid; Nephrotic Syndrome; Pregnancy; Estrogen; Diabetes Mellitus; Pancreatitis; Dysglobulinemia |
| V Uncommon | INCR. (40% NORMAL) | INCR. | 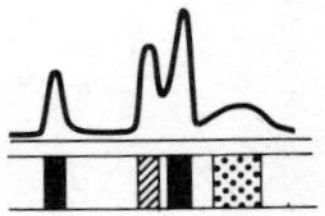 | PRE-BETA INCR. BETA AND ALPHA DECR. CHYLOMICRONS INCR. — Notes: 1. "Thick cream" layer 2. Cholest./TG ratio usually above 0.15 when plasma stands at 4° C. | Pancreatitis; Alcoholism; Diabetes Mellitus |

Fig. 12a.—Classification of lipoproteinemias.

If visual inspection discloses a cream-like precipitate of chylomicrons, normal cholesterol and triglycerides signify Frederickson type I whereas elevation of either points toward type V. Likewise, if serum has normal chylomicron content, elevation of cholesterol with normal triglyceride is type II, whereas the opposite means type IV. If both cholesterol and triglyceride are significantly abnormal, this may be type II or type III. Type II has recently been subdivided into IIa and IIb. IIa has increased beta and cholesterol but normal pre-beta and triglyceride. Type IIb has elevated cholesterol, triglyceride, beta, and pre-beta. Type III is uncommon; it is similar to IIb in that both cholesterol and triglyceride are elevated, but it frequently has a slightly different electrophoretic pattern ("broad beta") and always has a peculiar "floating beta" component (a beta-mobility protein which floats at 1.006 density instead of 1.013) which can only be demonstrated by ultracentrifugation. Types II and IV constitute the majority of lipoproteinemias; V is less common, and I and III are uncommon.

Type IV is probably more common than II. Most type IV patients have the acquired form. Type II is more frequently congenital than is type IV; however, the majority of type II patients have the acquired form, the most common etiology being a high cholesterol diet.

Some specimens from patients with types IIb, III, or IV may be somewhat cloudy or faintly milky in appearance; this must be differentiated from the thicker, cream-like precipitate of increased chylomicrons.

Lipoprotein electrophoresis is not absolutely necessary to categorize many patients; however, it is useful to confirm the diagnosis and to help separate types IIa, IIb, III, and some cases of IV. In classic cases, type III displays a "broad beta" band which obliterates the normal valley between beta and pre-beta peaks. Definitive diagnosis of type III must be done by ultracentrifugation.

Certain considerations affect interpretation of these lab results. Patients should be on a normal diet for several days previously and must be fasting at least 10 hours. If a test cannot be done the same day, the serum must be refrigerated but not frozen; freezing alters pre-beta and chylomicron fractions, although cholesterol and triglyceride determinations can be done. Certain lipoprotein types can be caused by specific diseases; in such a case, treatment must be directed primarily toward the etiologic disease. Normal range for cholesterol and triglyceride is age-related. Although there is no agreement as to what values are truly normal, Table 9a (above) lists normal ranges according to Frederickson. Because of laboratory technical limitations, one must be cautious in attributing significance to borderline results.

Plasma or serum may be used for lipoprotein analysis. Plasma collected with EDTA is preferred if the specimen cannot be tested the same day.

Two rare diseases display characteristic lipoprotein electrophoresis patterns. Tangier disease has no alpha peak. Bassen-
Kornsweg disease (associated with "pin-cushion" RBC called acantho-
cytes and neurologic abnormalities) lacks a beta peak.

## REFERENCES

Beaumont, J. L., et al.: Classification of hyperlipidaemias and
hyperlipoproteinaemias, Bull. World Health Organ. 43:891, 1970.
Bernier, G. M.: Adult hypogammaglobulinemia, Am. J. Med.
36:618, 1964.
Burgert, W., Jr.: Alpha-1 antitrypsin deficiency, Postgrad. Med.
47:63, 1970.
Cannon, D. C.: Immunoglobulin analysis in clinical diagnosis.
1. Quantitative methods, Postgrad. Med. 46:55, 1969.
Castelli, W. P., and Moran, R. F.: Lipid studies for assessing
the risk of cardiovascular disease and hyperlipidemia, Human
Path. 2:153, 1971.
Causey, J. Q.: IgG paraproteinemia associated with bronchogenic
carcinoma. Arch. Int. Med. 119:407, 1967.
Delaney, W. E.: Identification and quantitation of immunoglobulins,
Ann. Clin. Lab. Sc. 2:75, 1972.
Fessel, W. J., et al.: What is the albumin level? Arch. Int. Med.
114:547, 1964.
Fredrickson, D. S., et al.: Fat transport in lipoproteins—An inte-
grated approach to mechanisms and disorders, New England J.
Med. 276:34, 94, 148, 215, 273, 1967.
Frederickson, D. S., et al.: The Typing of Hyperlipoproteinemia:
A Progress Report (1968), in Holmes, W. L., et al. (eds.): Drugs
Affecting Lipid Metabolism (New York: Plenum Press, 1969).
Ishizaka, K.: Identification and significance of gamma E, Hosp.
Practice 4:70, 1969.
Kagan, B. M., and Stern, J. R.: Blood protein measurements in
diagnosis of disease, Pediat. Clin. North America 2:265, 1955.
Korngold, L.: Plasma Proteins: Methods in Study and Changes in
Diseases, in Stefanini, M. (ed.): Advances in Clinical Pathology
(New York: Grune & Stratton, Inc., 1966), Vol. 1, p. 340.
Kyle, R. A., and Bayrd, E. D.: "Benign" monoclonal gammopathy:
A potentially malignant condition? Am. J. Med. 40:426, 1966.
Kyle, R. A., et al.: Diagnosis of syndromes associated with hyper-
globulinemia, M. Clin. North America 54:917, 1970.
Leonardy, J. G.: Serum protein electrophoresis in office practice,
South. M. J. 64:129, 1971.
Lipo, J. F., and Preston, J. A.: Lipoprotein phenotyping, CRC
Critical Reviews in Clin. Lab. Sc. 2:461, 1971.
Martin, N. H.: The immunoglobulins: A review, J. Clin. Path.
22:117, 1969.

Mattioli, C., and Tomasi, T. B., Jr.: Human Serum Immuno-globulins, in Dowling, H. F. (ed.): Disease-a-Month (Chicago: Year Book Medical Publishers, Inc., April 1970).

Michaux, J., and Heremans, J. F.: Thirty cases of monoclonal immunoglobulin disorders other than myeloma or macroglobulinemia, Am. J. Med. 46:562, 1969.

Osserman, E. F., and Takatsuki, K.: Plasma cell myeloma: Gamma globulin synthesis and structure, Medicine 42:357, 1963.

Pruzansky, W., and Ogryzlo, M. A.: Changing pattern of diseases associated with M components, M. Clin. North America 56:371, 1972.

Ravel, R.: Serum protein electrophoresis in cirrhosis, Am. J. Gastroenterol. 52:509, 1969.

Ritzmann, S. E., and Levin, W. C.: Cryopathies: A review, Arch. Int. Med. 107:754, 1961.

Sharp, H. L.: Alpha-1 antitrypsin deficiency, Hosp. Practice 6:83, 1971.

Spiro, R. G.: Glycoproteins: Structure, metabolism, and biology, New England J. Med. 269:566, 616, 1963.

Terry, W. D., and Fahey, J. L.: Principles of Immunoelectrophoresis and Application to the Evaluation of Serum Gamma Globulins, in Sunderman, F. W., and Sunderman, F. W., Jr. (eds.): Serum Proteins and the Dysproteinemias (Philadelphia: J. B. Lippincott Company, 1964), p. 183.

Williams, R. C., Jr., et al.: Studies of "benign" serum M-components, Am. J. M. Sc. 257:275, 1969.

Zawadzki, Z. A., and Edwards, G. A.: Dysimmunoglobulinemia in the absence of clinical features of multiple myeloma and macroglobulinemia, Am. J. Med. 42:67, 1967.

Zawadzki, Z. A., and Edwards, G. A.: Pseudoparaproteinemia due to hypertransferrinemia, Am. J. Clin. Path. 54:802, 1970.

Zawadzki, Z. A., and Edwards, G. A.: Dysimmunoglobulinemia associated with hepatobiliary disorders, Am. J. Med. 48:196, 1970.

# CHAPTER 22

# Rheumatoid-Collagen Diseases

The relationship between the rheumatoid diseases and those of the so-called collagen-vascular group is both close and uncertain. Many of the clinical symptoms found classically in one disease or syndrome may be found in another; the difference is on emphasis of certain aspects over others. This similarity extends to laboratory tests, and makes even more difficult the separation of borderline or problem cases into one clear-cut group or the other. Until the exact etiology of each disease is known, things are likely to continue in this fashion. It may be that a common mechanism is operating which affects different target organs or tissues in different people; this would help to explain the spectrum of clinical and laboratory findings which become evident in large series of cases. Fortunately, most patients can be assigned to satisfactory categories using available clinical and laboratory data.

When disease primarily affects joints, the clinical history, age, pattern and location of the involved joint, and sometimes findings from direct joint aspiration, may all help. Gout usually involves single specific joints (usually including some of the small joints of the extremities), has an elevated serum uric acid, and responds specifically to colchicine. Septic arthritis is diagnosed by direct aspiration and culture of joint fluid. Pseudogout clinically somewhat resembles gout, but affects large joints such as the knee rather than small peripheral joints. Joint x-rays indicate some differences from classic gout.

In these three diseases, and rheumatoid arthritis in addition, joint aspiration may be a considerable aid in diagnosis. For cell counts and microscopic examination, some of the fluid should be placed in an anticoagulant. In septic arthritis, the fluid is characteristically purulent. In gout, urate crystals often are found within neutrophils or lying free. In pseudogout, calcium pyrophosphate crystals are found within phagocytes. Rheumatoid arthritis may also show small inclusions within phagocytes, and the joint fluid often gives a positive test for rheumatoid factor, sometimes even before the serum.

Although elevated uric acid is characteristic of gout, more uric acid elevations are due to other diseases than to gout. Perhaps the most frequent etiology in hospitalized patients is chronic renal disease with azotemia. Other conditions frequently associated with increased uric acid levels include tumors of blood cells (leukemia, polycythemia vera, and other myeloproliferative diseases), especially during treatment; therapy with thiazide diuretics; and eclampsia.

In active rheumatoid arthritis (RA), hemoglobin may be normal or mildly decreased. Uric acid is normal. The major advance in diagnosis during the past 15 years has been widespread use of serologic tests. It seems that in rheumatoid arthritis and related diseases, a medium-weight globulin is produced which is called the rheumatoid factor (RF). This has the ability to combine in vitro with normal gamma globulin. Complement is fixed during the reaction. Therefore, various types of serologic tests may be set up using this basic reaction, differing mainly in the type of indicator system used to visually demonstrate results. The original test was known as the sensitized sheep cell method, using antisheep RBC antibodies to combine with sheep RBC, then allowing the rheumatoid factor in the patient's serum to combine with the antibody gamma globulin coating the sheep cells. A positive result showed clumping of the RBC. It was found subsequently that synthetic particles such as latex could be coated with gamma globulin and the coated particles clumped by rheumatoid factor, thus giving a flocculation test. Just as happened with the STS for syphilis (p. 374), many combinations of ingredients have been tried with resulting variation in sensitivity and specificity—too many to discuss individually. However, one must make a distinction between tube tests and rapid slide tests, since the slide tests in general have a slightly greater sensitivity but correspondingly less specificity. They should be used mainly for screening purposes. The latex fixation tube test for rheumatoid arthritis, known also as the Plotz-Singer latex test, today is the most widely used and standard method. The average sensitivity in well-established clinical cases of adult RA is about 76% (range 53-94%). Normal controls average about 1% positive. For comparison, a widely used commercial latex slide test (Hyland "RA-test") averages about 89% positive in known adult RA cases, but reportedly averages about 10% positive in normal controls. Besides a certain small percentage of Plotz-Singer false positives in apparently normal persons, certain diseases give a significantly high number of reactions in a manner analogous to the "biologic false positive" of syphilis serology. These include collagen diseases, sarcoidosis, syphilis, various liver diseases including cirrhosis and hepatitis, and certain more rare diseases. The conditions mentioned average 10-40%, depending on the particular disease, the collagen-vascular group being highest (p. 446).

The opposite problem occurs in juvenile rheumatoid arthritis. Apparently rheumatoid factor takes some time to develop measurable activity, and even in patients with onset in adult age there is correlation both with duration and activity of the disease, most positive cases having active symptoms more than 6 months. There is no correlation with severity of symptoms. Standard rheumatoid arthritis tests yield from 5 to 40% positives in juvenile rheumatoid arthritis. Roughly the same percentages are reactive in the so-called RA variants, patients with certain diseases such as psoriasis, ulcerative colitis, and Reiter's syndrome, who have symptoms identical to rheumatoid arthritis in a certain proportion of cases.

Collagen-Vascular Diseases: This is an ill-defined collection of syndromes which have certain points of similarity, among which the most striking are fibrinoid necrosis of collagenous tissue and involvement of various subdivisions of arteries by an inflammatory process. Some diseases emphasize one of these aspects and some the other. The main connection between these often quite dissimilar syndromes is the probability that basic etiology of them all is some manifestation of an immunologic hypersensitivity disorder. Since the three most common diseases in this group are disseminated lupus erythematosus, polyarteritis nodosa, and scleroderma, these three will be briefly discussed from the laboratory point of view.

Lupus erythematosus features various combinations of facial skin rash, arthritis, nephritis, systemic symptoms such as fever and malaise, and inflammation of serous membranes such as the pericardium. The disease is by far most frequent in women, predominantly young or middle-aged adults. Hepatomegaly is found in about 30% of patients, splenomegaly in nearly 20%, and adenopathy in nearly 50%. There is anemia in up to 80% of patients, mostly of moderate degree, but which uncommonly is severe and hemolytic. WBC are classically slightly to moderately lower than normal, but not always. Thrombocytopenia is present in a large minority of cases. There are often one or more manifestations of abnormal plasma proteins; these may include cold-precipitating cryoglobulins, circulating anticoagulants, autoantibodies, elevated gamma globulins, "false positive" rheumatoid arthritis and syphilis serology (STS) reactions, and certain even rarer phenomena.

The most useful test in lupus, and the one which a definitive diagnosis usually requires, is the lupus erythematosus (L. E.) cell preparation. This depends on the fact that a so-called antinuclear factor is produced in lupus which somehow reacts with nuclei of damaged cells, either of tissue or blood cell type. The nuclear material is converted to a homogeneous amorphous mass which stains basophilic with Wright's stain. This mass is then phagocytized by polymorphonuclear neutrophils and the presence of these neutrophils

containing the hematoxylin (blue staining) bodies are the so-called
L. E. cells. These L. E. cells are considered by many to be specific
for lupus erythematosus with one exception, a syndrome identical to
ordinary lupus which is produced by hypersensitivity to the drug
hydralazine (Apresoline). Nevertheless, one report indicates that
patients taking more than 1.5 Gm. of procainamide per day develop
positive L. E. preps in 50% of cases and antinuclear antibodies in
75%. Others believe that L. E. cells are not diagnostic of lupus—
only strongly suggestive. It is true that L. E. cells have been reported in certain other drug sensitivity cases, but some believe
these were not true L. E. cells. Certain patients with chronic liver
disease have occasionally demonstrated L. E. cells, but the possibility that these patients may in addition have had subclinical lupus
never has been completely ruled out. This has been made into a
syndrome called "lupoid hepatitis," although some of these patients
had cirrhosis rather than chronic hepatitis. The syndrome is not
universally accepted. Cases also are reported from time to time when
patients with classic rheumatoid arthritis or one of the other collagen
diseases produce a few L. E. cells. In rheumatoid arthritis, some
report an incidence which reaches 15-20%. Again, in some of these
patients it is almost a matter of philosophy whether one calls them
rheumatoid arthritis with L. E. cells, or lupus with predominantly
rheumatoid-type symptoms. Finally, artifacts may be confused with
true L. E. cells. To be definitive, the basophilic hematoxylin body
must be completely amorphous, without any remaining nuclear structure whatever. In many situations, one finds examples of neutrophils
with phagocytized nuclear material which still retains some identity
as a nucleus, such as residual chromatin pattern. These are not
true L. E. cells, and are called "tart cells." Increased numbers of
these may be seen in lupus, but do not have any diagnostic significance. Also confused by inexperienced persons are neutrophils
with ingested RBC.

L. E. preps may be done by different methods; their common
denominator is some way to traumatize a number of the WBC. After
this, there is an incubation period while the nuclei of the damaged
cells are converted to hematoxylin bodies and then ingested by some
of the living neutrophils. The preparation is centrifuged; smears of
the neutrophil layer are made and, after Wright's stain, are searched
for L. E. cells. When hematoxylin bodies are formed, sometimes
groups of neutrophils are found surrounding one of the bodies preparatory to one neutrophil phagocytizing it. These groupings are
called rosettes, and are considered by some as equal in importance
to true L. E. cells; others insist on finding classic L. E. cells for
definite diagnosis. It must be emphasized that the L. E. phenomenon
is often very intermittent, sometimes present for varying periods,
and sometimes absent. There is some correlation to the activity of
the disease, but not entirely. It is possible (although not usual) to
have positive L. E. preps one day and not the next, and sometimes

several preps done the same day may have both positive and negative results.  This seems due to the nature of the disease, the
strictly empirical nature of the test, and, to some extent, the technical aspects of the test itself.  Adrenocortical steroid treatment
often suppresses L. E. cell production.

The antinuclear factor responsible for the L. E. cell phenomenon is not the only autoantibody or "factor" demonstrable in systemic lupus.  A wide variety of such factors has been demonstrated,
reactive against either nuclear or cytoplasmic constituents with
varying degrees of tissue and cellular constituent specificity.  Fluorescent tests for antinuclear antibodies (ANA) have been devised,
using a variety of methods to obtain suitable nuclei.  Most of these
tests are positive in over 95% of lupus patients, whereas the L. E.
prep is positive in 60-80% of patients, depending on several factors
such as duration, activity, and severity of disease (p. 447).  The
L. E. prep is currently still the most specific test for systemic
lupus erythematosus, although there is some dispute as to how specific the L. E. prep actually is.  Nevertheless, the high sensitivity
of the fluorescent antinuclear antibody test makes it much more efficient for screening than the L. E. prep.  If the fluorescent ANA
test is negative, chances of a positive L. E. prep are very low.
Since any test has the possibility of technical error, a negative
ANA in a patient with high suspicion of lupus should be repeated.

Polyarteritis nodosa features inflammation of small and me-
dium-sized arteries.  Single organs or multiple systems may be involved, although usually the lungs are spared.  The kidney is the
most frequent to show abnormalities, with hematuria the main sign.
Hypertension is fairly common.  Laboratory studies usually show a
moderate leukocytosis having neutrophilic increase and immaturity
of the ordinary type seen with infections.  Mild anemia is also common.  There often is an increase in serum gamma globulin.  The
main diagnostic procedure is biopsy.  The most common type is
muscle biopsy and the usual region is the gastrocnemius because it
is easy to reach.  However, if biopsy is done, it should be from
some muscle with a painful area if any are present; random samples
give poor results.  The biopsy should be generous, since the lesions
of polyarteritis lie in small arteries.  The incidence of positive
single muscle biopsies in fairly definite cases of polyarteritis ranges
from 20 to 40%; obviously, it will be on the lower side in mild or
questionable cases.  Another difficulty is that occasionally patients
with classic RA may have arteritis nearly identical to polyarteritis.
Lupus also may have arteritis, but the lesions tend to be more in
arterioles.  Other more rare syndromes of the collagen-vascular
group may create histologic difficulty.  Therefore, the clinical picture has as much importance as the biopsy report.

Scleroderma (progressive systemic sclerosis) leads to progressive dense connective tissue replacement of certain areas which
normally contain only small amounts of loose collagen.  These in-

clude the dermis of the skin, the submucosa of the esophagus or
other parts of the gastrointestinal tract, and the heart. The lungs
frequently develop a slowly progressive type of diffuse fibrosis,
radiologically most prominent in the lung bases. In addition, the
kidneys are often affected by a somewhat different histologic process, similar to malignant hypertension. The disease is most common in middle-aged women. Clinically, the skin changes produce
tautness and lack of elasticity; this most often occurs in the hand
and is often accompanied by Raynaud's phenomenon. Esophageal
involvement leads to dysphagia, while small bowel changes may produce localized dilatation. Laboratory tests show the hemoglobin to
be most often normal. There may be an increased erythrocyte sedimentation rate, and there may be associated hypergammaglobulinemia of a diffuse type, although this is not a constant feature.
Scleroderma produces a relatively high incidence of positive rheumatoid factor tests and also of biologic false positive syphilis serologies.
Diagnosis usually can be made clinically, but may be suggested by
barium swallow esophageal x-rays in patients who have esophageal
symptoms. Biopsy of an affected skin area is the procedure of
choice if the diagnosis cannot be made clinically.

Acute rheumatic fever (ARF) is a disease which has a specific
etiologic agent and yet demonstrates some similarity with the rheu-
matoid-collagen-vascular group. The etiologic agent is the beta hemolytic Lancefield group A streptococcus. Apparent hypersensitivity
or other effect of this organism causes connective tissue changes
manifested by focal necrosis of collagen and the development of peculiar aggregates of histiocytes, "Aschoff bodies." Symptoms of
ARF include fever, a migratory type of polyarthritis, and frequent
development of cardiac damage manifested either by symptoms or
only by electrocardiographic changes. Diagnosis or confirmation of
diagnosis often rests on appropriate laboratory tests. Throat culture should be attempted; the finding of beta hemolytic streptococci,
Lancefield group A, would be a strong point in favor of the diagnosis,
if the clinical picture is highly suggestive. However, throat cultures
are often negative. Blood cultures are almost always negative. Beta
streptococci produce an enzyme known as streptolysin-O. About 7-
10 days after infection, antibodies to this material begin to appear.
Highest incidence of positive tests is during the third week after onset of ARF. At this time, 90-95% abnormal results are obtained;
thereafter, the antibody titer drops steadily. At the end of 2 months
only 70-75% are positive; at 6 months, 35%; at 12 months, 20%.
Therefore, since the streptococcus most often cannot be isolated,
antistreptolysin titers of over 200 Todd units may be helpful evidence
of a recent infection. However, this does not actually prove that the
disease in question is ARF or that the streptococcal infection which
produced the antibodies was recent enough to cause the present symptoms. The erythrocyte sedimentation rate (ESR) is usually elevated
during the clinical course of ARF and is a useful indication of cur-

rent activity of the disease. However, the ESR is very nonspecific and only indicates an active inflammatory process somewhere in the body. In a minority of ARF patients, peculiar subcutaneous nodules develop, most often near the elbows. These are composed of focal collagen necrosis surrounded by palisading of histiocytes. In some cases, therefore, biopsy of these nodules may help confirm the diagnosis of ARF. However, biopsy is not usually done if other methods make the diagnosis reasonably certain. Also, the nodules are histologically similar to those of rheumatoid arthritis. During the acute phase of the disease there usually is a moderate leukocytosis, and most often there is a mild-to-moderate anemia.

## REFERENCES

Alarcon-Segovia, D. , et al. : Significance of the lupus erythematosus phenomenon in older women with chronic hepatic disease, Mayo Clin. Proc. 40:193, 1965.

Bianchi, F. A. , and Keech, M. K. : Comparison of two slide tests in rheumatoid arthritis, J. A. M. A. 185:318, 1963.

Bloch, K. J. : Recent modifications in serological tests for rheumatoid arthritis, Bull. Rheumat. Dis. 9:185, 1959.

Caplan, H. I. : The use of latex fixation tests in non-rheumatic states, Ann. Int. Med. 59:449, 1963.

Feinstein, A. R. : The natural histories of acute rheumatic fever, Bull. Rheumatic. Dis. 17:423, 1966.

Goldgraber, M. B. , and Kirsner, J. B. : Scleroderma of the gastrointestinal tract: A review, A. M. A. Arch. Path. 64:255, 1957.

Hall, A. P. : Serologic tests in rheumatoid arthritis, M. Clin. North America 45:1181, 1961.

Hoffbauer, F. W. : Lupoid hepatitis, Postgrad. Med. 38:376, 1965.

Hollander, J. E. (ed.): Arthritis (7th ed. ; Philadelphia: Lea & Febiger, 1966).

Holman, H. R. : The L. E. Cell Phenomenon, in Rytand, D. H. and Creger, W. P. (eds.): Annual Review of Medicine (Palo Alto, Calif. : Annual Reviews, Inc. , 1960), Vol. 11, p. 231.

Lane, J. J. , Jr. , and Decker, J. L. : Latex particle slide tests in rheumatoid arthritis, J. A. M. A. 173:982, 1960.

Maxeiner, S. R. , Jr. , et al. : Muscle biopsy in the diagnosis of periarteritis nodosa: An evaluation, S. Clin. North America 32:1225, 1952.

Mills, L. C. , and Moyer, J. H. (eds.): Inflammation and Diseases of Connective Tissue (Philadelphia: W. B. Saunders Company, 1961).

Primer on the Rheumatic Diseases (6th ed. ; New York: The Arthritis Foundation, 1964).

Rothfield, N. F. : The role of antinuclear reactions in the diagnosis of systemic lupus erythematosus: A study of 53 cases, Arthritis & Rheumat. 4:223, 1961.

Rothfield, N. F. : Serologic tests in rheumatic diseases, Postgrad.
    Med. 45:116, 1969.
Singer, J. M. : The latex fixation test in rheumaticoid diseases. A
    review, Am. J. Med. 31:766, 1961.
Stevens, M. B. , et al. : The clinical significance of extracellular
    material (ECM) in LE-cell preparations, New England J. Med.
    268:976, 1963.
Symposium on Periarteritis Nodosa, Proc. Staff Meet. Mayo Clin.
    24:17, 1949.
Wilkinson, M. , and Sacker, L. S. : The lupus erythematosus cell
    and its significance, Brit. M. J. 2:661, 1957.

# CHAPTER 23

# Acid-Base and pH

Fluid and electrolyte problems are common in hospitalized patients. In general, most of these situations are produced secondary to other disease processes or as undesirable side effects of therapy. In addition, a few diseases characteristically lead to certain electrolyte alterations which are important for diagnosis and treatment.

Fluid and electrolytes in one form or another comprise nearly all of the human body. It is useful to think of these constituents as though they were contained in three separate compartments among which are variable degrees of communication: individual cells, containing intracellular fluid; vascular channels, containing blood or lymph; and the extracellular nonvascular tissue components, the interstitial fluid. Shifts of fluid and electrolytes between and within these compartments take place continually as the various activities concerned with hemostasis, cell metabolism, and organ function go on. These changes can, to some degree, be monitored clinically by their effects on certain measurable parameters, including the pH and concentration of certain ions ("electrolyes") in a fairly accessible substance, the blood. This chapter will cover blood pH and its disturbances, while the next chapter will take up certain electrolyte and fluid disorders.

Blood pH comes from the French words puissance hydrogen, meaning the strength or power of hydrogen. The hydrogen ion concentration of blood expressed in terms of gram molecular weights of hydrogen per liter (mols/liter) is so much less than 1 (for example, 0.0000001) that it is easier to communicate this information in terms of logarithms (thus the previous example becoming $1 \times 10^{-7}$). The symbol pH simplifies this even more, because pH is defined as the negative logarithm of the hydrogen ion concentration (in the preceding example, $1 \times 10^{-7}$ becomes $10^{-7}$ which then becomes 7.0). In this way, a relatively simple scale is substituted for very cumbersome tiny numbers. In the pH scale, therefore, a change of 1.0 pH unit means a tenfold change in hydrogen ion concentration (7.0 to 6.0 means $10^{-7}$ to $10^{-6}$ mols/liter).

The normal pH of arterial blood is 7.4, with a normal range between 7.36 and 7.44. It seems that blood pH must be maintained within relatively narrow limits, because pH outside the range 6.8 to 7.8 is incompatible with life. Therefore, hydrogen ion content is regulated by a series of buffer substances. A buffer is a substance which can bind hydrogen ions to a certain extent without developing marked change in pH. Among substances which act as buffers are hemoglobin, plasma protein, phosphates, and the bicarbonate-carbonic acid system. Bicarbonate is by far the body's most important buffer substance; it is present in large quantities and can be controlled by the lungs and kidneys.

A brief review of the bicarbonate-carbonic acid system recalls that carbon dioxide in aqueous solution exists in potential equilibrium with carbonic acid ($CO_2 + H_2O \rightleftharpoons H_2CO_3$). The enzyme carbonic anhydrase catalyzes this reaction toward attainment of equilibrium; otherwise, the rate of reaction would be minimal. Carbon dioxide is produced by cellular metabolism and released into the blood stream. There, most of it diffuses into the red blood cells where carbonic anhydrase catalyzes its hydration to carbonic acid ($H_2CO_3$). Carbonic acid readily dissociates into H+ and $HCO_3^-$ ions. Eventually, only a small amount of dissolved $CO_2$ and a much smaller amount of undissociated carbonic acid remain in the plasma. Therefore, the great bulk of the original $CO_2$ (amounting to 75%) is carried in the blood as bicarbonate, with only about 5% still in solution (as dissolved $CO_2$ or undissociated $H_2CO_3$), and about 20% coupled with hemoglobin as a carbamino compound or, to a much lesser extent, with other buffers such as plasma proteins.

This situation can best be visualized by means of the Henderson-Hasselbalch equation. This states that pH = pK + log $\dfrac{Base}{Acid}$, where pK is the dissociation constant (ability to release hydrogen ions) of the particular acid chosen, such as carbonic acid. The derivation of this equation will be disregarded in order to concentrate on the clinically useful parts, the relationship of pH, base, and acid. If the bicarbonate-carbonic acid system is to be interpreted by means of the Henderson-Hasselbalch equation, then $\dfrac{Base}{Acid} = \dfrac{HCO_3^-}{H_2CO_3}$ since bicarbonate is the base and carbonic acid is the acid. Actually, most of the so-called carbonic acid represented in the equation is dissolved $CO_2$, which is present in plasma over 100 times the quantity of undissociated carbonic acid. Therefore, the formula should really be $\dfrac{HCO_3^-}{H_2CO_3 + CO_2}$, but it is customary to let $H_2CO_3$ stand for the entire denominator. The next step is to note from the Henderson-Hasselbalch equation that pH is proportional ($\cong$) to $\dfrac{Base}{Acid}$. This means that in the bicarbonate-carbonic acid system, $pH \cong \dfrac{HCO_3^-}{H_2CO_3}$.

The kidney is the main regulator of bicarbonate manufacture (the numerator) and the lungs primarily control $CO_2$ excretion (the equation denominator).

The kidney has several means of excreting hydrogen ions. One is the conversion of monohydrogen phosphate to dihydrogen phosphate ($HPO_4^=$ to $H_2PO_4^-$). Another is the formation of ammonia in renal tubule cells by deamination of certain amino acids such as glutamine. Ammonia ($NH_3$) then diffuses into the urine, where it combines with hydrogen ion to form ammonium ion ($NH_4^+$). A third mechanism is the one with which there is most concern now, the production of bicarbonate in the renal tubule cells. These cells possess carbonic anhydrase, which catalyzes the formation of carbonic acid ($H_2CO_3$) from $CO_2$. The carbonic acid dissociates, leaving bicarbonate ($HCO_3^-$) and hydrogen ion ($H^+$). The hydrogen ion is excreted in the urine by the phosphate or ammonium pathways or combined with some other anion. The bicarbonate goes into the blood stream where it forms part of the pH buffer system, as was already mentioned. Not only does bicarbonate assist in buffering hydrogen ions within body fluids, but bicarbonate which is filtered at the glomerulus into the urine can itself combine with urinary hydrogen ions (produced by the renal tubule cells from the carbonic acid cycle and excreted into the urine).

The lungs, on the other hand, take carbonic acid, change it to $CO_2$ and water with the aid of carbonic anhydrase, and blow off the $CO_2$. In this process, a mechanism for excreting $H^+$ ions exists, because the bicarbonate in the plasma can combine with free $H^+$ ions to form carbonic acid, which can then be eliminated from the lungs in the form of $CO_2$, as was just described. This process can probably handle excretion of most normal and mildly abnormal hydrogen ion quantities. However, when large excesses of free $H^+$ are present in body fluids, the kidney plays a major role, because not only are $H^+$ ions excreted directly in the urine, but bicarbonate is formed which helps buffer additional amounts of $H^+$ in the plasma.

Going back to the Henderson-Hasselbalch equation, which is now modified to indicate that pH is proportional ($\cong$) to $\dfrac{HCO_3^-}{H_2CO_3}$, it is easy to see that variations in either the numerator or denominator will change pH. If $HCO_3^-$ is increased without corresponding increase in $H_2CO_3$, the ratio will be increased and the pH will rise. Conversely, if something happens to increase $H_2CO_3$ or dissolved $CO_2$, the denominator will be increased, the ratio will be increased, the pH will fall, and so on. Clinically, an increase in normal plasma pH is called alkalosis and a decrease is called acidosis. The normal ratio of bicarbonate to carbonic acid is 20:1.

Next will be described the laboratory tests used in pH problems, which, incidentally, are often called acid-base because of the importance of bicarbonate and carbonic acid changes involved.

$CO_2$ combining power has been the usual laboratory test done because it is the easiest to obtain and to perform. Venous blood is drawn aerobically with an ordinary syringe and the serum is removed after clotting and centrifugation. The $CO_2$ tension of this serum is then equilibrated to normal alveolar levels of 40 mm. Hg by simply having the technician blow his own alveolar air into the specimen through a tube arrangement. This maneuver adjusts the amount of dissolved carbon dioxide to the normal amounts found in normal arterial blood. The bicarbonate of the serum is then converted to $CO_2$ by acid hydrolysis in a vacuum and the released gas is measured. The released $CO_2$ thus consists of the dissolved $CO_2$ of the specimen already present plus the converted bicarbonate (and thus the denominator plus the numerator of the Henderson-Hasselbalch equation). Subtraction of the known amount of dissolved $CO_2$ and $H_2CO_3$ in normal blood from this measurement gives what is essentially a value for serum bicarbonate alone (the so-called combining power since bicarbonate combines with $H^+$ ions). The inaccuracy that may be caused by these manipulations should be obvious. However, most laboratories continue to do this test because of convenience.

$CO_2$ content (total $CO_2$ content) is determined from heparinized arterial or venous blood which is drawn anaerobically. This may be done in a vacuum tube or a syringe which is quickly capped (mineral oil is not satisfactory for sealing). The blood is centrifuged and the plasma removed. At this point, all the carbon dioxide present is still at the same $CO_2$ tension or partial pressure of dissolved gas that the patient possessed. Next, the plasma is analyzed for $CO_2$ in a method which converts bicarbonate and carbonic acid to the gas form. Thus, $CO_2$ content measures the sum of bicarbonate, carbonic acid, and dissolved $CO_2$. Since the amount of dissolved $CO_2$ and $H_2CO_3$ in blood is very small, normal values for $CO_2$ content are quite close to those of the $CO_2$ combining power (which measures only bicarbonate). Since the specimen has been drawn and processed with little or no contact with the outside air, the result is obviously more accurate than that obtained from the $CO_2$ combining power.

A third method is one popularized by Astrup. This is based on the fact that most of the denominator of the Henderson-Hasselbalch equation is dissolved $CO_2$; since the partial pressure of $CO_2$ (the $pCO_2$) of the specimen is proportional to the amount of dissolved $CO_2$, the $pCO_2$ is therefore proportional to the denominator of the Henderson-Hasselbalch equation and may be used as a measure of the denominator. In practice, a small amount of whole blood (plasma can be used), collected anaerobically, is analyzed in a special apparatus for pH and for $pCO_2$. The bicarbonate may then be calculated (from the Henderson-Hasselbalch equation), or the $pCO_2$ value itself may be used in conjunction with pH to differentiate acid-base abnormalities.

pH has been quite a problem as far as laboratory technique is concerned. Most instruments measure the difference in electrical charge between two electrodes placed into the unknown solution, which in this case is plasma or whole blood. Unfortunately, the pH changes of blood are relatively very small, so that the instrument must be very sensitive. The more sensitive it is made, the more difficult to gain stability and reliability of results, since only a small error in the equipment may show up as a significant pH change. More recently, better machines have been put on the market, and direct pH reading should become a more routine laboratory test than it is now. On the technical side, it should be noted that at room temperature, plasma pH decreases at the rate of about 0.015 pH unit every half hour. Unless measurement is done within 1/2 hour after drawing, the blood should be refrigerated where it can be kept up to 4 hours. Venous specimens are nearly as accurate as arterial blood for pH if blood is drawn before the tourniquet is released, without motion of the patient's hand or arm after tourniquet application. Room air contact must be avoided.

With this background, one may proceed to the various clinical disturbances of pH. These have been classically known as the state of acidosis when pH is decreased toward the acid side of normal, and alkalosis, when pH is elevated toward the alkaline side of normal. Acidosis, in turn, is usually subdivided into metabolic and respiratory etiology, and the same for alkalosis.

Metabolic acidosis may be due to at least three main causes:

1. Acid-gaining acidosis: Hydrogen ions not included in the $CO_2$ system are added to the blood. The common situations are:

   a) Direct administration—such as treatment with ammonium chloride, or the late effects of salicylate poisoning. Ammonium chloride ($NH_4Cl$) releases $H^+$ ions and $Cl^-$ ions as the liver utilizes this compound for $NH_3$ in order to synthesize urea. Aspirin is acetylsalicylic acid, which in large quantities will eventually add enough $H^+$ ions to cause acidosis, even though in the early stages there is respiratory alkalosis (to be discussed later).

   b) Excess metabolic acid formation—found in diabetic ketoacidosis, starvation, or severe dehydration. These conditions cause utilization of body protein and fat for energy instead of carbohydrate, with production of ketone bodies and various metabolic acids.

The results of acid-gaining acidosis are a decrease in free bicarbonate which is used up trying to buffer the excess hydrogen ions. Thus, the numerator of the Henderson-Hasselbalch equation is decreased, the normal 20:1 ratio is decreased, and the pH is therefore decreased. The $CO_2$ content (or $CO_2$ combining power) is also decreased because the bicarbonate which it measures has been decreased as a primary response to the addition of excess acid.

2. Base-losing acidosis: This situation is caused by severe intestinal diarrhea, especially if prolonged or in children. Diseases such as cholera, or possibly ulcerative colitis or severe dysentery might do this. The mechanism is direct loss of bicarbonate from the lumen of the small intestine. Normally, bicarbonate is secreted into the small intestine, so that the contents of the small intestine are alkaline in contrast to the acidity of the stomach. Most of the bicarbonate is reabsorbed; however, prolonged diarrhea or similar conditions could mechanically prevent intestinal reabsorption enough to cause significant bicarbonate loss in the feces. In addition, the $H^+$ ions which were released from $H_2CO_3$ in the formation of bicarbonate by carbonic anhydrase are still present in the blood stream, and add to the effect. However, the primary cause is the direct loss of bicarbonate; the numerator of the Henderson-Hasselbalch equation is decreased, the 20:1 ratio is decreased, and the pH is decreased. Naturally, the $CO_2$ content is also decreased.

3. Renal acidosis: This occurs in kidney failure which produces the clinical syndrome of uremia. As mentioned previously, the kidney has the major responsibility for excreting large excesses of hydrogen ions. In uremia, hydrogen ions from metabolic acids which normally would be excreted this way are retained in the blood stream due to loss of renal tubular function. Just as in acid-gaining acidosis, these excess hydrogen ions must be buffered, so part of the available body fluid bicarbonate is used up. This decreases the numerator of the Henderson-Hasselbalch equation, decreases the normal 20:1 ratio, and therefore decreases pH. Again, the $CO_2$ content is decreased.

The second major category of acidosis is that called respiratory acidosis. This may be due to any condition which causes pulmonary $CO_2$ retention. These include the respiratory muscle paralysis of polio, respiratory brain center depression sometimes seen in encephalitis or due to large doses of such drugs as morphine, primary lung disease such as pulmonary fibrosis or severe emphysema which destroy oxygen-exchange ability, and sometimes heart diseases, such as chronic congestive heart failure. The basic problem here is carbonic acid excess, produced by the $CO_2$ retention. Thus, the denominator of the Henderson-Hasselbalch equation is increased, the normal 20:1 ratio is decreased, and the pH is decreased. The $CO_2$ content is sometimes normal but is usually increased, because of kidney attempts to handle the excess $CO_2$ by forming more bicarbonate and excreting more $H^+$ ions.

Alkalosis may also be divided into metabolic and respiratory types. In metabolic alkalosis, there are three relatively common situations which should be discussed.

    a) Alkali administration: Usually when sodium bicarbonate is taken in large quantities for the treatment of peptic ulcer symptoms. In this case, excess bicarbonate is absorbed above the amount needed to neutralize stomach hydrochloric acid. The numerator of the Henderson-Hasselbalch equation is increased, the normal 20:1 ratio is increased, and the pH therefore rises. $CO_2$ content will naturally also rise because of the additional bicarbonate. Lactate, citrate, or acetate in sufficient quantities may also produce alkalosis, since they are oxidized to $HCO_3^-$.

b) Acid-losing alkalosis: This most frequently happens due to severe or protracted vomiting, such as may occur with pyloric stenosis. Gastric HCl is lost in vomiting. This was originally produced by conversion of carbonic acid to bicarbonate and $H^+$ ions, mediated by carbonic anhydrase of the gastric mucosa. The bicarbonate is kept in the blood stream, but the $H^+$ ions are secreted into the gastric lumen as HCl. When HCl is lost through vomiting, the $H^+$ ions are continually being lost, causing the $CO_2$ content to be increased, because the bicarbonate released when HCl is produced is still in the blood stream and increases when HCl is being formed at an increased rate. Therefore, the 20:1 ratio is increased and the pH is increased. Since $H_2CO_3$ is decreased as it is being continually used to produce more HCl, the lungs tend to retain $CO_2$ in order to compensate. Therefore, $pCO_2$ may actually increase, although not enough to prevent increase of the 20:1 ratio.

c) Hypokalemic alkalosis: This is most commonly due to excess $K^+$ loss by the kidney, such as might happen with overuse of certain diuretics which cause $K^+$ as well as $Na^+$ loss. Normally, most body $K^+$ is intracellular, whereas the majority of $Na^+$ and $H^+$ ions are extracellular. When excess $K^+$ is lost in the urine, intracellular $K^+$ diffuses out of the cells to replace some of that being lost from plasma. $Na^+$ and $H^+$ ions move into the cells to replace the $K^+$ that has moved out. Thus, $H^+$ ions are lost from extracellular fluid and plasma. A second mechanism depends on the fact that sodium is reabsorbed from the urine into the renal distal tubule cells by an active transport mechanism. This transport mechanism involves excretion of $H^+$ and $K^+$ ions into the urine to replace the reabsorbed $Na^+$ ions. $H^+$ and $K^+$ compete with each other in this exchange (or transport) system. Therefore, if an intracellular deficit of $K^+$ exists (in the tubule cells), more $H^+$ is excreted into the urine to allow the reabsorption of the same quantity of sodium. The result of renal $H^+$ loss and extracellular fluid $H^+$ loss is an acid-losing type of alkalosis. Therefore, more $H^+$ ions are manufactured by the kidney from $H_2CO_3$ in order to replace lost extracellular $H^+$ ions; more $HCO_3^-$ ions are thereby formed; and the numerator of the Henderson-Hassalbalch equation is increased. The denominator is eventually increased if the lungs attempt to compensate by increasing $CO_2$ retention by slower breathing. However, respiratory compensation is frequently minimal or insignificant in hypokalemic alkalosis, so that the $pCO_2$ frequently remains normal. Also, the urine pH is decreased because of the excess $H^+$ ions being excreted in the urine. This is the opposite of what one would ordinarily expect, because, in acidosis, the kidney usually attempts to compensate by excreting more $H^+$ ions (acid urine), whereas in alkalosis it would normally try to conserve $H^+$ ions and thus produce a urine of higher pH (alkaline urine).

The other major subdivision of alkalosis is that of respiratory alkalosis. This happens when the respiratory mechanism blows off more $CO_2$ than normally, due to respiratory center stimulation from some cause. The main conditions in which this happens are the so-called hyperventilation syndrome, caused by hysteria or anxiety; high fever; and direct stimulation of the respiratory center by drugs. Overdose of aspirin can cause this in the early stages, although later, after more of the aspirin is absorbed, there develops a metabolic acidosis. In hyperventilation, from whatever cause, respirations are increased and deeper, blowing off more $CO_2$. This creates a carbonic acid deficit, since carbonic acid is being used up in order to replenish $CO_2$ by the lung carbonic anhydrase enzymes. Therefore, the denominator of the Henderson-Hasselbalch equation is decreased, the 20:1 ratio is increased, and plasma pH increases. $CO_2$ content will decrease, because when $H_2CO_3$ is lost due to formation of $CO_2$ in the lungs, bicarbonate is converted to $H_2CO_3$ in the kidney in order to secondarily compensate for or replace the decreasing plasma carbonic acid.

To summarize plasma pH problems: In metabolic acidosis there is eventual bicarbonate deficit leading to decreased plasma pH and decreased $CO_2$ content (or $CO_2$ combining power). In respiratory acidosis there is primary carbonic acid excess which causes decreased plasma pH, but the $CO_2$ content is increased due to renal attempts at compensation. In metabolic alkalosis there is eventual bicarbonate excess leading to increased plasma pH and increased $CO_2$ content. In respiratory alkalosis there is primary carbonic acid deficit which causes increased plasma pH, but the $CO_2$ content is decreased due to renal attempts at compensation. The urine pH usually reflects the status of the plasma pH except in hypokalemic alkalosis, where there is acid urine pH despite plasma alkalosis.

As noted, $CO_2$ content or combining capacity essentially constitutes the numerator of the Henderson-Hasselbalch equation. $pCO_2$ is essentially a measurement of the equation denominator, and can be used in conjunction with pH to indicate acid-base changes. This is the system popularized by Astrup and Siggaard-Andersen. $pCO_2$ follows the same direction as the $CO_2$ content in classic acid-base syndromes.  In metabolic acidosis, the $pCO_2$ is decreased, because acids other than $H_2CO_3$ accumulate, and $CO_2$ is blown off by the lungs in attempts to decrease body fluid acidity.  In metabolic alkalosis, the $pCO_2$ is increased if the lungs compensate by hypoventilation; in mild or acute cases, $pCO_2$ may remain normal.  In respiratory alkalosis, the $pCO_2$ is decreased, because increased ventilation blows off more $CO_2$.  In respiratory acidosis, the $pCO_2$ is increased, because of $CO_2$ retention due to decreased ventilation.

Acid-base data interpretation has always been one of the least understood areas of medicine.  Use of the Henderson-Hasselbalch equation makes it simple, in classic noncorrected cases.  The equation numerator ($HCO_3^-$ or $CO_2$ content) and denominator ($pCO_2$) usually follow each other; as one increases or decreases, so does the other, and therefore the direction of change for one can be predicted from the behavior of the other.  pH follows the same direction of abnormality as $pCO_2$ and $CO_2$ content in metabolic acidosis or alkalosis; it goes in the opposite direction in cases of respiratory acidosis or alkalosis.  Therefore, if pH is known and either $HCO_3^-$ or $pCO_2$ is known, it can be surmised whether the disorder is respiratory or metabolic in origin.  Normal values for $pCO_2$ are roughly 35-45 mm. Hg and for $CO_2$ content approximately 20-30 mEq. / L.  In metabolic acid-base disorders, the numerator ($HCO_3^-$) of the Henderson-Hasselbalch equation is primarily affected, while the denominator ($pCO_2$) attempts to compensate by means of regulating the breathing rate.  In respiratory acid-base disorders, the denominator ($pCO_2$) is primarily affected, while the numerator ($HCO_3^-$) attempts to compensate by kidney action.

The above explanations refer to uncomplicated noncorrected cases with attempts at compensation.  Since attempts at compensation may, for some reason, not be adequate, or even may be impossible, changes in the compensatory component may not be as marked as the primary change or may even be confined to population normal range.  This is more likely to occur in metabolic alkalosis, especially the hypokalemic type.  On the other hand, compensatory changes may substantially succeed in correcting pH to normal range.  Finally, attempts at therapy or the presence of one physiologic abnormality superimposed on a disease with others may complicate matters.

Two other concepts which form an integral part of the Astrup system should be defined.  The term "buffer base" refers to all substances in the buffering system of whole blood which are able to bind excess hydrogen ions.  Bicarbonate forms slightly over half of total buffer base; hemoglobin comprises about one third of total buffer base, consisting of three quarters of the nonbicarbonate buffer system.  Normal buffer base values for any patient are therefore calculated on the basis of the actual hemoglobin concentration as well as normal figures for pH and bicarbonate.  The term "base excess" refers to any difference in the measured total quantity of blood buffer base from the patient's calculated normal value.  Thus, an increase

in total buffer base (such as an increase in $HCO_3^-$) is considered a
"positive" base excess; a decrease in total buffer base from calculated normal (such as a decrease in $HCO_3^-$) is considered a "negative" base excess.

In many cases involving acid-base disturbances, the diagnosis
is obvious, and the only reason for obtaining $CO_2$ studies is to gauge
the severity of the disorder.  pH determination would not be needed.
This would be the situation in diabetic acidosis, for example.  However, in other patients, the underlying disorder is not obvious;
there may be intervening attempts at therapy, or compensatory
mechanisms may obscure a classic picture.  In these cases, pH
measurement is essential in order to interpret values of $pCO_2$ or
$CO_2$ content.  The problem is one of diagnosis rather than simple
estimation of severity.

## REFERENCES

Bigger, J. T., Jr., et al.: Management of cardiac problems in the
    intensive care unit, M. Clin. North America 55:1183, 1971.
Blumentals, A. S. (ed.): Symposium on acid-base balance, Arch.
    Int. Med. 116:647-742, 1965.
Christensen, H. N.: Diagnostic Biochemistry (New York: Oxford
    University Press, 1959).
Davis, R. P.: Logland: A Gibbsian view of acid-base balance, Am.
    J. Med. 42:159, 1967.
Elkinton, J. R.: Renal acidosis: Diagnosis and treatment, M. Clin.
    North America 47:935, 1963.
Filley, G. F.: Acid-Base and Blood Gas Regulation (Philadelphia:
    Lea & Febiger, 1971).
Kaufman, H. E., and Rosen, S. W.: Clinical acid-base regulation—
    The Bronsted schema, Surg., Gynec. & Obst. 103:1, 1956.
Nahas, G. G. (ed.): Current concepts of acid-base measurement,
    Ann. New York Acad. Sc. 133:1-274, 1966.
Simmons, D. H., and Shkolnick, S.: Acid-base alterations in pul-
    monary disease, Dis. Chest 45:175, 1964.
Still, G., and Rodman, T.: The measurement of the content of car-
    bon dioxide in plasma, Am. J. Clin. Path. 38:435, 1962.
Sunderman, F. W., and Sunderman, F. W., Jr. (eds.): Clinical
    Pathology of the Serum Electrolytes (Springfield, Ill.: Charles C
    Thomas, Publisher, 1966).
Weisberg, H. F.: A better understanding of anion-cation ("acid-
    base") balance, S. Clin. North America 39:1, 1959.
Weisberg, H. F.: pH of venous blood (Questions and Answers),
    J. A. M. A. 194:688, 1965.
Winters, R. W., et al.: Acid-Base Physiology in Medicine: A Self-
    Instruction Program (Westlake, Ohio: The London Company, 1967).
Zaroda, R. A.: Effect of various anticoagulants on carbon dioxide-
    combining power of blood, Am. J. Clin. Path. 41:377, 1964.

# CHAPTER 24

# Serum Electrolytes

Chapter 23 discussed pH and its clinical variations. The present chapter will attempt to cover the most frequent conditions associated with abnormalities of the major body electrolytes: sodium, potassium, and chloride.

Before going further, a clear distinction must be made between total body electrolyte concentration and serum concentration. Total body concentration of any electrolyte such as sodium includes an intravascular component (comprising the concentration of the electrolyte within serum and within RBC), an interstitial fluid component, and an intracellular component. Since most ions are diffusible to variable degrees between each of the three compartments, the serum concentration often does reflect the concentration in other fluid compartments. However, since the concentration of various electrolytes (such as sodium and potassium) is different between cells and extracellular fluid, in many situations the serum concentration does not accurately reflect intracellular electrolyte conditions. Furthermore, the serum electrolyte concentration depends on the amount of water present (plasma volume). A normal quantity of a particular electrolyte such as sodium may appear to have a low serum value if it is diluted by an excess of water. Likewise, an actual electrolyte deficit may show normal serum values if the plasma volume is decreased by excess water loss. Therefore, the serum levels of any electrolyte may or may not reflect the total body concentration, depending on the situation. Unfortunately, serum levels are the only electrolyte measurement which is readily available. A knowledge of what happens to total body levels as well as serum levels is essential to understand problems in certain situations.

The most frequent electrolyte abnormalities, from both clinical situations and abnormal laboratory values, are found with sodium. This is true because sodium is the most important cation of the body, both from a quantitative standpoint and from its influence on maintaining electrical neutrality. The most common causes of low or high serum sodium values are enumerated in Table 10. Some of the situations and the mechanisms involved require further explanation.

In protracted and severe vomiting, such as occurs with pyloric obstruction or stenosis, gastric fluid is lost in large amounts and a hypochloremic alkalosis develops, as described in Chapter 23. Serum sodium is usually within normal range, since gastric contents have a relatively low sodium content. Occasional patients may even show a hypernatremia if fluid loss exceeds loss of electrolytes. Despite normal serum levels, total body sodium is somewhat depleted, so replacement therapy should also include some sodium. Serum potassium is most often low, due to direct loss and to the alkalosis which develops when so much HCl is lost. Similar findings are produced by continuous gastric tube suction if continued over 24 hours.

In severe or long-standing diarrhea, the most common acid-base abnormality is a base-losing acidosis. Serum sodium, chloride, and potassium values are most often normal, despite considerable depletion of total body stores of these electrolytes, especially of potassium. The normal serum findings are explained by the marked loss of water which is characteristic of diarrhea. The diarrhea seen in sprue differs somewhat from the electrolyte pattern of other diarrhea etiologies in that hypokalemia is a somewhat more frequent finding. Regardless of the serum values, known deficits of water and electrolytes must be cautiously replaced.

Diabetic acidosis and its treatment provide very interesting electrolyte problems. Lack of insulin causes metabolism of protein and fat to provide energy which normally is available from carbohydrates. Ketone bodies and other metabolic acids accumulate; the blood sugar level is also elevated, and both sugar and ketones are excreted in the urine. Glucosuria produces an osmotic diuresis; a certain amount of serum sodium is lost with the sugar and water, and other sodium ions accompany the strongly acid ketone anions.

The effects of diuresis, as well as accompanying electrolyte loss, are manifested by severe dehydration. The serum sodium and chloride are often low in untreated diabetic acidosis, although (because of water loss) less often they may be within normal range. The serum potassium is usually normal. Nevertheless, even with normal serum levels, considerable total body deficits exist for all these electrolytes. The treatment for severe diabetic acidosis is insulin and large amounts of intravenous fluids. Sodium and chloride usually are given with the fluid to replace their deficits. After insulin administration, potassium ions tend to move into body cells, being no longer needed to combine with ketone acid anions. Also, potassium is apparently taken into liver cells when glycogen is formed from plasma glucose under the influence of insulin. In most patients,

TABLE 10.—CLINICAL SITUATIONS FREQUENTLY ASSOCIATED
WITH SERUM SODIUM ABNORMALITIES

Hyponatremia

1. Sodium and Water Depletion (Deficit Hyponatremia)
   a) Loss of GI secretions with replacement of fluid but not elec-
      trolytes
      i) Vomiting
      ii) Diarrhea
      iii) Tube drainage
   b) Loss from skin with replacement of fluids but not electrolytes
      i) Excessive sweating
      ii) Extensive burns
   c) Loss from kidney
      i) Diuretics (mercurial, chlorothiazide)
      ii) Chronic renal insufficiency (uremia) with acidosis
   d) Metabolic loss
      i) Starvation with acidosis
      ii) Diabetic acidosis
   e) Endocrine loss
      i) Addison's disease (or long-term steroid therapy sudden
         withdrawal)
   f) Iatrogenic loss from serous cavities
      i) Paracentesis or thoracentesis

2. Excessive Water (Dilution Hyponatremia)
   a) Congestive heart failure
   b) Cirrhosis
   c) Acute or chronic renal insufficiency (oliguria)
   d) Excessive water administration
   e) Diabetic acidosis (therapy without adequate sodium replace-
      ment)

3. Intracellular Loss (Tired Cell Syndrome)
   a) Cachexia and severe malnutrition
   b) Cirrhosis
   c) Carcinomatosis

Hypernatremia

Dehydration is the most frequent over-all clinical finding in hypernatremia

1. Deficient water intake (either orally or intravenously)
2. Excess water output (excess sweating, diabetes insipidus)
3. Occasional cases of severe protracted vomiting or diarrhea
4. Some cases of cerebral disease with ADH control loss

the serum potassium falls to nearly half admission values after 3-4 hours of fluid and insulin therapy (if adequate urine output is present), due to continued urinary potassium loss, shifts into body cells, and rehydration. After this time, potassium supplements should be added to the other treatment.

Sweat consists of water with a small but significant sodium chloride content. In extensive sweating, especially in a patient with fever, large amounts of water are lost. In addition, enough sodium and chloride loss occurs so as to produce total body deficits, sometimes of surprising degree. However, because of even more severe water deficit, the serum electrolyte values are normal or elevated.

In extensive burns, plasma and extracellular fluid leak into the damaged area in large quantities. If the affected area is extensive, hemoconcentration becomes noticeable and enough plasma may be withdrawn from the circulating blood volume to bring the patient close to or into shock. Plasma electrolytes accompany this loss from the circulation. The serum sodium may be normal or decreased. If the patient is supported over the initial reaction period, fluid will begin to return to the circulation after about 48 hours. Therefore, after this time, fluid and electrolyte requirements should be much less, so as not to overload the circulation. Silver nitrate treatment for extensive burns may itself cause clinically significant hyponatremia (due to electrolyte diffusion into the hypotonic silver nitrate solution).

Thus far, electrolyte disturbances have been relatively straightforward. In other common or well-organized syndromes, abnormality is closely tied to the role of the kidney in water and electrolyte physiology. A brief résumé of current information on this subject may be helpful in understanding clinical situations discussed later. Formation of urine begins with the glomerular filtrate which is similar to plasma, except that plasma proteins are too large to pass the glomerular capillary membrane. In the proximal convoluted tubules, about 85% of filtered sodium is actively reabsorbed by the tubule cells. The exchange mechanism is thought to be located at the tubule cell inner border (the side opposite from the tubule lumen); sodium is thus actively pumped out of the tubule cell into the renal interstitial fluid. Sodium from the urine passively diffuses into the tubule cell to replace that which is pumped out. Chloride and water passively accompany sodium from the urine into the cell and from thence into the interstitial fluid. Most of the filtered potassium is also reabsorbed, probably by passive diffusion. At this time, some hydrogen ion is actively secreted by tubule cells into the urine, but not to the extent that occurs farther down the nephron (electrolyte pathways and mechanisms are substantially less well known for the proximal tubules than for the distal tubules).

In the ascending (thick) loop of Henle, sodium is still actively reabsorbed, except that the tubule cells are now impermeable to water. Therefore, since water cannot accompany reabsorbed so-

dium and remains behind in the urine, the urine at this point becomes relatively hypotonic (the excess of water over what would
have been present had water reabsorption continued is sometimes
called "free water," and purely from a theoretical point of view is
sometimes spoken of as though it were a separate entity, almost
free from sodium and other ions).

In the distal convoluted tubules, three processes go on.
First, sodium ions continue to be actively reabsorbed (in addition
to the sodium pump located at the interstitial side of the cell which
is pushing sodium out into the interstitial fluid, another transport
mechanism on the tubule lumen border now begins to actively extract
sodium from the urine into the tubule cells). Intracellular hydrogen
and potassium ions are actively excreted by the tubule cells into the
urine in exchange for urinary sodium. There is competition between
hydrogen and potassium for the same exchange pathway. However,
since hydrogen ions are normally present in much greater quantities
than potassium, most of the ions excreted into the urine are hydrogen. Second, the urinary acidification mechanisms other than bicarbonate reabsorption ($NaHPO_4$ and $NH_3$) are operable here. Third,
distal tubule cells are able to allow reabsorption of water in a selective fashion. Permeability of the distal tubule cell to water is altered by a mechanism under the influence of antidiuretic hormone
(ADH). There is a limit in possible quantity of water reabsorbed,
because reabsorption is passive; ADH simply acts on cell membrane
permeability, controlling the ease of diffusion. Therefore, only
"free water" (the theoretical excess of hypotonic water from iso-
tonic urine) is actually reabsorbed.

In the collecting tubules, the tubular membrane is likewise
under the control of ADH. Therefore, any "free water" not reabsorbed in the distal convoluted tubules plus water which constitutes
actual urine could theoretically be passively reabsorbed here. However, three factors act to control the actual quantity reabsorbed:
first, the state of hydration of the tubule cells and renal medulla in
general, which determines the osmotic gradient toward which any
reabsorbed water must travel; second, the total water reabsorption
capacity of the collecting tubules, which is limited to about 5% of
normal glomerular filtrate; and third, the amount of "free water"
reabsorbed in the distal convoluted tubules, which helps determine
the total quantity of water reaching the collecting tubules.

Whether collecting tubule reabsorption capacity will be ex-
ceeded and, if so, to what degree, is naturally dependent on the total
quantity of water available. The amount of water reabsorbed compared to degree of dilution (hypotonicity) of urine reaching the collecting tubules determines degree of final urine concentration.

Certain adrenal cortex hormones control sodium retention and
potassium excretion. Aldosterone is the most powerful, but cortisone and hydrocortisone do have some effect. In Addison's disease
there exists a state of adrenocortical insufficiency, so that normal

sodium-retaining influences on the kidney are lacking. Usually there is enough to just barely carry the person along; however, when placed under stress of any type, the remaining adrenal cortex cells cannot give a normal hormone response and prevent development of a critical situation. The so-called crisis of Addison's disease is simply the result of overwhelming fluid and salt loss from the kidneys, and responds to replacement. Serum sodium and chloride are low, serum potassium is usually high normal or elevated, and the patient is markedly dehydrated. The $CO_2$ content (or combining power) may be normal or may be slightly decreased due to the mild acidosis which accompanies severe dehydration. In the syndrome primary aldosteronism there is oversecretion of aldosterone leading to sodium retention and, therefore, potassium loss. The serum potassium is low and the serum sodium is often mildly elevated, although a substantial minority of patients have serum sodium values within normal range. For some reason, the low potassium levels do not seem to cause as severe symptoms as other more acute types of hypokalemia do, and the main clinical symptom of this disease is hypertension. Sodium retention usually is not sufficient to produce edema. In Cushing's syndrome, there is overproduction of hydrocortisone, which in some cases may lead to hypokalemia and/or hypernatremia. If this occurs, however, it usually is mild, and the patient does not have clinical symptoms directly referable to his serum electrolyte abnormalities. Hypertension is fairly common in Cushing's syndrome.

In cirrhosis, hyponatremia and hypokalemia are frequent, separately or concurrently. There is a variety of etiologies: ascitic fluid sequestration; attempts at diuresis, often superimposed on poor diet or sodium restriction; paracentesis therapy; and hemodilution. Electrolyte abnormalities are more likely to appear when ascites is present, and to become most severe if azotemia complicates liver disease. Hemodilution is a frequent finding in cirrhosis, especially with ascites; this may be due to increased activity of aldosterone, which is normally deactivated in the liver, or sometimes is attributable to "inappropriate" secretion of ADH.

Congestive heart failure is frequently associated with hyponatremia (and, much less frequently, hypokalemia). The most frequent cause of hyponatremia is overtreatment with diuretic therapy, usually in the presence of dietary sodium restriction. However, sometimes the hyponatremia may be dilutional, due to retention of water as glomerular filtration rate is decreased by heart failure, or by "inappropriate" secretion of ADH. If hypokalemia is present, it usually is a side effect of diuretics.

Iatrogenic electrolyte disturbances most often result in decreased concentration of one or more serum electrolyte values. This may be due to treatment administered by a physician, or by conscious or unconscious attempts at therapy by the patient or his relatives. For example, marked sweating leads to thirst; ingestion of large quantities of water alone would dilute body fluid sodium, already depleted, even further.  A baby with diarrhea may be treated at home with water or sugar water; this replaces water without adequate replacement of electrolytes and has the same dilutional effect as the preceding example.  On the other hand, the infant may be given boiled skimmed milk or soup, which are high-sodium preparations; the result may be hypernatremia if fluid intake is not adequate. On the physician's side, the effects of excessive diuretic therapy have been mentioned.  Probably even more common is dilutional hyponatremia induced by intravenous infusion of electrolyte-free solutions such as 5% dextrose in water.  Superimposed on inadequate oral intake or previous deficits, this may lead to a dilutional effect. If renal water excretion is impaired, normal maintenance fluid quantities may lead to dilution, whereas excessive infusions may produce actual water intoxication or pulmonary edema.  There may also be problems when excessive losses of fluid or various electrolytes occur due to any reason, and replacement therapy is attempted but either is not adequate or is excessive.  The net result of any situation mentioned above is a fluid and/or electrolyte problem, which must be carefully and logically reasoned out, beginning from the primary deficit (the etiology of which may still be active) and proceeding through subsequent events.  Adequate records of fluid and electrolyte administration are valuable in solving the problem.

Recognition of dilutional syndromes is often difficult.  Three laboratory procedures may be of help.  The first is a plasma volume determination, most often done using albumin tagged with iodine-131 (RISA).  The second is a serum water determination.  Serum water value elevation in the presence of normal plasma protein levels is good evidence in favor of a dilutional syndrome.  Measurement of substances that are relatively constant in blood, such as hemoglobin, total protein, or creatinine, may be useful to indicate hemodilution or concentration.  These are most helpful when previous baseline values exist.  An obvious drawback is that values for any serum constituent may change due to disease rather than from water shifts.

Speaking of iatrogenic dilutional syndromes, it should be mentioned that the normal physiologic response to surgery is that of moderate fluid and electrolyte retention.  In the first 24 hours after surgery there tends to be decreased urine output, with fluid and electrolytes remaining in the body which would normally be excreted. Because of this, care should be taken not to overload the circulation with too much intravenous fluid on the first postoperative day.  Incidentally, in certain cases such as extensive surgical procedure and patients admitted originally for other problems, it is often useful to have preoperative serum electrolyte values so that subsequent electrolyte problems can be better evaluated.

Antidiuretic hormone (ADH) has been mentioned as one regulator of plasma volume, via its action on renal distal tubule water reabsorption.  ADH is produced by the posterior pituitary under control of the hypothalamus. Several factors influence ADH production: blood osmotic changes (concentration and dilution, acting on osmoreceptors in the hypothalamus), blood volume changes, certain neural influences such as pain, and certain drugs, such as morphine and alcohol. Lack or insufficient production of ADH leads to the syndrome known as diabetes insipidus. Water cannot be retained normally by the kidney; a continual diuresis of dilute urine is produced, and marked dehydration results. Pitressin given parenterally corrects the defect. Another syndrome involving ADH is now being well recognized, although it is not frequent. This is so-called inappropriate secretion of ADH, or "inappropriate ADH" (IADH). Basically, this syndrome results from water retention by ADH in situations in which one would not expect ADH to be secreted. The criteria for IADH syndrome includes hyponatremia with serum hypoosmolality, continued renal excretion of sodium despite hyponatremia, urine osmolality which shows a significant degree of concentration (instead of the maximally dilute urine one would expect), and no evidence of blood volume depletion. In other words, ADH is secreted despite hemodilution and/or decreased serum osmolality. The reason for increased sodium excretion is not definitely known; it is thought that increase of interstitial fluid volume by water retention may lead to suppression of sodium reabsorption (in order not to reabsorb even more water). Blood volume often is in normal range (since sodium is not retained) and there usually is no edema (since interstitial fluid expansion usually is only moderate).

A problem may arise concerning what urine osmolality value qualifies as a significant degree of concentration in order to diagnose IADH. If the serum and urine specimens are obtained "together" and if the serum demonstrates significant hyponatremia and hypo-osmolality, a urine osmolality value greater than that of the serum specimen would be considered more concentrated than usual. However, in some cases of IADH the urine does not necessarily have to possess higher osmolality than the serum if it can be demonstrated that water retention is taking place in spite of a hypotonic plasma. Also, since some patients with IADH may have low urine sodium due to low body intake of sodium, the diagnosis of IADH may be assisted by administering a test dose of sodium. In IADH, infusion of saline does not correct the hyponatremia; most of the sodium will appear in the urine as long as the patient does not restrict fluids (fluid restriction will cause sodium retention in IADH). Water restriction is the treatment of choice.

This syndrome in its classic form has been reported mainly with some cases of intracranial injury or cerebral infection, and in a few patients with bronchogenic carcinoma (especially the undifferentiated "oat-cell" type).

There are, however, somewhat more frequent situations which have many features of IADH without its classic syndrome. The dilutional hyponatremia of cirrhosis and congestive heart failure may

TABLE 11.—CLINICAL SITUATIONS COMMONLY ASSOCIATED
WITH SERUM POTASSIUM ABNORMALITIES

Hypokalemia

1. Inadequate intake (cachexia or severe illness of any type)
2. Intravenous infusion of potassium-free fluids
3. Protracted vomiting
4. Renal loss (primary aldosteronism; diuretics)
5. Treatment of diabetic acidosis without potassium supplements
6. Treatment with large doses of ACTH or cortisone
7. Cirrhosis

Hyperkalemia

1. Renal failure with oliguria ("renal shutdown")

sometimes be of this type, although usually other mechanisms can better account for hyponatremia, such as overuse of diuretics. However, in some cases, IADH seems to contribute; these patients differ from the classic IADH syndrome in that edema is often present, and the urine contains very little sodium. In other words, the main feature is water retention with dilutional hyponatremia. This has been called the "refractory dilutional syndrome"; treatment with sodium can be dangerous; therapy consists of water restriction.

Another syndrome involving hyponatremia is without any really good explanation, although here again IADH may contribute in part. These persons have chronic wasting illness such as carcinomatosis, chronic malnutrition, or simple old age. Serum sodium levels are mildly or moderately decreased. As a rule, these persons do not have symptoms from their hyponatremia and seem to have physiologically adjusted to the lower serum level. Treatment with salt does not raise the serum values. Apparently the only cure is to improve the patient's state of nutrition, especially his body protein, which takes considerable time and difficulty. This situation has been called the "tired cell syndrome."

The situation with abnormal potassium values is in many respects comparable to that of sodium (Table 11). Some of these situations are also tied to sodium and were discussed earlier. These include diabetic acidosis with treatment, adrenal disease such as primary aldosteronism and Addison's disease, certain cardiac patients, and the effect of diuretics, particularly the chlorothiazide group. Hypokalemia is frequent in cirrhosis. There are, likewise, similarities in that dilution with potassium-free fluids such as glucose water or saline may lead to potassium deficit. Besides the effect of outright dilution, there is in addition an element of continued renal loss. The kidney is apparently set up best to conserve sodium and to excrete potassium (since one way to conserve sodium is to excrete potassium ions in exchange), so that when normal intake of potassium stops, it takes time for the kidney to adjust and stop losing normal amounts of potassium ions. In the meantime, a deficit may be created. The potentiality for gastrointestinal hypokalemia should be mentioned again. Although potassium is present in GI tract secretions only in relatively small amounts, continued loss of these secretions will eventually lose enough potassium to require replacement. This is especially true for diarrhea.

Hypokalemia has a close relationship to alkalosis. Increased plasma pH (alkalosis) results from decreased extracellular fluid hydrogen ion concentration; the extracellular fluid deficit draws hydrogen from body cells, leading to decreased intracellular concentration and therefore less hydrogen ion available in renal tubule cells for exchange with urinary sodium. This means increased potassium excretion in exchange for urinary sodium, and eventual hypokalemia. Besides being produced by alkalosis, hypokalemia can itself lead to alkalosis—or, at least, a tendency toward alkalosis. Hypokalemia results from depletion of intracellular potassium (the largest body store of potassium). Hydrogen ion diffuses into body cells to partially replace the intracellular cation deficit caused by potassium deficiency; this tends to deplete extracellular fluid hydrogen levels. In addition, more hydrogen is excreted into the urine in exchange for sodium, since the potassium which normally would participate in this exchange is no longer available. Both mechanisms tend to eventually deplete extracellular fluid hydrogen. As noted in Chapter 23, in alkalosis due to hypokalemia an acid urine is produced, contrary to the usual situation in alkalosis. This incongruity is due to the intracellular acidosis which results from hypokalemia.

High potassium values are found in relatively few diseases. Of these, the only common situation is renal shutdown with failure to produce adequate urine quantities and therefore inability to excrete enough potassium.

Serum calcium is an important body electrolyte which is covered further in Chapter 28. A list of the most common diseases associated with disorders of calcium metabolism has been included there, along with typical laboratory findings.

Before concluding this material, it might be useful to describe some of the clinical symptoms of electrolyte imbalance. Interestingly enough, they are very similar for low sodium, low potassium, and high potassium. They include muscle weakness, nausea, anorexia, and mental changes which usually tend toward drowsiness and lethargy. The electrocardiogram in hypokalemia is very characteristic, and with serum values below 3.0 mEq./L. usually shows depression of the S-T segment and flattening or actual inversion of the T wave. In hyperkalemia, the opposite happens; the T wave becomes high and peaked; this usually begins with serum potassium values over 7 mEq./L. (normal values being 4.0-5.5 mEq./L.). One final note on hypokalemia—potassium antagonizes the action of digitalis, and hypokalemia may allow digitalis toxicity with doses which would ordinarily be nontoxic.  Conversely, very high concentrations of potassium are toxic to the heart, so that intravenous infusions should never give more than 20 mEq./hr. even with good renal function.

In the clinical laboratory, the four commonly used "electrolyte" determinations include serum sodium, chloride, $CO_2$, and potassium.  Serum chlorides have not been specifically mentioned because, in general, they follow the serum sodium (except in a few situations such as the hyperchloremic alkalosis of vomiting).  Usually it is sufficient to get all four of these tests initially and after that to follow only the important ones, namely sodium and potassium.  If the $CO_2$ is normal (or close to it), there usually is no need to keep reordering it unless something specific is in mind.  Serum chlorides, as mentioned, usually parallel the sodium levels and are useful mainly as a rough check on the sodium values.  Therefore, chlorides also can generally be omitted or only spot checked after the initial values are received.  It usually is not necessary to get repeat determinations on chloride or $CO_2$ except in special circumstances or when the initial $CO_2$ is markedly abnormal.

Serum and urine osmolality may assist in diagnosis of certain fluid and electrolyte problems.  Osmolality (pp. 144-145) is the measure of the number of osmotically active particles in a solution. It is determined by the degree of induced freezing point change in a special machine.  Units are milliosmoles (mOsm.) per liter of water.  Therefore, osmolality depends not only on the quantity of solute particles but also on the quantity of water in which they are dissolved.  Sodium is by far the major constituent of serum osmolality.  Plasma proteins have little osmotic activity and are essentially noncontributory to serum osmolality.  Serum (or plasma) osmolality may be estimated from the formula mOsm. = (1.86 x sodium) $+ \frac{BS}{18} + \frac{BUN}{2.8} + 5$, with blood sugar (BS) and BUN in mg./100 ml. and Na (sodium) in mEq./L.  A quick approximation is 2Na $+ \frac{BS}{20} + \frac{BUN}{3}$.  Normal adult range is 275-300 mOsm.  The ratio of serum sodium concentration to serum osmolality (Na/Osm. ratio) is normally 0.43-0.50.

Decreased serum osmolality is always caused by hyponatremia. Increased osmolality may be produced by water deficit (dehydration), sodium overload, hyperglycemia, uremia, unknown metabolic products, or various drugs or chemicals, especially ethyl alcohol.  The difference between calculated and measured osmolality gives a clue to the presence of unusual solutes.  Many substances do not affect osmolality; those which do are potentially dialyzable.  Osmolality is one of the criteria for diagnosis of hyperosmolar nonketotic acidosis. The technique is widely used in renal dialysis to make certain the electrolyte composition of the solution is within acceptable limits.

Low serum sodium is most often accompanied by low osmolality in dilution syndromes, salt (without water) depletion, and the
"tired cell" syndrome. Some patients lose salt and water concurrently; some of the extracellular water loss is replaced from intracellular water, with the final result being a relative sodium deficit.
Another cause of sodium deficit is a low-salt diet in patients with
chronic renal disease whose kidneys cannot retain sodium. Differentiation between hyponatremia caused by dilution and that by depletion is frequently not easy. Establishing proof that dehydration
exists may also be difficult. Plasma volume determination is the
most accurate way to prove dilution or dehydration, but may not be
available. Measurement of hemoglobin (or hematocrit) and total
protein may help. Increase from previous values suggests water deficit, especially if accompanied by hypernatremia. If hematocrit and
total protein elevation is accompanied by hyponatremia, this suggests
sodium depletion, whereas hyponatremia plus decreased hematocrit
and total protein (from previous levels) is more suggestive of a dilution component. In this situation, decrease in plasma proteins is
not as reliable as hematocrit, due to the frequency of albumin decrease in many serious illnesses. In the case of decreased hematocrit, occult bleeding must be ruled out. Serum water determination
has been suggested as an aid in diagnosis of dilution syndrome (p. 421).

In hyponatremia without coincident increase in the other solutes, the Na/Osm. ratio is said to be normal (i.e., there is a decrease both in sodium and in osmolality). An appreciable minority
of patients with hyponatremia have osmolality in the normal population range. Some of these patients may be dehydrated; others may
have cardiac, renal, or hepatic disease. These diseases characteristically reduce the Na/Osm. ratio, this being partially attributed
to the effects of increased blood sugar, urea, or unknown metabolic
substances. Especially in uremia, osmolality changes cannot always
be accounted for by effects of BUN alone. Patients in shock may develop disproportionately elevated measured osmolality compared to
calculated osmolality; again, this points toward circulating metabolic
products. Besides elevating osmolality, these substances displace
a certain amount of sodium from serum, thus lowering sodium
levels. One milliequivalent of sodium will be displaced by each 35
mg./100 ml. blood sugar or each 5 mg./100 ml. BUN increase over
normal limits. Elevated serum lipids will also displace sodium,
but without elevating osmolality.

## REFERENCES

Bland, J. H.: Clinical Metabolism of Body Water and Electrolytes
(Philadelphia: W. B. Saunders Company, 1963).
Boyd, D. R., and Baker, R. J.: Osmometry: A new bedside lab-
oratory aid for the management of surgical patients, Surg. Clin.
North America 51:241, 1971.

Butcher, H. R. ,. Jr. :  The pathophysiology of sodium depletion in
man, S. Clin. North America 45:345, 1965.

Epstein, F. H. , et al. :  Cerebral hyponatremia, New England J.
Med. 265:513, 1961.

Finkel, R. M. :  Hyponatremia, M. Clin. North America 56:645,
1972.

Goldberger, E. :  A Primer of Water, Electrolyte, and Acid-Base
Syndromes (3rd ed. ; Philadelphia:  Lea & Febiger, 1965).

Leaf, A. :  The clinical and physiologic significance of the serum
sodium concentration, New England J. Med. 267:24, 77, 1962.

Lobdell, D. H. :  Freezing-point osmometry—Simple and valuable
procedure, Lab. Med. 1:43, 1970.

Mansberger, A. R. , et al. :  Refractometry and osmometry in clinical surgery, Ann. Surg. 169:672, 1969.

Martin, H. E. , et al. :  Fluid and electrolyte therapy of severe
diabetic acidosis and ketosis, Am. J. Med. 24:376, 1958.

Parenteral Water and Electrolyte Solutions, Med. Letter Drugs &
Therapeutics 12:77, 1970.

Scheiner, E. , et al. :  Water and electrolyte disturbances in cancer
patients, M. Clin. North America 50:711, 1966.

Takasu, T. , et al. :  Hyponatremia in congestive heart failure, Ann.
Int. Med. 55:368, 1961.

# CHAPTER 25

# Diagnosis of Malabsorption

The function of the gastrointestinal tract is to perform certain mechanical and enzymatic procedures on food and then to absorb necessary constituents into the blood stream and excrete the remainder. When the usual dietary constituents are not absorbed normally, symptoms may develop which form part of the syndrome known as malabsorption (Table 12). There are three basic types of malabsorption. The first concerns the interruption of one of the stages in fat absorption (indicated in Table 12 by I, II, and III); this primarily concerns fat absorption and also those substances dependent on the presence of lipid. Another broad category is intrinsic defect of the small bowel mucosa, listed in the classification as IV, A-D. This type shows interference with not only fat and fat-soluble substances but also carbohydrates and many other materials. The third category is represented by IV, E and also by the deficiency disease called pernicious anemia. In these cases, lack of one specific substance normally produced by the gastrointestinal tract leads to malabsorption of other substances dependent on them for absorption.

Steatorrhea, meaning the appearance of excess quantities of fat in the stool, is the major manifestation of most of the malabsorption syndromes from most causes. Many patients with steatorrhea also have diarrhea, but the two are not synonymous; a patient can have steatorrhea without diarrhea. In children, the principal diseases associated with steatorrhea and malabsorption are celiac disease and cystic fibrosis of the pancreas. In adults, the most common causes are tropical sprue, nontropical sprue (the adult form of celiac disease), and pancreatic insufficiency. The clinical picture is roughly similar for all these diseases, but varies according to the cause, severity, and duration of the etiology. The most common chief complaints of severe malabsorption, in general,

294

TABLE 12.—CLASSIFICATION OF MALABSORPTIVE DISORDERS
(With Comments on Occurrence and Associated Abnormalities)

I.  Inadequate mixing of food with bile salts and lipase.  Mild chem-
    ical steatorrhea common, but clinical steatorrhea uncommon.
    Actual diarrhea uncommon.  Anemia in approximately 15-35%;
    most often iron deficiency, rarely megaloblastic
    A.  Pyloroplasty
    B.  Subtotal and total gastrectomy (occasional megaloblastic
        anemias reported)
    C.  Gastrojejunostomy

II. Inadequate lipolysis—lack of lipase or normal stimulation of
    pancreatic secretion.  Steatorrhea only in far-advanced pan-
    creatic destruction, and diarrhea even less often
    A.  Cystic fibrosis of the pancreas
    B.  Chronic pancreatitis
    C.  Cancer of the pancreas or ampulla of Vater
    D.  Pancreatic fistula
    E.  Severe protein deficiency
    F.  Vagus nerve section

III. Inadequate emulsification of fat—lack of bile salts.  Clinical
     steatorrhea uncommon, sometimes occurs in very severe
     cases.  Usually no diarrhea
     A.  Obstructive jaundice
     B.  Severe liver disease

IV. Primary absorptive defect—small bowel
    A.  Inadequate length of normal absorptive surface.  Unusual
        complication of surgery
        1.  Surgical resection
        2.  Internal fistula
        3.  Gastroileostomy
    B.  Obstruction of mesenteric lymphatics (rare)
        1.  Lymphoma
        2.  Hodgkin's disease
        3.  Carcinoma
        4.  Whipple's disease
        5.  Intestinal tuberculosis
    C.  Inadequate absorptive surface due to extensive mucosal dis-
        ease.  Except for Giardia infection and regional enteritis,
        most of these diseases are uncommon.  Steatorrhea only if
        extensive bowel involvement
        1.  Inflammatory
            a.  Tuberculosis
            b.  Regional enteritis or enterocolitis (diarrhea very
                common)
            c.  Giardia lamblia infection (diarrhea common; rare
                to get malabsorption)

2.  Neoplastic
3.  Amyloid disease
4.  Scleroderma
5.  Pseudomembranous enterocolitis (diarrhea frequent)
6.  Radiation injury
7.  Pneumatosis cystoides intestinalis
D.  Biochemical dysfunction of mucosal cells
1.  "Glutin-induced" (steatorrhea and diarrhea very common)
a.  Celiac disease (childhood)
b.  Nontropical sprue (adult)
2.  Enzymatic defect
a.  Disaccharide malabsorption (rare—diarrhea frequent symptom)
b.  Pernicious anemia (deficiency of "gastric" intrinsic factor)
3.  Cause unknown. Uncommon except for tropical sprue (which is itself common only in the tropics)
a.  Tropical sprue (diarrhea and steatorrhea very common)
b.  Severe starvation
c.  Diabetic visceral neuropathy
d.  Endocrine and metabolic disorder (e. g., hypothyroidism)
e.  Zollinger-Ellison syndrome
f.  Miscellaneous
E.  Malabsorption associated with altered bacterial flora (diarrhea fairly common)
1.  Small intestinal blind loops, diverticula, anastomoses (rare)
2.  Drug (oral antibiotic) administration (infrequent but not rare)

---

are diarrhea and weakness, weight loss, and mild functional gastrointestinal complaints (anorexia, nausea, mild abdominal pain). Physical findings and laboratory results tend to differ in the various etiologies. In severe cases of sprue, tetany, bone pain, tongue surface atrophy, and even bleeding may be found. Physical examination may show abdominal distention and also peripheral edema in nearly half of the patients. In pancreatic insufficiency, physical examination may be normal or show malnutrition. Neurologic symptoms are found with moderate frequency in pernicious anemia, but may be present in other etiologies. Laboratory examination varies again according to severity and etiology, but in sprue most often includes one or more of the following: anemia, steatorrhea, hypoproteinemia, hypocalcemia, and hypoprothrombinemia. In pancreatic insufficiency, the main abnormalities are steatorrhea and decreased carbohydrate tolerance (sometimes overt diabetes).  Pernicious anemia is different and has only anemia without diarrhea, steatorrhea, or the other test abnormalities.  The majority of stomach operations do not cause diarrhea or abnormalities of fat absorption.

Steatorrhea is due to excess excretion of fat in the stools from inability to absorb this substance.  Anemia is most often macrocytic, but sometimes is of the iron deficiency type due to various degrees of deficiency of folic acid, vitamin $B_{12}$, and iron.  Calcium may be deficient because of gastrointestinal loss due to the diarrhea usually present.  Prothrombin formation by the liver is often impaired to various degrees because of lack of vitamin K.  This is the fat-soluble vitamin which is produced by bacteria in the small bowel.  Long-term oral antibiotics may reduce the bacterial flora by killing these bacteria and thus interfere with vitamin K formation; inability to absorb fat will secondarily prevent vitamin K and vitamin A, which are dependent on fat solubility for intestinal absorption, from entering the blood stream.  Malnutrition resulting from lack of fat and carbohydrate absorption leads to hypoproteinemia, mainly secondary to lack of normal production of albumin by the liver.  This also contributes to the peripheral edema that many patients show.

Generally speaking, the patients usually present in one of two ways.  In some cases, the major finding on admission is anemia, and once malabsorption is suspected, either by the finding of megaloblastic bone marrow changes or by other symptoms or signs suggestive of malabsorption, then the problem becomes one of differentiating between pernicious anemia and other types of malabsorption.  The other major picture is the patient who presents with one or more local symptoms of malabsorption, either mild or marked in severity, in whom the diagnosis has to be firmly established and the etiology investigated.  There are several basic tests for malabsorption which, if used intelligently, usually can lead to the diagnosis and in some cases to the responsible etiology.

Qualitative fecal fat in the stool may be stained by Sudan III dye, whereby neutral fat will appear as bright orange droplets.  The fatty acids normally do not stain.  These fatty acids and the original neutral fat may then be converted to stainable fatty acids by heat and acid hydrolysis.  The preparation is then stained and examined a second time to determine if the droplets are increased from the first examination.  The reliability of this type of procedure is debated in the literature, but it seems fairly accurate if the technician is experienced.  Naturally, there will be difficulty in distinguishing normal from only low-grade degrees of steatorrhea.  It is possible to get some idea of etiology by estimating the amount of neutral fat versus fatty acid; lack of fatty acid suggests pancreatic disease.

The basic diagnostic test for presence of steatorrhea is quantitative fecal fat.  Stool collections are taken over a minimum of 3 full days.  The patient should be on a diet containing approximately 50-150 Gm. of fat a day (average 100 Gm.) beginning 2 days before

the test collection.  It is necessary to make sure that the patient is
actually eating enough of this diet to take in at least 50 Gm. of fat a
day; it is also obviously important to make sure that all the stools
are collected and the patient is not incontinent of feces.  If the patient has constipation, which some do have, it may be necessary to
use a bedtime laxative.  Normal diet shows an average excretion of
less than 7 Gm. of fat per 24 hours.  Five to 7 Gm. excretion for
24 hours is equivocal, since many patients with minimal steatorrhea
and a small but significant percentage of normal persons fall into
this range.  Finally, it should be noted that some patients with partial or complete malabsorption syndromes may have normal fecal
fat excretion.  This seems most common in cases of tropical sprue.

    Plasma Carotene: Carotene is the fat-soluble precursor of
vitamin A and is adequately present in most normal diets which contain green or yellow vegetables.  Normal values are considered 70-
300 micrograms/100 ml.  Thirty to 70 micrograms/100 ml. are
usually considered moderately decreased levels and less than
30 micrograms/100 ml. means severe depletion.  Other causes of
low plasma carotene besides malabsorption are poor diet, severe
liver disease, and high fever.  There is considerable overlap between carotene values in malabsorption and in normal control patients, but this usually is over the 30 microgram level.  However,
this test is valuable mostly as a screening procedure.

    X-Ray Examination: A "small bowel series" is done by letting
barium pass into the small intestine.  There are several changes in
the normal radiologic appearance of the small bowel which are suggestive of malabsorption.  These changes appear in 70-90% of cases,
depending on the severity of disease, the etiology, and the particular investigator.  The radiologic literature agrees that many chronic
diseases, especially when associated with fever and cachexia, may
cause an interference with digestion of such severity as to produce
a pattern which may be confused with sprue.  Secondary malabsorption cannot be distinguished from primary unless certain rare causes
such as tumor happen to be the etiology.  The so-called diagnostic
patterns of sprue are thus characteristic of, but not specific for,
primary small intestine absorption, and are not present in probably
20% of the cases.

    Radioisotope Techniques: In order to test for fat malabsorp-
tion, a neutral fat named triolein combining glycerol and fatty acid
has been tagged with radioactive $I^{131}$.  It is also possible to tag a
simple fatty acid such as oleic acid with $I^{131}$.  This radioactive fat
can be administered in several ways, usually as a capsule or as
part of a fatty meal.  After a certain period, a specimen of blood
can be drawn and measured for radioactivity.  The stool also can
be measured for radioactivity, with either procedure giving an idea
of how much fat was either absorbed or rejected by the intestinal
mucosa.  In malabsorption due to pancreatic disease, radioactive
fatty acid (oleic acid) is absorbed normally, but not radioactive

neutral fat (triolein). In primary small bowel malabsorption, both types of fat show abnormal absorption. There have been many reports on this subject. The main problem with the test is a technical one, and this concerns the way the radioactive fat is administered. Apparently results differ quite markedly according to whether the radioisotope is given as a capsule or as an integral part of a fatty meal, and even the type of fatty vehicle has some influence on absorption. This test is promising but is not yet standardized. At present, it is probably better to avoid using radioactive fat techniques, since the same information generally can be obtained in other ways, and the accuracy of these procedures is open to considerable question.

Schilling Test: Pernicious anemia is an interesting disease in which a combination of specific (anatomic) lesions and factor deficiency lead to a characteristic clinical picture. This is discussed more fully under the macrocytic anemias. Briefly, the pernicious anemia patients have atrophic gastritis, a complete lack of gastric hydrochloric acid (known as achlorhydria), and a partial or complete deficiency of so-called intrinsic factor. This is produced by the stomach and it is necessary for the absorption of vitamin $B_{12}$ which normally takes place in the ileum. Laboratory findings vary according to the duration and severity of the disease, but classically consist of a macrocytic anemia in which the average red cell size is slightly larger than normal, a megaloblastic bone marrow in which the normal red cell series is distorted into peculiar appearance which is characteristic and which is called megaloblastic change, and often by secondary abnormality in the white cells and platelets leading to low blood levels (leukopenia and thrombocytopenia) and certain white cell morphologic changes. In true pernicious anemia, oral administration of usual dietary amounts of vitamin $B_{12}$ will have no measurable effect on the clinical course or the hematologic picture. This is of the order of 1-2 micrograms per day. A few patients will respond to a dose of as little as 5 micrograms, and nearly all to 100 micrograms, presumably by the effect of mass action on the small intestine mucosa despite intrinsic factor deficiency. The Schilling test consists of oral administration of 0.5 micrograms of vitamin $B_{12}$ which has been tagged with radioactive cobalt. At the same time, 1,000 micrograms of nonisotopic vitamin $B_{12}$ is given intramuscularly to saturate tissue-binding sites and to allow a portion of any labeled $B_{12}$ absorbed from the intestine to be excreted or flushed out into the urine. In the normal person, approximately 33% of the absorbed radioactive $B_{12}$ will thus appear in the urine and the total normal 24-hour urinary excretion is 8-40% of the original oral dose. Since poor renal function may delay excretion, a 48-hour collection may be necessary if the BUN is elevated. In classic pernicious anemia, the Schilling test will be positive, meaning less than 8% urinary excretion of the radioisotope for 24 hours, if no intrinsic factor has been given with the test dose.

The test is then completely repeated after 3 days, using adequate amounts of intrinsic factor. The test will then show normal values since the added intrinsic factor will now allow normal vitamin $B_{12}$ absorption. The Schilling test with and without intrinsic factor is extremely helpful in distinguishing pernicious anemia from various other malabsorption syndromes, which may show part or all of the classic "PA" clinical and laboratory findings. A considerable number of patients with sprue and a few with some of the other malabsorption diseases may have positive Schilling tests without intrinsic factor, but $B_{12}$ malabsorption will not be corrected by the addition of intrinsic factor. This differential procedure is especially helpful because other laboratory tests may be confusing. For example, some cases of primary malabsorption may fail to have steatorrhea and some may have achlorhydria, especially in the older age groups. In fact, about 30% of normal patients over age 70 apparently do not produce hydrochloric acid. Finally, occasional patients with classic pernicious anemia also show impaired absorptive function tests which one would expect in other malabsorption syndromes. The Schilling test both with and without intrinsic factor can thus be very helpful and, incidentally, can be done even if the patient already has been started on treatment, as long as intrinsic factor is not being given.

One additional caution: some PA patients may exhibit abnormal Schilling test results with added intrinsic factor, but then revert to a typical normal absorption response with intrinsic factor after treatment with parenteral vitamin $B_{12}$.

False positive tests may be produced by incomplete urine collection (normal output is greater than 800 ml./24 hours and usually is over 1,000 ml.). False negative results may be produced by fecal contamination of the urine.

Besides quantitative (fecal) fat studies, the most important test for malabsorption is the D-xylose test. Rather than a screening test for malabsorption per se, it is a test that identifies the sprue-type diseases and differentiates them from other malabsorption etiologies. Originally, an oral glucose tolerance test was used in malabsorption since it was found that most patients with sprue showed a flat curve. However, some patients with obvious malabsorption had a normal curve and it was also found in several large series that up to 20% of normal patients had a so-called flat curve, so this test was abandoned. D-xylose is a pentose isomer which is absorbed in much the same manner as glucose from the jejunum. The standard test dose is 25 Gm. of D-xylose in 250 ml. of water, followed by another 250 ml. of water. The patient is fasted overnight, since xylose absorption is delayed by other food. After the test dose, the patient is kept at bed rest for 5 hours without food. The normal person's peak blood levels are reached in approximately 2 hours and fall to fasting levels in approximately 5 hours. Xylose is excreted mostly in the urine with approximately 80-95% of the excretion in the first 5

hours and the remainder in 24 hours. Side effects of the oral xylose
are mild diarrhea and abdominal discomfort in a small number of
patients. Normal values for (2 hour) blood xylose levels are over
25 mg./100 ml.; 20-25 mg./100 ml. is equivocal, and less than 20
mg./100 ml. is strongly suggestive of malabsorption. The 5-hour
urine xylose normal values are greater than 5 Gm.; 4-5 Gm. is
equivocal, and less than 4 Gm. is suggestive of malabsorption.
Values for 24-hour urine collection are normally greater than 5 Gm.
It is obviously very important to make sure that the urine collection
is complete and that there is no fecal contamination of the urine. A
catheter may have to be used if the patient is incontinent of urine, or
if there is a question of fecal contamination, but catheterization
should be avoided if at all possible. Two main physiologic circumstances may affect the 5-hour urinary excretion—renal insufficiency
and advanced age. It was found that there may be abnormally low 5-
hour urine excretion of xylose in persons over age 65. However, one
study claims that the 24-hour urine collection is normal in these
cases unless actual malabsorption is present. If the serum creatinine level is borderline or elevated, the 5-hour urine xylose excretion is also likely to be abnormally low, and again the 24-hour urine
may be useful. In these cases, however, the 2-hour blood levels
may help, for they should be normal and are not affected by the two
conditions mentioned. Otherwise, the 5-hour urine excretion is
more reliable than the blood levels, which tend to fluctuate.

The xylose test may be helpful in differential diagnosis and
etiology of malabsorption. Most patients with cystic fibrosis and
pancreatic insufficiency are said to have normal urine values. This
is also true of most patients with liver disease. Classic pernicious
anemia has a normal xylose test, although it must be remembered
that many of these patients are aged and may have low urine results
from this cause. In megaloblastic anemia of pregnancy some patients have abnormal xylose tests although probably the majority
show normal values. A minor percentage of patients with partial
gastrectomy are reported to have abnormal urine values. Patients
with functional diarrhea and duodenal ulcer have normal tests.

In malabsorption diseases, there is excellent D-xylose correlation with proved cases of sprue and celiac disease. The urine
results are more often clear-cut than the blood levels. There is no
correlation between the amount of steatorrhea present. Cases of
regional enteritis involving extensive areas of the jejunum may have
abnormal tests, while normal results are associated with this disease when it is localized to the ileum. Patients with Whipple's disease and multiple jejunal diverticula may also be abnormal. Finally,
there are certain diseases other than malabsorption which for some
reason sometimes have abnormal urinary xylose excretion. Myxedema shows this quite often. There are reports that this may occur in diabetic neuropathic diarrhea, rheumatoid arthritis, acute or
chronic alcoholism and occasionally in severe congestive heart fail-

ure. Ascites is reported to produce abnormal urine excretion with normal plasma levels. Although probably not common in the diseases just mentioned, abnormal results still occur often enough that one must be aware of this fact.

Small Intestine Biopsy: It has been shown that in classic cases of sprue, both tropical and nontropical, the mucosa of the small intestine shows characteristic histologic abnormalities. Instead of the normal monotonous finger-like villous pattern, the villi are thickened and blunted with flattening of the cuboidal epithelium and eventual fusion and often disappearance of the villi altogether. Depending on the degree of change in the villi, these biopsies may be classified as moderate or severe changes. These same changes to a much lesser degree may be found in many of the other conditions causing malabsorption, including even subtotal gastrectomy. However, these usually are not of the severity seen in sprue and generally can be differentiated by the clinical history or other findings. Other causes of malabsorption, such as Whipple's disease, which characteristically shows many PAS-positive macrophages in the mucosa, may be detected on biopsy.

This chapter has considered certain tests for intestinal malabsorption. In my opinion, the most useful tests for an initial screening for malabsorption syndromes are the D-xylose, plasma carotene, and qualitative fecal fat. (Some institutions do not do the plasma carotene, however.) If all of these are normal, chances of demonstrating steatorrhea by other means would be very low. If one or all are abnormal, it may be necessary to do a quantitative fecal fat study. X-ray studies may show compatible abnormalities and may also reveal some of the secondary causes of steatorrhea. A careful history, physical examination, and appropriate laboratory studies usually can rule out many of the causes of malabsorption, including most of those in categories I to III in Table 12. A Schilling test with and without intrinsic factor may be necessary to differentiate pernicious anemia from malabsorption diseases with a similar clinical picture. Jejunal biopsy may occasionally be necessary, but the diagnosis usually can be made by routine methods. In patients over age 60 it might be useful to obtain both a 5-hour and 24-hour D-xylose urine collection, with the 5-hour value added to the next 19 hours to give the total 24-hour figure. If pernicious anemia is suspected, a bone marrow to show megaloblastic changes and a gastric analysis for free acid should be done. If no free acid (after stimulation) is found, a Schilling test without intrinsic factor is needed. If the Schilling test without intrinsic factor is positive, it is followed by a Schilling test with intrinsic factor.

REFERENCES

Adlersberg, D. , et al. : The roentgenologic appearance of the small intestine in sprue, Gastroenterology 26:548, 1954.

Bossak, E. T. , et al. : Clinical aspects of the malabsorption syndrome (idiopathic sprue): Observations in 94 patients, J. Mt. Sinai Hosp. 24:286, 1957.

Collins, J. R. : Small intestinal mucosal damage with villous atrophy: A review of the literature, Am. J. Clin. Path. 44:36, 1965.

di-Sant'-Agnese, P. S. , and Jones, W. O. : The celiac syndrome (malabsorption) in pediatrics, J. A. M. A. 180:308, 1962.

Drummey, G. D. , et al. : Microscopical examination of the stool for steatorrhea, New England J. Med. 264:85, 1961.

Etheridge, C. L. : Protein-losing enteropathy, M. Clin. North America 48:75, 1964.

Gardner, F. H. : A malabsorption syndrome in military personnel in Puerto Rico, A. M. A. Arch. Int. Med. 98:44, 1956.

Gardner, F. H. : Hematologic aspects of sprue, Am. J. Clin. Nutrition 8:179, 1960.

Gordon, R. S. , et al. : Protein-Losing Gastroenteropathy, in Disease-a-Month (Chicago: Year Book Medical Publishers, Inc. , August, 1966).

Jeffries, G. H. , et al. : Malabsorption, Gastroenterology 46:434, 1964.

Joske, R. A. , and Curnow, D. H. : The D-xylose absorption test, Australasian Ann. Med. 11:4, 1962.

Laster, L. , and Ingelfinger, F. J. : Intestinal absorption: Aspects of structure, function and disease of the small-intestine mucosa, New England J. Med. 264:1138, 1192, 1246, 1961.

McIntire, P. A. , et al. : Pathogenesis and treatment of macrocytic anemia: Information obtained with radioactive vitamin B$_{12}$, A. M. A. Arch. Int. Med. 98:541, 1956.

Oxenhorn, S. , et al. : Malabsorption syndrome: Intestinal absorption of vitamin B$_{12}$, Ann. Int. Med. 48:30, 1958.

Raskin, H. F. , et al. : Selected practical tests of gastrointestinal function, M. Clin. North America 43:341, 1959.

Ruffin, J. M. , and Roufail, W. M. : Whipple's disease: Evolution of current concepts, Am. J. Digest. Dis. 11:580, 1966.

Shiner, M. : Problems in interpretation of intestinal mucosal biopsies, J. A. M. A. 188:165, 1964.

Summerskill, W. H. J. , and Moertel, C. G. : Malabsorption syndrome associated with anicteric liver diseases, Gastroenterology 42:380, 1962.

Texter, E. C. , et al. : Laboratory procedures in the diagnosis of malabsorption, M. Clin. North America 48:117, 1964.

Thaysen, E. H. , and Mullertz, S. : The D-xylose absorption tolerance test, Acta med. scandinav. 171:521, 1962.

Wenger, J. : Blood carotene in steatorrhea and the malabsorption syndrome, Am. J. Med. 22:373, 1957.

Wilson, F. A. , and Dietschy, J. M. : Differential diagnostic approach to clinical problems of malabsorption, Gastroenterology 61:911, 1971.

Wollaeger, E. E., and Scudamore, H. H. : Spectrum of diseases
    causing steatorrhea, Arch. Int. Med. 113:819, 1964.

# CHAPTER 26

# Gastrointestinal Function

## I. GASTRIC ANALYSIS

Gastric analysis has two main uses: to determine gastric acidity, and to obtain material for exfoliative cytology.

When gastric aspiration is performed for gastric acidity, the major concern is free acid and the major problem is whether or not any is present. To determine this, alcohol or caffeine stimulation by mouth may be used, but only histamine (or Histalog) by subcutaneous injection gives a strong enough stimulation to be sure of the results. If the other methods fail to show free acid, histamine will be necessary. The only reason for not using histamine exclusively (many clinicians do) is that many persons get troublesome side effects from it. The easiest procedure is to test the first material aspirated from the stomach after the tube is put down; if this has free acid, then histamine will not be needed.

Presence of free acid is useful clinically in the diagnosis of pernicious anemia, where it is always absent, and may be helpful in differential diagnosis of gastric carcinoma versus peptic ulcer. Absence of free acid after histamine is a strong point against ulcer and in favor of cancer (given the presence of a suspicious stomach lesion). Presence of free acid may occur in a smaller but still considerable percentage of gastric carcinoma and is usually, but not always, found with ulcer. High gastric free acid (50 units or over in any one specimen) tends to suggest ulcer rather than cancer (but again, not 100%). The amount of acid, therefore, is not too helpful unless very high or entirely absent; even then, it is not absolutely diagnostic. Incidentally, about one third of all persons over age 70 have no demonstrable free acid, and even a small percentage of otherwise normal young people. Duodenal ulcer patients tend to have hyperchlorhydria (above-normal HCl secretion), while gastric ulcer patients as a group often have normal or even low rates.

The amount of free acid is sometimes helpful in the surgical treatment of duodenal ulcer. Some surgeons prefer to do a hemigastrectomy (removal of half the stomach) rather than a subtotal gastrectomy (two thirds resection) because the postoperative complications are less in the former. If, however, the free acid is over 50 units (hyperchlorhydria), they may in addition perform vagotomy to lessen stimulation of the remaining HCl-producing cells.

Gastric acidity used to be reported in degrees or units; this is the same as milliequivalents per liter. Most authorities today recommend timed collection and report in milliequivalents per hour. A 1-hour basal specimen is collected; normal is 1-6 mEq./hour. Duodenal ulcer overlaps with normal, but almost 50% of cases have elevated levels. Values of over 10 mEq./hour are suspicious for Zollinger-Ellison syndrome (p. 386). Histamine (or better, Histalog) is then given, and four 30-minute consecutive specimens are collected. Maximum acid output (MAO) is the sum of all four 30-minute collections. MAO over 45 mEq./HCl/hour is suspicious for duodenal ulcer. If the disease in question is pernicious anemia rather than ulcer, the basal collection should have a pH over 6, and poststimulation pH should not drop more than 1 pH unit.

A method of tubeless gastric analysis called Diagnex Blue is available. A blue dye is coupled to a cation exchange resin. Free HCl in the stomach replaces the indicator dye, which is absorbed, then excreted and tested in the urine. Caffeine stimulation by mouth is used in the test. This is a fairly reliable test, but useful mostly as a screening procedure, since about 50% of those showing no free acid by the caffeine Diagnex procedure will have some demonstrated by histamine. If positive, however, there obviously is no need for histamine.

## II.  DIFFERENTIAL TESTS IN DIARRHEA

As mentioned previously, besides anemia, chronic diarrhea is a prominent symptom of the various malabsorption diseases and may be the chief complaint. There are many conditions which cause a chronic diarrhea, which must be differentiated from the relatively common types which last only a few days and which usually respond to the ordinary treatment. Diarrhea in infants will not be specifically discussed, since this is a special problem peculiar to that age group.

In all age groups with long-term or chronic diarrhea, a stool should be obtained for culture to rule out the presence of Salmonella or Shigella bacteria. A stool should also be obtained for ova and parasites, with special emphasis on the possibility of amebas being present. As discussed above, one of the malabsorption syndromes may be the etiology, either in children or in young and middle-aged adults; in children, this would be due to either cystic fibrosis of the pancreas or celiac disease. In an adult, the various forms of sprue and more rarely some of the secondary malabsorption causes might be considered. In children and young and middle-aged adults, ulcerative colitis is a possibility, especially if there is blood in the stools. This would call for a sigmoidoscopic examination. In adults over age 40, carcinoma of the colon has been found to cause diarrhea in a significant proportion of cases. A barium enema and signoidoscopic examination are necessary. In the aged, in addition to carcinoma, fecal impaction is a frequent cause of diarrhea and this usually can be determined easily by ordinary rectal examination. In many cases, no organic etiology for persistent diarrhea can be found. This situation is often called "functional diarrhea" and is attributed to psychiatric causes. The organic diseases listed above must be ruled out before deciding that a patient has a psychosomatic disorder.

### III.  OTHER PROCEDURES

The most frequent major diseases affecting the gastrointestinal tract may be divided into benign and malignant and localized into upper GI (stomach and duodenum) and lower GI (colon). The major benign disease of the upper GI tract area is peptic ulcer; those of the lower GI are diverticulosis and mucosal polyp. The malignant disease usually affecting either area is the same—adenocarcinoma. As a general rule, GI carcinoma is not common under age 40 (although it can occur), and increases steadily in probability after that age (many other types of cancer do likewise). The major clinical symptom of peptic ulcer is epigastric pain which classically occurs between meals and is relieved by food or antacids. Gastric carcinoma may have similar pain, nonspecific pain, or simple gastric discomfort. The major symptom of colon carcinoma is change in bowel habits, either toward chronic diarrhea or constipation. However, either upper or lower GI carcinoma may be relatively asymptomatic until very late.

Laboratory tests for these GI lesions may be divided into three categories: screening tests, x-ray, and direct visualization techniques. The most useful screening test is examination of the feces for blood. Usually this blood is occult (not grossly visible), sometimes it is grossly visible; if from the upper GI tract it is often black ("tarry"), while lower GI bleeding may still show unchanged blood and color the stool red. Anemia of the chronic iron deficiency type is often present, although not always, and sometimes may be severe. Occult blood in the feces can be demonstrated by simple chemical tests for hemoglobin. The two most popular tests for this purpose are guaiac and Hematest (orthotoluidine). Many studies have evaluated these (and other) methods. Guaiac is considered by the majority to combine adequate sensitivity and specificity. Hematest is said to be slightly more sensitive than guaiac, but whereas guaiac can be

used with patients on regular diet, Hematest is reported to give a
significant number of false positive results if the patient is eating
meat. The stool obtained by rectal examination is adequate for
testing by either method. Besides ulcer, polyp, or malignancy,
other serious GI diseases such as ulcerative colitis, regional enteritis, and diverticulitis may give guaiac-positive stools.

Gastric analysis may be helpful in screening peptic ulcer from
cancer of the stomach, as mentioned earlier. Low free acid or
achlorhydria (with histamine) is suspicious for cancer, if a stomach
lesion is known to be present. X-ray procedures include upper GI
series for stomach and duodenum, and barium enema for the colon.
In the upper GI series, the patient swallows a barium mixture, and
a series of x-ray films shows this radiopaque material filling the
stomach and duodenum. Barium enema means barium washed into
the colon through a tube, after all feces are eliminated by laxatives
and regular enemas. The major cause of poor barium enema studies is inadequate colon preparation. If feces remain in the colon
after preparation for this procedure, obviously the barium cannot
fill these areas, and small lesions may be missed. Direct visualization techniques include gastroscopy for stomach and proctoscopy
and sigmoidoscopy for rectal and sigmoid colon lesions. Biopsy
and specimens for cytology (Papanicolaou smears) can be obtained
at the same time. Simple rectal examination allows many rectal
and prostate cancers to be detected by the doctor's finger. For this
reason, rectal examination is always included as a part of any good
physical examination. In summary, rectal examination and stool
tests for occult blood are the best simple screening procedures for
GI tumors. If these are positive, or with strong clinical suspicion,
one can proceed to x-ray studies of the area indicated. When possible, direct visualization techniques are extremely helpful, especially proctoscopy.

## IV. PANCREATIC FUNCTION

The pancreas is an important gastrointestinal accessory organ and may be involved in disease from both its exocrine and endocrine aspects. Pancreatic enzymes consist mainly of starch-digest-
ing amylase, fat-digesting lipase, and protein-digesting trypsin, as
well as bicarbonate and certain other substances. These are secreted through the pancreatic duct, which enters the duodenum close
by the common bile duct. Intrinsic diseases of the pancreatic parenchyma or obstruction of the pancreatic duct by tumor or edema
of the common bile duct, ampulla of Vater, or the surrounding areas
may cause diminution or complete absence of pancreatic secretions
and secondarily lead to symptoms from lack of these important digestive enzymes. The diseases of the endocrine system which involve the islands of Langerhans in the pancreas will be discussed in
the next chapter.

The most important parenchymal diseases are acute and chronic pancreatitis and carcinoma of the pancreas. Acute pancreatitis classically is manifested by sudden onset of severe epigastric pain which may radiate elsewhere, often to the back. There may be nausea and vomiting. If severe, there may be abdominal distention, rigidity of the abdomen, and shock. In the most severe and classic cases, the diagnosis is obvious. However, in the cases of mild or moderate degree or in patients with a chronic low-grade or intermittent type of pancreatitis, symptoms may be vague or atypical. Even in some severe cases the clinical picture may be mimicked by certain other diseases. The most common diseases which are confused with acute or sometimes chronic pancreatitis are perforated peptic ulcer, gallbladder inflammation or stones, and infarction of the bowel due to mesenteric artery occlusion. Myocardial infarcts may sometimes be confused, since, in a few cases, the pain may radiate to the upper abdomen; in addition, the SGOT may be elevated in more than half of acute pancreatitis patients. In acute pancreatitis, the most important laboratory test is the serum amylase. Serum levels will become abnormal between 2 and 12 hours after onset in up to 80% of the cases and within 24 hours in up to 90%. Thereafter there is a relatively early return to normal, with most cases reaching a peak by 24 hours and returning to normal in 48-72 hours. In some patients the serum amylase will remain elevated longer due to continued pancreatic cell destruction, but a fair number will not. In certain situations there may be falsely low or normal serum amylase. The administration of glucose will cause decreased serum amylase, so that one should wait at least 1 hour and preferably 2 after the patient has eaten to get a serum amylase. One should realize that values taken during intravenous fluid therapy containing glucose may be unreliable. In massive hemorrhagic pancreatic necrosis there may not be any serum amylase elevation at all because no functioning cells are left to produce it. These cases are very few, however. Other conditions besides pancreatitis may cause an elevated serum amylase, although classically they do not reach the level of values found in severe acute pancreatitis. These include perforated peptic ulcer (which may perforate near the pancreas and cause a chemical pancreatitis), the administration of morphine or Demerol, intestinal obstruction, acute diseases of the salivary gland (since these also secrete amylase), and occasional cases of ruptured ectopic pregnancy, uremia, acute cholecystitis, and for approximately 72 hours after some cases of cholecystography using radiopaque dyes. Serum lipase is more specific for pancreatic damage and rises slightly later than the amylase, although usually within 24 hours, and tends to remain abnormal longer, with most cases returning to normal in 7-10 days after onset. However, it is elevated less frequently than amylase. Other laboratory findings in acute pancreatitis vary according to the severity of the disease. In the severe cases there may be a moderate leukocytosis with a shift to the left.  Moderate hyperglycemia may be present, and in the very severe cases outright diabetes may develop.  There may be a mild jaundice probably due to edema around the ampulla of Vater.  Serum calcium may be decreased, sometimes to quite low values.  This usually appears within 3-14 days after onset of symptoms, most frequently on the 4th or 5th day.  This is attributed to the liberation of pancreatic lipase into the peritoneal cavity, with resulting digestion of fat and the combination of fatty acids with calcium which we see grossly as fat necrosis.  Again, in the very severe cases there may be hemorrhagic phenomena due either to release of proteolytic enzymes such as trypsin into the blood, or else from release of blood into the abdominal cavity from a hemorrhagic pancreas.

Chronic pancreatitis on the other hand and its resulting pancreatic insufficiency may often be very difficult to diagnose.  This depends again on the degree of pancreatic destruction and whether it occurs acutely or in a low-grade fashion.  The serum amylase in chronic pancreatitis is still important, although much more unreliable than in the acute cases.  In about half the patients it is within normal range.  Repeated determinations are necessary at intervals of perhaps 3 days.  Moreover, the values may be borderline or only slightly elevated, leading to confusion with the other causes of elevated amylase mentioned previously.  In this situation, the urine amylase may be helpful.  This usually rises within 24 hours after the serum amylase and as a rule remains abnormal 7-10 days after the serum concentration returns to normal.  Various investigators have used 1-, 2-, and 24-hour collection periods with roughly equal success.  The shorter collections have to be very accurately timed, while the 24-hour specimen may involve problems in complete collection.  It is important to have the results reported as units per 24 hours.  Frequently, the values are reported as units per 100 ml. which is inaccurate because it is influenced by fluctuating urine volumes.  One drawback of both serum and urine amylase is their relation to kidney function.  When significant BUN elevation is present, either transiently or permanently, neither the serum nor the urine amylase gives reliable information except when greatly elevated.  That is to say, the serum amylase may be falsely elevated, and the urine amylase falsely decreased by inability of the kidney to excrete the amylase.  However, in these cases, the urine amylase may be of some help if it is elevated at all.  Also, by the time shock and the azotemia have subsided, the serum amylase may have returned to normal, whereas the urine amylase may still be elevated.

Chronic pancreatic insufficiency may occur as a result of pancreatitis or hemochromatosis in adults and in the disease known as cystic fibrosis of the pancreas in children.  The diagnosis may be quite difficult, since the disease either represents an end stage phenomenon with no acute process going on, or else may take place slowly and subclinically over a long period.  The classic case of chronic pancreatitis has diabetes, pancreatic calcification on x-ray, and steatorrhea. The diagnosis of diabetes will be discussed in the next chapter. Steatorrhea may be demonstrated by quantitative fecal fat studies as described earlier. Either of these parameters may be normal or borderline in many patients. It may be desirable to attempt to assess pancreatic function by several methods. One of these is the measure of pancreatic trypsin excreted in the stools. A diluted portion of stool is placed on a photographic film with the presence of trypsin indicated by digestion of the gelatin covering of the film. However, this test is inaccurate because proteolytic bacteria exist in the colon which may themselves digest the gelatin. The stool may be examined directly and useful information obtained. Theoretically, in pancreatic insufficiency, there should be a large amount of neutral fat and very little fatty acid. However, a variable amount of fatty acid may in reality be present because some of the colon bacteria apparently are able to convert neutral fat to fatty acid. In the presence of demonstrable steatorrhea, a normal D-xylose test is usually found in pancreatic insufficiency or cystic fibrosis. Reports have appeared advocating measurement of serum amylase after injection of the pancreatic-stimulating hormone secretin. There is still controversy over the usefulness of this procedure. Also possible is direct measurement of pancreatic fluid constituents after secretin stimulation by means of duodenal tube drainage. This technique would have to be done by an experienced gastroenterologist and is not widely available.

Pancreas scanning using selenomethionine, an amino acid analog, is helpful in certain situations. In order to produce worthwhile results, a stationary imaging device such as the Anger scintillation camera must be used. The patient fasts overnight, and the scan is begun shortly after a high-protein meal to stimulate the organ. Under these conditions, a normal scan is effective in ruling out serious pancreatic disease. Abnormal scans may be produced by a variety of conditions, including nonfasting, active peptic ulcer, gastric surgery or vagotomy, chronic pancreatitis, pancreatic tumor, and malnutrition. Usual degrees of acute pancreatitis tend to produce abnormal scan image. Islet cell tumors are usually too small to be demonstrated, and most often exist with a normal scan.

Finally, a few words should be said about the diagnosis of cystic fibrosis of the pancreas. This classically occurs in children, but may not be manifested until adolescence or even occasionally in adults. It is a hereditary disease carried by a recessive gene. The disease affects the mucous glands of the body, but for some reason seems to affect those of the pancreas more than any other. The pancreatic secretions become thickened and eventually block the pancreatic acini, leading to secondary atrophy of the pancreatic cells. The same process may be found elsewhere such as in the lungs, where inspissated secretions may lead to recurrent bronchopneumonia, and in the liver, where thickened bile may lead to plugging of the small ducts and to a secondary cirrhosis in very severe cases. These patients usually do not have a watery type of diarrhea, but this is not always easy to ascertain by the history. The diagnosis is made because the sweat glands of the body are also involved in the disease. Although these patients excrete normal volumes of sweat, the sodium and chloride concentration of the sweat is abnormal in that much higher values of these electrolytes are lost. Cystic fibrosis and its diagnosis are discussed in Chapter 33.

Cystic fibrosis in children should be differentiated from so-called celiac disease. Celiac disease is basically the childhood form of nontropical sprue seen in adults, both of which in many cases seem due to hypersensitivity to a substance known as glutin. This substance is found in wheat, oats, and barley, and causes both histologic changes and clinical symptoms which are indistinguishable from tropical sprue, which is not influenced by glutin. These patients have normal sweat electrolytes, often will respond to a glutin-free diet, and behave like ordinary cases of the malabsorption syndrome.

## REFERENCES

Ambromovage, A. M. , et al. : The twenty-four hour excretion of amylase and lipase in the urine. Ann. Surg. 167:539, 1968.

Anderson, M. C. : Review of pancreatic disease, Surgery 66:434, 1969.

Bockus, H. L. (ed.): Gastroenterology (2d ed. ; Philadelphia: W. B. Saunders Company, 1963-1965).

Bolt, R. J. , et al. : A clinical evaluation of tubeless gastric analysis, Gastroenterology 32:34, 1957.

Cooley, R. W. : The diagnostic accuracy of radiologic studies of the biliary tract, small intestine, and colon, Am. J. M. Sc. 246:610, 1963.

Dreiling, D. A. , and Greenstein, A. J. : Enzymes in Pancreatic Disease, in Coodley, E. L. (ed.): Diagnostic Enzymology (Philadelphia: Lea & Febiger, 1970), p. 171.

Gambill, E. E. , and Mason, H. L. : One-hour value for urinary amylase in 96 patients with pancreatitis. Comparative diagnostic value of tests of urinary and serum amylase and serum lipase, J. A. M. A. , 186:24, 1963.

Gilbertson, V. A. , and Knatterud, G. L. : Gastric analysis as a screening measure for cancer of the stomach, Cancer 20:127, 1967.

Ginsberg, A. L. : Alterations in immunologic mechanisms in diseases of the gastrointestinal tract, Am. J. Digest. Dis. 16:61, 1971.

Gorden, H. E. , et al. : Diagnosis and management of gastrointestinal bleeding, Ann. Int. Med. 71:993, 1969.

Greegor, D. H.: Detection of silent colon cancer in routine examination, CA 19:330, 1969.

Henke, W. J., et al.: Evaluation of pancreatic function tests in confirmed pancreatic disease, Gastroenterology 41:233, 1961.

Katz, D., et al.: Sources of bleeding in upper gastrointestinal hemorrhage: A re-evaluation, Am. J. Digest. Dis. 9:447, 1964.

Mendeloff, A. I.: Selection of a screening procedure for detecting occult blood in feces, J. A. M. A. 152:798, 1953.

Morgan, T. E., and Roantree, R. J.: Evaluation of tests for occult blood in the feces, J. A. M. A. 164:1664, 1957.

Piper, D. W., et al.: The assessment of gastric secretion in man, M. J. Australia 57:549, 1970.

Raskin, H. F., et al.: Selected practical tests of gastrointestinal function, M. Clin. North America 43:341, 1959.

Rogers, A.: Immunoglobulins and the gastrointestinal tract, Postgrad. Med. 48:75, 1970.

Ruzicka, F. F., and Rossi, P.: Normal vascular anatomy of the abdominal viscera, Radiol. Clin. North America 8:3, 1970.

Schindler, R.: Critical evaluation of biopsy techniques for the diagnosis of gastritides, Am. J. Digest. Dis. 7:167, 1962.

Sparberg, M., and Kirsner, J. B.: Gastric secretory activity with reference to HCl, Arch. Int. Med. 114:508, 1964.

Stefanini, P., et al.: Diagnosis and management of acute pancreatitis, Am. J. Surg. 110:866, 1965.

Steigmann, F., and Hyman, S.: Acute gastrointestinal bleeding, Postgrad. Med. 41:252, 1967.

Toffler, A. H., and Spiro, H. M.: Shock or coma as the predominant manifestation of painless acute pancreatitis, Ann. Int. Med. 57:655, 1962.

Van Goidsenhoven, G. E., et al.: Pancreatic function in cirrhosis of the liver, Am. J. Digest. Dis. 8:160, 1963.

Williams, L. F.: Gastrointestinal hemorrhage as a postoperative phenomenon, Am. J. Surg. 116:375, 1968.

# CHAPTER 27

# Tests for Diabetes and Hypoglycemia

Besides exocrine digestive enzymes secreted into the duodenum, the pancreas has endocrine functions centered in the islands of Langerhans. Their location is primarily in the tail and body of the pancreas; their hormones are glucagon and insulin, and their secretion is directly into the blood stream. True diabetes mellitus results from hypofunction of the pancreatic islands of Langerhans, specifically the islet beta cells which produce insulin. This may be idiopathic, or secondary to pancreatic involvement by carcinoma, pancreatitis, or hemochromatosis. The idiopathic type is by far the most common. Its clinical features will not be discussed except to point out that there are two general categories of diabetics—those whose disease begins relatively early in life, is more severe, requires insulin for management, and shows severe insulin deficiency on assay, and a second group whose disease begins in late middle age or afterward, is less severe, can be treated with small doses of insulin or with oral medication, and shows some degree of insulin production.

Most laboratory tests for diabetes attempt to reflect pancreatic islet hypofunction, qualitative or quantitative, by measuring insulin production. Direct insulin assay was once technically too difficult for any but a few research laboratories. Therefore, emphasis in clinical medicine has been on indirect methods, whose end point usually demonstrates the action of insulin on a relatively accessible and measurable substance, the blood sugar. This necessity for indirect measurement of insulin makes certain flaws inherent in all laboratory procedures based on blood sugar determination. These problems derive from any technique which attempts to assay one substance by monitoring its action on another.

Ideally, one should measure a substrate which is specific for the reaction or enzyme in question under test conditions which eliminate the effects on utilization by any other factors. The blood sugar level does not meet any of these criteria. The blood sugar level depends primarily on the liver, which exerts its effect on blood glucose homeostasis via its reversible conversion of glucose to glycogen as well as gluconeogenesis from fat and protein. Next most important is tissue utilization of glucose which is mediated by pancreatic insulin, but is affected by many factors in addition to insulin.

The actual mechanisms involved in the regulation of blood sugar levels are complex, and in many cases only partially understood. Insulin is thought to act primarily on tissues at the cellular level, but its mode of action still has not been definitively established. The most accepted current theory involves alteration of cell membrane permeability to glucose. Others have suggested some influence on the hexokinase enzyme system which mediates the conversion of glucose to glucose-6-phosphate; also, there is some evidence that insulin enhances glycogen, protein, and fat synthesis. In addition, insulin may have a direct effect on the liver, possibly by suppressing glucose formation from glycogen (glycogenolysis). The liver is affected by at least three important hormones: epinephrine, glucagon, and hydrocortisone (cortisol). Epinephrine from the adrenal medulla stimulates breakdown of glycogen to glucose, apparently by converting inactive hepatic cell phosphorylase to active phosphorylase which mediates the conversion of glycogen to glucose-1-phosphate. In addition, there is evidence that gluconeogenesis from lactate is enhanced via the enzyme adenosine 3, 5-monophosphate. Glucagon is a hormone which is produced by the pancreatic alpha cells and released by the stimulus of hypoglycemia. It is thought to act on the liver in a manner similar to that of epinephrine. Hydrocortisone (cortisol), cortisone, and similar 11-oxygenated adrenocorticosteroids also influence the liver, but in a different manner. One fairly well documented pathway is enhancement of glycogen synthesis from amino acids. This increases the carbohydrate reserve available to augment blood sugar levels; thus, steroids like cortisol essentially stimulate gluconeogenesis. In addition, cortisol deficiency leads to anorexia, and also causes impairment of carbohydrate absorption from the small intestine.

The technique of blood sugar determination must be considered because different methods vary in specificity and sensitivity to glucose. The blood specimen itself is important; for each hour of standing at room temperature glucose values of whole blood decrease 10 mg./100 ml. unless a preservative is added. Fluoride is considered the best preservative at present. Plasma or serum are more stable than whole blood; if serum can be removed from the cells before 2 hours, serum glucose values remain stable up to 24 hours at room temperature (some authors report occasional decreases). Refrigeration assists this preservation. Serum or plasma values are about 10-15% higher than those of whole blood. This is important, because normal values quoted in the literature are mostly those from whole blood, while most present-day automated equipment uses serum. Normal values mentioned in this chapter will be those for serum. The two nonautomated analytical methods in common use are the Somogyi-Nelson and the Folin-Wu. Somogyi-Nelson is a reasonably accurate determination for blood sugar of any type, although blood sugar is composed essentially of glucose under most conditions. Normal serum values are usually 70-110 mg./100 ml. Folin-Wu measures various reducing substances such as creatinine, glutathione, and ergothianine, in addition to sugar. Therefore, Folin-Wu runs 20-30 mg./100 ml. above Somogyi values but can fluctuate widely, as much as 10-70 mg./100 ml. Many laboratories have automated blood glucose determinations; one of the most popular of the machines is the Autoanalyzer, which utilizes a ferricyanide sugar method that corresponds reasonably closely to Somogyi-Nelson. The widely used Technicon SMA-12/60 is based on a neocuproine reducing-substance method which is actually 10% above the company's stated 110 mg./100 ml. fasting upper limit of normal for serum. Venous blood is generally used; capillary (arterial) blood gives values which are approximately 30 mg./100 ml. higher but which vary considerably with sometimes as much as 100 mg./100 ml. difference. This venous-capillary divergence may be negligible when fasting. Most investigators prefer the so-called true blood sugar procedures, so that blood sugar values mentioned hereafter will be those of the Somogyi-Nelson method.

A more recent test for blood glucose is a rapid semiquantitative paper dipstick method named Dextrostix. A portion of the paper strip is impregnated with glucose oxidase, an enzyme specific for glucose, plus a color reagent. One drop of whole blood is used; the color which develops is compared to a reference color chart. Evaluations of this test to date provide a consensus that, with experience, values between 40 and 130 mg./100 ml. usually agree within at least $\pm$ 30-40% with values obtained from standard methods. Persons without much familiarity with the technique may obtain more erratic results. Dextrostix tends to underestimate to varying degrees any concentration of glucose over approximately 130 mg./100 ml. The method has been found useful to differentiate between hypoglycemia and hyperglycemia, and to provide a gross approximation of diabetic blood sugar control for outpatients. Additional considerations are possible differences between capillary (fingerstick) blood and venous blood values, alluded to previously; also, the fact that fluoride blood preservatives will inactivate the glucose oxidase enzyme.

The diagnosis of diabetes is made by demonstrating abnormally increased blood sugar under certain controlled conditions. If insulin deficiency is large, carbohydrate homeostatic mechanisms are unable to compensate and the fasting blood sugar is consistently elevated. If insulin deficiency is smaller, abnormality is noted only when an unusually heavy carbohydrate load is placed on the system. In uncompensated insulin deficiency, a fasting blood sugar reveals abnormality; in equivocal cases or in compensated insulin deficiency, a variety of carbohydrate tolerance test procedures are available to unmask the defect. In order to properly use and interpret these procedures, the various factors involved must be thoroughly understood.

## Glucose Tolerance Test (GTT)

This is a provocative type of test in which a relatively large dose of glucose challenges the body homeostatic mechanisms. All other variables being normal, it is assumed that the subsequent rise and fall of the blood sugar is due mainly to production of insulin in response to hyperglycemia, and that the degree of insulin response is mirrored in the behavior of the blood glucose. Failure to realize that this assumption is predicated on all other variables being normal explains a good deal of confusion which exists in the literature and in clinical practice.

The most important factor in the GTT is the need for careful standardization of the test procedure. Without these precautions any type of glucose tolerance test yields such varied results that an abnormal response cannot be interpreted. Previous carbohydrate intake is very important. If diet has been low in both calories and carbohydrates for as little as 3 days preceding the test, glucose tolerance may be diminished temporarily and the GTT may shift more or less toward diabetic levels. This has been especially true in starvation, but the situation does not have to be this extreme. Even a normal caloric diet which is low in carbohydrates may influence the GTT. A preparatory diet has been recommended which includes approximately 300 Gm. of carbohydrates per day for 3 days preceding the test, although others believe that 100 Gm. for each of the 3 days is sufficient. The average American diet contains approximately 100-150 Gm. of carbohydrates; it is obviously necessary in any case to be sure the patient actually eats at least 100 Gm. a day for 3 days. Inactivity has been reported as a significant influence on the GTT, also toward the diabetic side. One study found almost 50% more diabetic GTT response in bedridden patients compared to ambulatory patients otherwise identical in most other respects. There is a well-recognized trend toward decreasing carbohydrate tolerance with advanced age. Although the degree of abnormality is not enough to affect fasting sugar normal range, glucose tolerance upper limits increase about 1 mg./100 ml. per year beyond age 50. There are three schools of thought as to the interpretation of this fact. One group feels that effects of aging either unmask latent diabetes or represent true diabetes due to impairment of islet cell function in a manner analogous to subclinical renal function decrease through arteriosclerosis. Another group applies arbitrary correction formulas to decrease the number of abnormalities to a predetermined figure based on estimates of diabetes incidence in the given population. The most widely accepted viewpoint regards these changes as physiologic rather than pathologic; and, in order to avoid labeling these persons diabetic, it extends the upper limits of normal by adding 1 mg./100 ml. to each GTT value for each year over age 50. Fasting values are not affected. The effect of <u>obesity</u> is not certain. Some believe that obesity per se has little influence on the GTT. Others believe that obesity decreases carbohydrate tolerance; they have found significant differences after weight reduction, at least in obese mild diabetics. <u>Fever</u> tends to produce a diabetic-type GTT response; this is true regardless of the etiology, but more so with infections. <u>Diurnal variation</u> in glucose tolerance has been reported, with significantly decreased carbohydrate tolerance during the afternoon in many persons whose GTT curves were normal in the morning. This suggests that tests for diabetes should be done in the morning.

### The Oral Glucose Tolerance Test

The oral dose of glucose has been fairly well standardized at 100 Gm. of dextrose. Some have used as little as 50 Gm. with equally good results. This is administered as a 50% solution or dissolved in 300-500 ml. of water, in either case flavored by some substance such as lemon juice. The dose may be calculated from body weight.

Blood specimens are taken fasting, then 1/2 hour, 1, 2, and 3 hours after dextrose ingestion. Fajans and Conn advocate an additional specimen at 1 1/2 hours. After ingestion and a lag period, the blood sugar curve rises sharply to a peak, usually in 15-60 minutes. In one study, 76% had maximal values at 1/2 hour, 17% at 1 hour. The curve then falls steadily but more slowly, reaching normal levels at 2 hours. These may be fasting values or simply within normal blood sugar ranges.

Occasionally, after the fasting level is reached, there may follow a transient dip below the fasting level, usually not great, then a return to fasting values. This relative hypoglycemic phase of the curve (when present) is thought due to a lag in the ability of the liver to change from converting glucose to glycogen (in response to previous hyperglycemia) to its other activity of supplying glucose from glycogen. In some cases, residual insulin may also be a factor. This "hypoglycemic" phase, if present, is generally between the second and fourth hours. Several reports indicate that so-called terminal hypoglycemia, which is a somewhat exaggerated form of this phenomenon, occurs in a fairly large number of patients with GTT indicative of mild diabetes. They believe that an abnormally marked hypoglycemic dip often appears in mild diabetics 3-5 hours after meals or a test dose of carbohydrates, and may be one of the earliest clinical manifestations of the disease.

Criteria for interpretation of the oral GTT have varied widely. This situation is brought about because of the absence of a sharp division between diabetics and nondiabetics, variations in methodology, and variations in adjustment for the many conditions which may affect the GTT quite apart from diabetes mellitus; some of these factors have been mentioned previously and others will be discussed later. The criteria of Fajans and Conn are probably the most widely accepted, at least by investigators in the field. Normal oral GTT values follow (mg./100 ml. true glucose):

| Time | Serum (mg./100 ml.) | Whole Blood (mg./100 ml.) |
|---|---|---|
| Fasting | 70-110 | 60-100 |
| 1 hour | Less than 185 | Less than 160 |
| (1 1/2 hours) | (Less than 160) | (Less than 145) |
| 2 hours | Less than 140 | Less than 120 |

NOTE: Add 1 mg./100 ml. per year over age 50 to each nonfasting value.

For the diagnosis of diabetes mellitus, at least two of these figures must be abnormal (assuming all other factors which could influence the GTT are eliminated). If only one single value on the curve is abnormal, it is considered suspicious, but not diagnostic, of diabetes. Other authorities suggest slightly different criteria. Taking a representative sample of the literature, normal values for (whole blood) fasting blood sugar (FBS) range from 100 to 120 mg./100 ml.; 1-hour levels from 150 to 170 mg./100 ml.; and 2-hour values from "FBS" to 120 mg./100 ml. Nevertheless, the criteria of Fajans and Conn correlate well enough with the clinical course of diabetes to warrant acceptance in the interest of diagnostic uniformity.

Screening tests for diabetes attempt to circumvent the multiple blood sugar determinations required for the GTT. The fasting blood sugar (FBS) and the 2-hour postprandial (2-hour pc) blood sugar level have been widely used. Since these methods constitute, in essence, isolated segments of the GTT, interpretation of their results must take several problems into consideration in addition to those inherent in the GTT.

An abnormality in the FBS, for example, raises the question of whether a full GTT is needed for confirmation of diabetes. Most authors believe that if the FBS is elevated, there is no need to do the full glucose tolerance test. Whatever the etiology for the abnormal FBS, the GTT will also be abnormal; since it is known in advance that the GTT will be abnormal, no further information will be gained from performing the GTT. Most also agree that a normal FBS is not reliable in screening for diabetes. In one study, 63% of those with diabetic GTT had normal FBS; and others have similar experiences, although perhaps with less striking figures.

Most investigators believe that of all the GTT values and criteria, the 2-hour level is the most crucial. The 2-hour value alone has therefore been proposed as a screening test. This recommendation is based on the fact that the helpfulness of blood sugar levels prior to the 2-hour time point is open to some question. Fajans and Conn state that "the diagnosis of diabetes mellitus cannot be made with confidence on the basis of an abnormal elevation of blood sugar level at 1/2 or 1 hour if it is accompanied by a normal 2-hour blood sugar level in the GTT." The main reason for this lies in the effect of gastric emptying on glucose absorption. It has been fairly well proved that normal gastric emptying does not deliver a saturation dose. Therefore, slow gastric emptying tends to produce a low or "flat" GTT. On the other hand, either unusually swift gastric transit or delivery of a normal total quantity of glucose to the small intestine within a markedly shortened time span results in abnormally high amounts of glucose absorbed during the initial phases of the tolerance test. Since homeostatic mechanisms are not instantaneous, the peak values of the tolerance curve reach abnormally high tolerance test. Since homeostatic mechanisms are not instantaneous, the peak value of the tolerance curve reach abnormally high figures before the hyperglycemia is brought under control. An extreme example of this situation occurs in the "dumping syndrome" produced by gastrojejunostomy.

If previous time interval specimens are considered unreliable, the question then is justified as to whether the 2-hour value alone is sufficient. In many cases, if the 2-hour level is definitely abnormal, then a full GTT would not add any useful information, although an FBS would provide some further indication of the severity of derangement in carbohydrate homeostasis. If the 2-hour level is equivocal (140 mg./100 ml. $\pm$ 10 mg./100 ml.), then a GTT should be done, since abnormalities in other areas of the curve would give added support to the suspicion of diabetes. This assumes also that nonpancreatic diabetogenic influences are ruled out. There are several provisos to this situation which must be kept in mind. If the 2-hour postprandial specimen follows an ordinary meal rather than as part of a standard tolerance test, the problem of adequate carbohydrate preparation may obscure results as well as possible variations in the amount and type of sugar ingested. Also, Fajans and Conn, as well as others, report one variation of the normal oral GTT which drops relatively swiftly to normal at approximately 1 1/2 hours and then rebounds above 140 mg./100 ml. by 2 hours. In one report this phenomenon occurs in as many as 5-10% of cases. This is the basis for the suggested inclusion of a 1 1/2-hour specimen into the oral GTT procedure. Finally, Fajans and Conn call attention to their follow-up data on persons with normal 2-hour values but abnormal or borderline levels elsewhere in the GTT curve. Subsequent retesting over periods of years frequently revealed progression to a degree of carbohydrate impairment diagnostic of diabetes. With these limitations, the 2-hour postprandial blood sugar is a very useful screening test. It is definitely more sensitive than the FBS, and

its specificity could be increased by utilizing the standard carbohydrate preparation and a standard oral glucose test dose.

Besides the intrinsic and extrinsic factors which modify response to the oral glucose tolerance test procedure, other diseases
besides diabetes mellitus regularly produce diabetic-type GTT patterns or curves.  Among these are adrenal, thyroid, and pituitary
hormone abnormalities which influence liver or tissue response to
blood glucose levels.  Cushing's syndrome results from hypersecretion of hydrocortisone.  Since this hormone stimulates gluconeogenesis, among its other actions, 70-80% of these patients exhibit
decreased carbohydrate tolerance, while 25% of those with Cushing's
syndrome demonstrate overt diabetes.  Pheochromocytomas of the
adrenal medulla (or elsewhere) have been reported to produce hyperglycemia in nearly 60% of the affected patients, and glycosuria in a
lesser number.  These tumors produce norepinephrine or epinephrine,
either continually or intermittently.  The diabetogenic effects of
epinephrine were mentioned earlier, and it has been noted that those
pheochromocytomas which secrete norepinephrine rather than epinephrine are not associated with abnormalities of carbohydrate metabolism.  Primary aldosteronism leads to the overproduction of aldosterone, the chief electrolyte-regulating adrenocortical hormone.
This increases renal tubular excretion of potassium and retention of
sodium.  Patients with primary aldosteronism frequently may develop decreased carbohydrate tolerance.  According to Conn, this is
most likely due to potassium depletion, which in some manner adversely affects the ability of pancreatic beta cells to respond normally to a hyperglycemic stimulus.  Parenthetically, there may be
some analogy in the reports that chlorothiazide diuretics may cause
added decrease in carbohydrate tolerance in diabetics, thus acting
as a diabetogenic agent.  Some say no such effect exists in normal
persons, but others maintain that it does in a few.  Chlorothiazide
often leads to potassium depletion as a side effect; indeed, one report indicates that potassium supplements will reverse the diabetogenic effect.  However, other mechanisms have been postulated.

Thyroid hormone has several effects on carbohydrate metabolism.  First, thyroxine acts in some way on small intestine mucosal cells to increase hexose sugar absorption.  In the liver, thyroxine causes increased gluconeogenesis from protein and increased
breakdown of glycogen to glucose.  The metabolic rate of peripheral
tissues is increased, resulting in an increased rate of glucose utilization.  Peripheral tissue glycogen is depleted.  Nevertheless, the
effect of hyperthyroidism on the GTT is variable.  Apparently the
characteristic hyperthyroid curve is one that peaks unusually high,
sometimes with glucosuria, but which returns to normal ranges by
2 hours.  However, in one extensive survey, as many as 7% were
reported to have diabetic curves and another 2% had actual diabetes
mellitus.  Surprisingly, the type of curve found in any individual
case was without relation to the severity of the hyperthyroidism.  In

myxedema, a "flat" oral GTT (defined as a peak rise of less than 25 mg./100 ml. above FBS) is common. However, in hypothyroidism a normal or even a diabetic type curve may be found, since absorption defects vary in degree and are counterpoised against decreased tissue metabolism.

Hyperpituitarism, especially acromegaly, may produce a diabetic or pseudodiabetic GTT. Growth hormone (somatotropin) is thought to have its own ability to stimulate gluconeogenesis. Actually, the influence of the pituitary on carbohydrate metabolism has been mainly studied in conditions of pituitary hypofunction; in hypopituitarism, a defect in gluconeogenesis was found which was due to a combination of thyroid and adrenocorticosteroid deficiency rather than to either agent alone.

In acute pancreatitis, perhaps 25-50% of patients may develop transient hyperglycemia. In chronic pancreatitis, abnormal glucose tolerance or outright diabetes mellitus is extremely common.

A variety of nonendocrine disorders may produce diabetogenic effects on carbohydrate tolerance. Chronic renal disease with azotemia frequently demonstrates a diabetic curve of varying degree, sometimes even to the point of fasting hyperglycemia. The reason is not definitely known. It is said that the tolbutamide test (to be discussed later) is normal in nondiabetics with azotemia. Hyperglycemia with or without glycosuria occurs from time to time in patients with cerebral lesions. These may include tumors, skull fracture, cerebral infarction, intracerebral hemorrhage, and encephalitis. The mechanism is not known, but experimental evidence suggests some type of center with regulatory influence on glucose metabolism located in the medulla and the hypothalamus, and perhaps elsewhere. Similar reasoning applies to the transient hyperglycemia, sometimes accompanied by glucosuria, seen in severe carbon monoxide poisoning. This is said to appear in 50% of these patients, and seems to be due to a direct toxic effect on the cerebral centers responsible for carbohydrate metabolism. One subgroup of lipoproteinemia (p. 259) is also said to frequently elicit some degree of decreased carbohydrate tolerance which sometimes may include fasting hyperglycemia.

Malignancies of varying types are reported to produce decreased carbohydrate tolerance in varying numbers of cases, but the true incidence or the mechanism involved is difficult to ascertain due to the presence of other diabetogenic factors such as fever, cachexia, liver dysfunction, and inactivity.

Liver disease often affects the oral GTT; this is not surprising in view of the importance of the liver in carbohydrate homeostasis. Abnormality is most often seen in cirrhosis; the degree of abnormality has a general (although not exact) correlation with degree of liver damage. In well-established cirrhosis, the 2-hour postprandial blood sugar is usually abnormal. FBS is variable, but is most often normal. Fatty liver may produce GTT abnormality similar to that of cirrhosis. Infectious hepatitis has less abnormality than cirrhosis, becomes normal during convalescence, and may be normal throughout in mild disease.

Myocardial infarction has been shown to precipitate temporary hyperglycemia, glucosuria, or decreased carbohydrate tolerance. In one representative study, 75% had abnormal GTT during the acute phase of infarction, with 50% of these being frankly diabetic curves; follow-up showed that about a third of the abnormal curves persisted. Besides the well-known increased incidence of atherosclerosis (predisposing to infarction) in overt or latent diabetics, emotional factors in a stress situation and shock with liver damage may be contributory. Emotional hyperglycemia is considered a well-established entity and probably is secondary to epinephrine effect.

Oral glucose tolerance tests in pregnancy are the subject of dispute. Some investigators believe that the oral GTT in gravid women does not differ from that of nulliparas, and thus any abnormalities in the curve are suspicious of latent diabetes. Others believe that pregnancy itself, especially in the last trimester, tends to exert a definite diabetogenic influence. This view is reinforced by observations that various synthetic estrogen-progesterone combinations used for contraception often mimic the diabetogenic effects of pregnancy. This may occur in 18-46% of cases, and, as in pregnancy, the FBS is most often normal. The exact mechanism is not clear; some offer an explanation of altered intestinal absorption.

Salicylate overdose in children frequently produces a clinical situation which closely resembles diabetic acidosis. Salicylate in large quantities has a toxic effect on the liver, leading to decreased glycogen formation and to increased breakdown of glycogen to glucose. Therefore, there may develop a mild-to-moderate elevation in blood sugar, accompanied by ketonuria. Plasma ketone tests may even be positive, although usually only to mild degree. Salicylic acid metabolites give positive results using tests for reducing substances such as Clinitest (p. 118), so that such tests will falsely suggest glucosuria. In addition, salicylate stimulates the central nervous system respiratory center in the early phases of overdose, so that increased respiration may suggest the Kussmaul breathing of diabetic acidosis. The $CO_2$ content (or combining power) is decreased. Later on, a metabolic acidosis develops.

Differentiation from diabetic acidosis can be accomplished using simple tests for salicylate in plasma or urine. A dipstick test called Phenistix (p. 125) is very useful for screening purposes. A positive plasma Phenistix reaction for salicylate is good evidence of salicylate poisoning. A positive test in urine is not conclusive, since in urine the procedure will detect nontoxic levels of salicylate, but a negative urine test would be strong evidence against the diagnosis. Definitive chemical quantitative or semiquantitative tests for blood salicylate levels are available. It is important to ask about a history of medication given to the patient or the possibility of accidental ingestion in children with suspicious clinical symptoms.

Salicylate intoxication is not frequent in adults. When it occurs, there is much less tendency toward development of a pseudo-diabetic acidosis syndrome. In fact, in adults, salicylate in nontoxic dose occasionally produces hypoglycemia, which tends to occur 2-4 hours postprandially.

Dilantin is reported to decrease glucose tolerance; and overdose occasionally produces a type of nonketotic hyperglycemic coma.

Complete discussion of the oral GTT must include reference to other studies which attack the clinical usefulness of the procedure. These comprise reports of large series of normal persons showing up to 20% "flat" GTT results, studies which showed different curves in repeat determinations after time lapse, and others which were able to obtain various types of curves on repeated tests in the same individual. Therefore, sensitivity, specificity, and reproducibility have all been challenged, even under standardized test conditions. However, it is the opinion of most that the oral GTT is still the standard parameter of carbohydrate tolerance. Fajans and Conn believe that it is still the most sensitive test for diabetes in routine use.

## Intravenous Glucose Tolerance Test (IV-GTT)

This test was devised to eliminate some of the objections to the oral GTT. Standard procedure is as follows: The patient has a 3-day high carbohydrate preparatory diet. After an FBS is obtained, a standard solution of 50% glucose is injected intravenously over a 3-4 minute period. Blood samples are obtained at 1/2, 1, 2, and 3 hours, although it would seem more informative to omit the 1/2-hour specimen and substitute a 1 1/2-hour sample. The curve reaches a peak immediately after injection (300-400 mg./100 ml. accompanied by glucosuria) then falls steadily but not linearly toward fasting levels. Criteria for interpretation are not uniform. However, most believe that a normal response is indicated by return to fasting levels by 1-1 1/4 hours. The height of the curve has no significance. Most agree that the IV-GTT is adequately reproducible. In diabetes, fasting levels are not reached in 2 hours and often not even by 3. The curve in liver disease is most characteristically said to return to normal between 1 1/4 and 2 hours; however, some patients with cirrhosis have a diabetic-type curve. Many of the same factors which produce a diabetogenic effect on the oral GTT do likewise to the intravenous procedure; these include carbohydrate deprivation, inactivity, old age, fever, uremia, stress, neoplasms, and the various steroid-producing endocrine diseases. There are, however, several differences from the oral GTT. Alimentary problems are eliminated. The IV-GTT is said to be normal in pregnancy, also in hyperthyroidism, although one report found occasional abnormality in thyrotoxicosis. The IV-GTT is conceded to be somewhat less sensitive than the oral procedure, although, as discussed above, a little more specific.

## Cortisone Glucose Tolerance Test (C-GTT)

Fajans and Conn attempted to improve the sensitivity of the oral GTT. They found that the addition of adrenocortical steroids to the procedure magnified slight degrees of defective carbohydrate tolerance and produced an increased number of abnormal curves in a group of patients with a history or genetic background strongly predisposing toward diabetes. For example, of 17 persons with "suspicious" oral GTT, 88% had positive C-GTT. Their follow-ups tended to substantiate the test results, since they report that 25% of those with positive C-GTT and normal oral GTT developed outright diabetes and 10% probable diabetes. The procedure for the C-GTT is as follows: After standard 3-day carbohydrate diet, oral cortisone acetate is given at specified intervals; then the standard oral GTT is run. Normal values are approximately 20 mg./100 ml. above those of the standard oral GTT. The 2-hour value is the most crucial, just as in the standard GTT. Several reports have subsequently agreed with these findings regarding sensitivity and specificity. Others have not been enthusiastic. However, Fajans and Conn correctly point out that several misconceptions about C-GTT exist. The test does not disclose genetic susceptibility to diabetes, only a certain degree of decreased carbohydrate tolerance. The test and interpretation must be done as originally described, and, if comparison with standard oral GTT results is desired, the criteria of Fajans and Conn for the oral GTT must also be used. These authors further maintain that obesity per se does not seem to influence either the standard or C-GTT, although obesity in diabetics further decreased carbohydrate tolerance. Old age, inadequate carbohydrate diet, and most other diabetogenic factors which influence the standard oral GTT do likewise to the C-GTT. Cortisone priming seems to greatly increase the number of abnormal GTTs in pregnancy, and apparently the significance of this is not yet established. At present, the C-GTT is recommended by its originators mainly as a research tool; its usefulness lies in demonstrating probable diabetes in some persons with only minimally decreased carbohydrate tolerance.

## Plasma (or Serum) Insulin Assay

Insulin was the first substance used successfully in radioisotope immunoassay, and it is now available in most sizable reference laboratories. In general, juvenile diabetics have low fasting insulin levels, and an oral GTT using insulin determinations will usually produce a flat curve. Mild diabetics possess normal fasting insulin levels and display a GTT curve which has a delayed rise, either to normal height or to a point moderately above normal; in either case

the curve thereafter falls in a normal fashion.  Decreased tolerance
due to many other causes produces similar curves; an insulin GTT
has not been more efficient in uncovering subclinical diabetes than
blood sugar GTT.  Some maintain that the ratio of insulin values to
glucose values obtained on the same specimen during the oral GTT
is more reliable than insulin values alone.  At any rate, most investigators feel that, at present, plasma insulin levels should not be
used for diagnosis of diabetes mellitus.

A new classification of diabetes has been proposed and is gain-
ing considerable acceptance.  This is partially based on the various
laboratory tests discussed earlier.  The categories are:

1.  Prediabetes:  All laboratory tests normal; genetic predisposition.

2.  Subclinical diabetes:  Cortisone-GTT abnormal; oral GTT
normal.

3.  Latent (chemical) diabetes:  Oral GTT abnormal; FBS normal or abnormal; no clinical symptoms.

4.  Overt diabetes:  FBS abnormal; clinical diabetes.

Besides measurement of blood glucose or carbohydrate tolerance, certain other procedures are widely used or proposed for the
detection of diabetes mellitus.

## Glucosuria

The appearance of glucose in the urine has long been utilized
both for the detection of diabetes and as a parameter of treatment.
As a clue to diagnosis, urine sugar depends on hyperglycemia which
exceeds the renal tubular threshold for glucose.  This is usually
quoted as 170 mg./100 ml. (Somogyi values) for venous blood.  Of
some interest regarding the threshold concept in diabetics is evidence that some diabetics possess either low thresholds or, especially in the elderly, unusually high ones (up to 300 mg./100 ml.).
It has also been shown that arterial blood glucose levels are much
better correlated with glucosuria than venous ones.  Nevertheless,
routine urine testing provides a method for practical continuous outpatient monitoring of therapy and for the prevention of ketoacidosis.
This aspect provides another argument for more routine use of the
full GTT, since glucosuria can be correlated with degree of hyperglycemia.  Incidentally, many diabetic patients and many of those
involved in mass surveys take their urine sugar test before breakfast, which actually is the least likely time to produce glucosuria.
The problem of causes of hyperglycemia not due to diabetes mellitus was discussed earlier.  Renal threshold assumes importance
in another way because of the condition known as renal glucosuria.
This may be congenital or acquired; the acquired type may be idiopathic or secondary to certain diseases such as the Fanconi syndrome, acute tubular necrosis, or renal rickets.  In all types there
is glucosuria at lower blood sugar levels than normal.  Some report

that a significant number of those with the nonfamilial idiopathic variety of renal glucosuria eventually develop overt diabetes mellitus, although others do not agree.

Glucosuria of pregnancy occurs in the last trimester. Reported incidence depends on the sensitivity of the testing methods used, ranging from 5 to 35% or even 70%. The etiology seems to be a combination of increased glomerular filtration rate and temporarily decreased renal threshold. Lactosuria is even more common. Glucosuria without hyperglycemia occurs in 20% of patients with lead poisoning. This is due to a direct toxic effect on the renal tubule cells. Glucosuria of a transient nature has been reported in 24% of normal newborn infants. A study utilizing paper chromatography revealed galactosuria, usually in amounts too small for detection by routine techniques, to be even more common.

Mentioned here only for the sake of completeness are the two main types of urine sugar tests: the copper sulfate tests for reducing substances, and the glucose oxidase enzyme papers. The merits, drawbacks, and technical aspects of these tests, as well as a general discussion of glucosuria, are included in Chapter 12.

### Diagnosis of Diabetic Coma

Diabetic coma may occur without a history of diabetes or in circumstances where history is not available. Other major etiologies of coma have to be considered, including insulin hypoglycemia, meningitis or cerebrovascular accident, shock, uremia, and barbiturate overdose. Diabetic coma yields a clear-cut fast diagnosis by means of a plasma acetone test. Anticoagulated blood is obtained; a portion is centrifuged for 2 to 3 minutes and the plasma is tested for acetone. Diabetic acidosis severe enough to produce coma will be definitely positive (except for the rare cases of lactic acidosis or hyperosmolar coma). The other etiologies for coma will be negative, since they rarely produce the degree of acidosis found in diabetic coma. The findings of urinary glucose and acetone strongly suggest diabetes, but may occur in other conditions. Such findings would not entirely rule out insulin overdose (always a consideration in a known diabetic), since the urine could have been produced before the overdose. This would be unlikely, however, if urinary acetone were strongly positive. An elevated blood sugar also is strong evidence of diabetic coma, especially in marked degrees of elevation. Other conditions which might combine coma with hyperglycemia (cerebrovascular accident, acute myocardial infarction) have only mild or moderate hyperglycemia in those instances where hyperglycemia is produced. Besides blood sugar determination, a simple empirical test to rule out hypoglycemia is to inject some glucose solution intravenously. Cerebral damage is investigated by cerebrospinal fluid examination. Uremia is determined by means of the blood urea nitrogen, although other etiologies of coma besides primary renal disease may have an elevated BUN. Drug ingestion is established by careful history, analysis of stomach contents, and identification of the drug in blood samples (one anticoagulated and one clotted specimen are preferred). Shock is diagnosed on the basis of blood pressure; further laboratory investigation depends on the probable etiology.

Pancreatic Endocrine Hyperfunction: Whereas diabetes is caused by insulin deficiency, a syndrome is produced by insulin excess. The most well-known cause is islet cell adenoma (sometimes islet cell carcinoma). In these cases, symptoms are most often precipitated by fasting. The first effects are vague malaise and apathy, followed by hypoglycemia signs. These include nausea, weakness, nervousness, tachycardia, and sweating. If allowed to continue, fainting or even coma will follow, often with convulsions. Sometimes central nervous system symptoms predominate; these are identical to those of central nervous system hypoxia and produce bizarre behavior and blurring of consciousness. Differential diagnosis includes alcoholism, uremia, hyperventilation, barbiturate overdose, and diabetic coma. Hypoglycemia may be produced by other causes; the most important of these is called functional hypoglycemia. This condition is fairly common, and differs from organic hypoglycemia in that attacks are brought on by intake of carbohydrates. It represents an abnormal response of the pancreas to only moderately increased carbohydrate loads, resulting in oversecretion of insulin by the pancreas and the development of temporary hypoglycemia 1-3 hours later when the initial blood sugar elevation is eliminated and some of the excess insulin is still present. The initial blood sugar elevation is no greater than that of a normal person. Somewhat different conditions are found in certain postgastrectomy patients, where gastric emptying is swift and complete so that ingested carbohydrates are suddenly dumped into the duodenum, resulting in abnormally high blood sugar levels and temporary hypoglycemia after hastily produced insulin has overcome the initial hyperglycemia. This is called the dumping syndrome or alimentary hypoglycemia. The initial blood sugar elevation is definitely greater than that of a normal person.

Diagnosis of islet cell tumor is important, since the condition is surgically correctable, but accurate diagnosis is a necessity to avoid unnecessary operation. The basic criterion is Whipple's triad, which consists of:

1. Attacks of central nervous system or hypoglycemia symptoms while fasting.
2. An FBS of less than 10 mg./100 ml. below FBS normal lower limits at some time.
3. Relief of symptoms by glucose.

Diagnosis should be confirmed by either a 5-hour glucose tolerance test (Fig. 13) or a tolbutamide tolerance test. The tolbutamide test is preferred.

In the GTT, the patient fasts for 8-12 hours, unless symptoms are brought on sooner. The standard oral GTT is then given. Re-

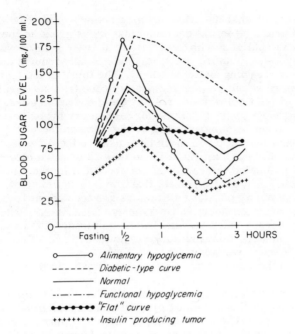

Fig. 13.—Representative oral glucose tolerance curves.

sults for insulin-producing tumors show normal or low FBS, the usual sharp rise after glucose, then a slower fall to hypoglycemic levels which do not rapidly return to normal range. If the curve has not reached 50 mg./100 ml. in 5 hours, 1 more hour is added. The curves for functional, hepatogenic, and alimentary hypoglycemia are different and reflect the mechanisms involved. The 5-hour curve is needed for these conditions unless a characteristic curve develops in less time. Unfortunately, a considerable minority of patients with pancreatic islet cell tumor are reported to show a "flat" curve, or sometimes even a diabetic-type curve, rather than the characteristic response just outlined. For this reason, and since many factors influence oral glucose tolerance, the tolbutamide test is considered more reliable and is easier to perform. In patients with insulin-producing tumors the fall in blood sugar is greater than that of most normals—down to the 40-65% of FBS range compared to normals who are usually over 50% of FBS.

Since there is occasional overlap, of greater significance is the fact that insulin tumor hypoglycemia persists for more than 3 hours, whereas, in most normals, the blood sugar level has returned to fasting values by 3 hours. In a few normals and in those with functional hypoglycemia, values return to at least 80% of FBS by 3 hours. Adrenal insufficiency also returns to at least 80% by 3 hours, although the initial decrease may be as great as the insulin tumor. Some patients with severe liver disease give curves similar to those of insulin tumor. However, this is not frequent and usually is not a real diagnostic problem. The tolbutamide test is apparently more sensitive than the oral glucose tolerance test for the diagnosis of islet cell tumor, but has the disadvantage that the characteristic responses of functional or alimentary hypoglycemia to the oral GTT cannot be demonstrated by the tolbutamide test.

Plasma insulin levels have been used in the diagnosis of islet cell tumor. Only two thirds of these tumors produce elevated fasting levels. The leucine tolerance test is abnormal in many insulinomas, but is significantly less accurate than the tolbutamide test.

The majority of islet cell tumors are located in the body or tail of the pancreas; about 90% are benign adenomas. Pancreatic artery angiography may be very helpful to pinpoint the exact location of the tumor. Most institutions, however, are able to detect less than 50% by arteriography.

Four other etiologies of hypoglycemia should be mentioned. They are:

1.  Certain nonpancreatic tumors: Presumably either by glucose utilization or by production of an insulin-like substance. The great majority have been intra-abdominal neoplasms of large size, usually described as fibrosarcoma or spindle cell sarcoma. Hepatoma is next most frequent.

2.  Leucine sensitivity of infancy and childhood: Symptoms produced by ingestion of cow's milk, which contains the amino acid leucine. Diagnosis is made by a leucine tolerance test, similar to the oral GTT but using oral leucine.

3.  Alcohol: May occur either in chronic alcoholics or occasional drinkers. Malnutrition, chronic or temporary, seems an important predisposing factor. Fasting for 12-24 hours precedes alcohol intake; symptoms may occur immediately, but most often follow 6-24 hours later.

4.  Overdose of insulin in a diabetic: Since the patient may be found in coma without any history available, insulin overdose must be a major consideration in any emergency-room comatose patient.

REFERENCES

Andres, R.: Aging and diabetes, M. Clin. North America 55:835, 1971.

Baker, R. J.: Newer considerations in the diagnosis and management of fasting hypoglycemia, Surg. Clin. North America 49:191, 1969.

Cohen, B. D.: Abnormal carbohydrate metabolism in renal disease, Ann. Int. Med. 57:204, 1962.

Conn, J. W.: Interpretation of the glucose tolerance test, Am. J. M. Sc. 199:555, 1940.

Conn, J. W.: Hypertension, the potassium ion, and impaired carbohydrate tolerance, New England J. Med. 273:1135, 1965.

Conn, J. W., and Seltzer, H. S.: Spontaneous hypoglycemia, Am. J. Med. 19:460, 1955.

Fajans, S.: What is diabetes? Definition, diagnosis, and course, M. Clin. North America 55:793, 1971.

Fajans, S. S., and Conn, J. W.: The early recognition of diabetes mellitus, Ann. New York Acad. Sc. 82:208, 1959.

Forsham, P.: Cushing's Syndrome, CIBA Clinical Symposia 15:49, 1965.

Frethem, A. A.: Clinics on endocrine and metabolic diseases. 10. Relation of fasting blood glucose level to oral glucose tolerance curve, Proc. Staff Meet. Mayo Clin. 38:110, 1963.

Gardner, F. H.: A malabsorption syndrome in military personnel in Puerto Rico, A. M. A. Arch. Int. Med. 98:44, 1956.

Glicksman, A. S., et al.: Diabetes mellitus and carbohydrate metabolism in patients with cancer, M. Clin. North America 40:887, 1956.

Grunt, J. A., et al.: Blood sugar serum insulin and free fatty acid interrelationships during intravenous tolbutamide testing in normal young adults and in patients with insulinoma, Diabetes 19:122, 1970.

Jackson, W. P. U.: The cortisone-glucose tolerance test with special reference to the prediction of diabetes, Diabetes 10:33, 1961.

John, J.: Hyperthyroidism showing carbohydrate metabolism disturbances, J. A. M. A. 99:620, 1932.

Kaplan, N. M.: Tolbutamide tolerance test in carbohydrate metabolism disturbances, Arch. Int. Med. 107:212, 1961.

Mackay, N., et al.: Observer error in Dextrostix estimations of blood-sugar, Lancet 2:269, 1965.

Madison, L. L.: Ethanol-Induced Hypoglycemia, in Levine, R., and Luft, R. (eds.): Advances in Metabolic Disorders (New York: Academic Press, 1968), Vol. 3, p. 85.

McDonald, G. W.: Reproducibility of the oral glucose tolerance test, Diabetes 14:473, 1965.

Medford, F. E.: An evaluation of the glucose oxidase skin test in the diagnosis of diabetes mellitus, West Virginia M. J. 60:255, 1964.

Milstein, J. M.: Hypoglycemia in the neonate, Postgrad. Med. 50:91, 1971.

Munch-Peterson, C. J.: Glycosuria of cerebral origin, Brain 54:72, 1931.

Raskin, T. J., et al.: Oral glucose tolerance as a test of liver function, Gastroenterology 25:548, 1953.

Schlicke, C. P., and Berghar, R.: Hypoglycemia due to islet cell
    tumor of the pancreas, Am. Surg. 36:646, 1970.
Seltzer, H.: Insights about diabetes and hyperinsulinism gained
    from the insulin immunoassay, Postgrad. Med. 46:73, 1969.
Smith, M.: The diagnosis of diabetes mellitus, M. Clin. North
    America 43:579, 1959.
Sowton, S.: Cardiac infarction and the glucose tolerance test,
    Brit. M. J. 1:84, 1962.
Spellacy, W. N.: A review of carbohydrate metabolism and the
    oral contraceptives, Am. J. Obst. & Gynec. 104:448, 1969.
Wolfe, W. G., et al.: Insulinoma of the pancreas, Arch. Surg.
    104:56, 1972.

# CHAPTER 28

# Thyroid and Parathyroid Function Tests

Thyroid tests make up an important segment of laboratory medicine. Many patients have at least one sign or symptom which suggests thyroid disease. On the other hand, thyroid dysfunction produces a wide variety of effects without any single one being diagnostic. There has been a continual search for a laboratory test which will provide a clear-cut diagnosis. Enumeration of the classic signs and symptoms of thyroid disease is the best way to emphasize the necessity for such a test.

Hyperthyroid (Thyrotoxicosis—Graves' Disease): Many patients have eye signs such as exophthalmos, lid lag, or stare. Other symptoms include tachycardia; warm, moist skin; heat intolerance; nervous hyperactive appearance; loss of weight; and tremor of fingers. Less frequent symptoms are diarrhea or congestive heart failure. Hemoglobin is usually normal; WBC are normal or slightly decreased. There is sometimes an increase in lymphocytes. Patients may have various combinations of these clinical symptoms or have only minimal changes. It is in clinically borderline cases that thyroid function tests are of especially great help.

Hypothyroid (Myxedema): Most common signs and symptoms include nonpitting edema of eyelids, face and extremities; loss of hair in outer one third of eyebrows; large tongue; cold, dry skin with cold intolerance; lethargic appearance and mental activity. Cardiac shadow enlargement on chest x-ray is common, with normal or slow heart rate. Anorexia and constipation are frequent. Laboratory tests show anemia in over 50%, with a macrocytic but nonmegaloblastic type in about 25% of myxedema cases. WBC are usually normal. The cerebrospinal fluid usually has elevated protein with normal cell counts, for unknown reasons. Again, the classic picture of myxedema is often completely missing or only partially developed; symptoms may be vague and misleading, or may suggest some other disease.

Conditions which superficially resemble or simulate hypothyroidism in the infant (cretinism) include mongolism and Hurler's disease (because of mental defect, facial appearance, and short stature); various types of dwarfism, including achondroplasia (because of short stature and retarded bone age); and nephrosis (because of edema, high cholesterol, and low PBI). Myxedema in older children and adults may be simulated by the nephrotic syndrome, mental deficiency (because of mental slowness), and sometimes simple obesity.

There is a comparatively large group of laboratory procedures which measure one or more aspects of thyroid function (Table 12a). The multiplicity of these tests implies that none is infallible or invariably helpful. In order to get best results, one must have a thorough knowledge of each procedure, including what aspect of thyroid function is measured, reliability in diagnosis of thyroid conditions, and false results caused by nonthyroid conditions. In certain cases, a brief outline of the technique involved when the test is actually performed helps clarify some of these points.

---

TABLE 12a.—THYROID FUNCTION TESTS
1.  Thyroid Uptake of Iodine
    RAI
2.  Thyroxine Tests
    a)  "Direct" measurement
        PBI
        BEI
        T-4 by column
        T-4 by isotope
            Competitive binding (Murphy-Pattee)
            Competitive binding—corrected
        Free thyroxine measurement (Stirling)
    b)  "Indirect" measurement
        T-3
        Free thyroxine index (Clark and Horn)
3.  Tissue Utilization of Thyroxine
    BMR
    Cholesterol
    Achilles tendon reflex
4.  Other
    T-3 suppression test
    T-3 by radioimmunoassay

---

Thyroid hormone production and utilization involves several steps (Fig. 14). Thyroid gland activity is under the control of thyroid-stimulating hormone (TSH), produced by the anterior pituitary under

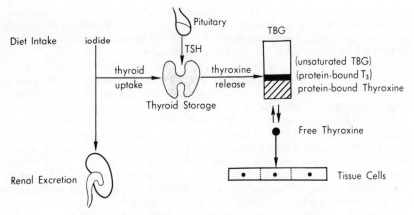

Fig. 14.—Iodine and thyroxine metabolism.

the guidance of the hypothalamus. The main raw material of thyroid hormone is inorganic iodide. Thyroid hormone synthesis begins when inorganic iodide is extracted from the blood by the thyroid. Within the thyroid, inorganic iodide is converted to organic iodine, and one iodine atom is incorporated into a tyrosine nucleus to form monoiodotyrosine. Monoiodotyrosine then incorporates a second iodine atom to form diiodotyrosine. Diiodotyrosine may condense with itself to form thyroxine ($T_4$) or with monoiodotyrosine to form triiodothyronine ($T_3$). Thyroxine is stored in the thyroid acini as thyroglobulin, to be reconstituted and released when needed. In the blood stream, thyroxine is the main component of thyroid hormone. The iodine of thyroxine accounts for about 95% of total serum iodine. Thyroxine is mostly bound to serum proteins. Alpha-1 globulin (thyroid-binding globulin, TBG) carries the majority; a lesser amount is bound to prealbumin and albumin molecules. A very small amount of thyroxine is present in the unbound or free form (free thyroxine, $T_F$); this amounts to less than 1%. The quantity of free thyroxine ($T_F$) depends to some extent on the degree of saturation of TBG. TBG saturation depends on the quantity of thyroxine available plus the total quantity of TBG available to bind thyroxine. TBG is normally about 15-30% saturated. Besides thyroxine, triiodothyronine ($T_3$) is present in small quantities. $T_3$ is much more active, weight for weight, than thyroxine ($T_4$); it is not yet established if $T_3$ is the metabolically active form of thyroxine or merely accompanies it from the thyroid storage depot. If $T_3$ is not the active substance, free thyroxine ($T_F$) probably is, because $T_F$ seems to have a better correlation with thyroid hormone activity than does total thyroxine.

Certain tests can monitor various stages in this cycle. Thyroid uptake of iodine is quantitated in the radioactive iodine uptake (RAI). Circulating thyroid hormone is measured directly by one of

the thyroxine tests (PBI, BEI, $T_4$, or $T_F$) or indirectly by determining the degree of TBG saturation ($T_3$ test). The end result of thyroid
hormone action can be estimated directly by the basal metabolic rate
(BMR) or indirectly by the serum cholesterol.

Radioactive Iodine Uptake (RAI): The degree of thyroid hormone production normally determines how much iodine will be extracted from the blood stream. A small tracer dose of $I^{131}$ can be
given, and the amount that enters the gland provides an indirect
measure of thyroid activity. The test is said to have a clinical accuracy of 70-95%, gives definitely better results in hyperthyroidism
than in the hypothyroid range, and is more accurate in Graves' disease than in thyrotoxicosis caused by hyperfunctioning ("toxic") nodule. In fact, 50-80% of patients with toxic nodular goiter are said to
have normal RAI. Thyroid uptake is usually measured 24 hours after
the test dose is administered. An occasional patient with thyrotoxicosis has unusually fast iodine turnover, so that maximal gland
iodine concentration is reached before 12 hours and thus falls into
normal range before 24 hours. In such cases, a 2-hour uptake is
recommended, although some investigators prefer a 4-hour or a 6-
hour determination.

Any condition which alters thyroid requirements for iodine will
effect the RAI. Iodine deficiency goiter will elevate the RAI results,
and excess organic or inorganic iodine will saturate the thyroid and
produce low RAI values. In cirrhosis, 25-50% of patients are said
to have abnormally high RAI uptake due to dietary deficiency of iodine, although the deficiency is not severe enough to produce clinical symptoms. The RAI is affected by most of the same diseases
that affect the PBI, but it differs in that some diseases, such as io-
dine-deficiency goiter, give abnormal RAI but not PBI, and hypoproteinemia gives abnormal PBI but not RAI. The RAI is affected
by many, but not all, of the same drugs, medications, and chemicals
which interfere with the PBI (p. 450). The RAI may be elevated
during the last trimester of pregnancy.

Normal values for the 24-hour RAI uptake are usually considered to be 15-40%; for the 2-hour uptake, 1.5-15%. Reports
from several areas in the last few years have noted a significant
drop in the normal 24-hour value (and presumably, in the early uptake level also); this has been attributed to iodine incorporated in
food or contaminating the environment. This makes it difficult to
interpret RAI results unless each laboratory periodically redeter-
mines its own normal values—a procedure which is hardly ever done
because of the nature of the test.

Thyroxine Tests: These procedures attempt to directly measure serum thyroxine and thus directly measure the actual hormonal
activity of the thyroid. In actuality, many of these tests measure
iodine, not thyroxine; but, since over 95% of serum iodine is normally part of thyroxine, iodine measurement approximates thyroxine
measurement unless something markedly increases serum free io-

dine.  The PBI was the first of these tests to be developed and is the best known and studied; the others were introduced subsequently in efforts to avoid some of the drawbacks of the PBI.

Protein-Bound Iodine (PBI): As mentioned previously, thyroxine normally contains most of the serum iodine and is mainly bound to certain serum proteins.  The PBI method precipitates serum proteins and measures the iodine present, thus providing a close but indirect estimation of thyroxine.  There are various modifications of the PBI, but all are very similar and have the same three basic steps:

1. Protein-bound iodine is removed from the serum by chemical precipitation of serum proteins.  The iodine of thyroxine is organic iodine, incorporated directly into the thyroxine molecule, rather than existing as inorganic ion (such as KI).
2. Protein is eliminated in order to isolate the iodine.  This may be accomplished by chemical ("wet") digestion or by incineration in a special furnace ("dry ash").  During either process, organic iodine is converted to iodide ion.
3. Iodide is measured by a chemical reaction whose color change is proportional to the amount of iodide present.

Because the PBI has been so extensively investigated, it has almost assumed the status of a reference method in thyroid disease, a technique against which all newer methods are compared.  Under ideal conditions, it has been pronounced the most reliable test for thyroid function, achieving a clinical accuracy of 90-95%.  There is some overlap between normal and hypo- or hyperthyroid ranges, since the normal range is relatively wide (4-8 mcg./100 ml.).  There are unfortunately several pitfalls for this otherwise extremely useful test, both clinically and in the laboratory.  Since thyroxine is carried to some extent by albumin and prealbumin proteins, any condition which leads to marked decrease of these proteins (such as the nephrotic syndrome or severe liver disease) will falsely decrease PBI.  However, contamination by organic or inorganic iodine is the main drawback of the PBI.  Inorganic iodine (iodide) is found mainly in medicines.  Organic iodine is located in many types of x-ray contrast media.  Contamination is a major headache in the laboratory, whether from unclean glassware, impurities in water, or from specimens with high iodine values influencing other tests done at the same time or later with the same equipment.  Values over 20 mcg./100 ml. are suspicious for contamination, and over 25 mcg./100 ml. are almost invariably due to iodine contamination.

Other factors which falsely influence PBI are a physiologic increase in pregnancy or with estrogen therapy (most commonly in the form of birth control pills), and treatment by thyroid hormone, antithyroid drugs, adrenocortical steroids, or various other medications.  The rule of thumb is: high estrogen situations elevate the PBI, while all other medications (excluding iodine or thyroid hor-

mone) decrease the PBI.  Many of these conditions and medications
exert effect by altering the serum level of thyroxine-binding globulin (TBG) rather than directly affecting thyroid function.  For example, if the amount of TBG is increased, then the amount of thyroxine bound to TBG must also increase in order to preserve the
normal degree of TBG saturation.  Besides drugs, abnormally high
or low levels of TBG may be congenital.

Another interesting situation is the treatment of hypothyroidism.  In treated hypothyroidism, therapeutically administered des-
iccated thyroid is measured along with endogenous thyroxine in the
PBI.  $T_3$ (Cytomel) therapy not only decreases endogenous thyroxine production and thus depresses PBI levels, but is used in amounts
too small to be itself measured in the PBI procedure.  Therefore,
the PBI cannot be used to follow $T_3$ therapy.  L-thyroxine (Synthroid)
treatment results in a PBI which usually is above normal range despite clinical euthyroid status.

Butanol-Extractable Iodine (BEI):  In most PBI procedures,
small amounts of inorganic iodide normally present in serum are
removed in the protein precipitation technique.  When large amounts
are present, some will combine with albumin and thus be included
in protein precipitation and falsely raise the PBI values.  Thyroxine
is more soluble in butanol than inorganic iodide or the precursors
mono- or diiodotyrosine, so that butanol extracts mostly thyroxine
and thus, essentially, is a way to remove contaminating inorganic
iodide.  BEI contamination by organic iodine is not eliminated, and
BEI is involved in the various other factors which influence PBI.  In
other words, the only difference between the PBI and BEI is elimination of inorganic iodide (except for a few special situations such
as lymphocytic thyroiditis, to be discussed later).

Thyroxine by Column ($T_4$ by Column):  Besides the BEI, a
simplified column chromatography technique has been introduced to
help meet the problem of iodine contamination.  In this procedure,
serum is placed on a special anion exchange resin which binds thy-
roxin and organic iodine.  Inorganic iodide, mono- and diiodotyro-
sines, and other proteins such as albumin are then washed off the
resin column.  Next, the thyroxine is released from the resin column in two or three elutions.  Each eluate sample is analyzed for
iodine in the same manner as the PBI.  In general, $T_4$ by column
gives results similar to those of the BEI.  The only significant difference is that one can often determine whether contamination by
organic iodine is present even in relatively smaller amounts, revealed by the percentages of iodine in each eluate fraction.  In the
BEI, one can recognize only major degrees of such contamination.
$T_4$ by column cannot prevent most false elevations due to organic
iodine, and is altered by all other factors which influence PBI.
Problems due to inorganic iodide are eliminated.

Thyroxine by Isotope:  Also called Murphy-Pattee, $T_4$ by
competitive binding, or $T_4$ by displacement, this test is available

in a variety of modifications and trade preparations. Isotope-labeled thyroxine is added to normal serum (a source of normal TBG) and equilibrium is established between bound and unbound labeled T4. If additional (nonlabeled) thyroxine is added to this system, the added (nonlabeled) thyroxine will also distribute itself between bound and free status, and this distribution will vary according to the total quantity of this added (nonlabeled) thyroxine. Since nonlabeled thyroxine will occupy some of the binding sites on the test system TBG, isotope-labeled T4 will be displaced. The amount of isotope displacement produced by addition of the patient's thyroxine (an extract of the patient's serum) is compared to the effect produced by a known amount of purified thyroxine, and this comparison is used to calculate the patient's T4 level. Since the end point of the test is not measurement of iodine, but instead involves only counting of radioactivity, T4 by isotope is not affected by either organic or inorganic iodine contamination. Since the level of protein-bound thyroxine is affected by the quantity of the patient's TBG, most of the factors beside iodine which affect the PBI do likewise to T4 by isotope. Another consideration is that certain commercial T4 kits provide a disturbing lack of reproducibility.

Besides the thyroxine test group, another technique is widely available for measuring serum thyroxine. Since the degree of TBG saturation reflects thyroid activity (assuming TBG levels are normal), if it were possible to determine the amount of unsaturated TBG (unsaturated TBG binding capacity) one could thus indirectly estimate the quantity of saturated protein (the PBI). This indirect procedure is the triiodothyronine (T3) test.

Triiodothyronine (T3) Test: This technique provides an estimate of the amount of unsaturated thyroxine-binding capacity of serum; in other words, the difference between protein-bound thyroxine (as measured in the PBI) and the total capacity of thyroxine-binding globulin (TBG) to bind thyroxine. In most individuals, the TBG total binding capacity for thyroxine is actually the sum of combined T4 and T3; therefore, a decrease in one means increased TBG avidity or binding capacity for the other. T3, however, is bound more loosely than is T4; therefore, T3 is more easily released from the carrier TBG and can be measured because of this fact. If one adds a substance which competes with TBG for T3, the amount of T3 which this substance takes away from the TBG depends on the degree to which TBG needs to keep T3; this, in turn, depends on the amount of T4 present, as mentioned earlier. T3 labeled with radioactive iodine is added to a serum sample from the patient. Synthetic resin particles or a resin sponge are also added; these substances compete with serum TBG for available T3. After a certain period, the resin is washed and the radioactivity in the resin (or the serum) is counted and compared to the original test dose total radioactivity. If the serum is saturated with T4 as one would expect in hyperthyroidism, much of the injected radioactive T3 has no place to go except onto the resin, and the resin uptake is increased over normal values. In hypothyroidism, less thyroxine is present, the plasma proteins are relatively unsaturated, and most of the test dose of $T_3$ is taken up by the serum TBG, leaving a decreased resin uptake of radioactive $T_3$. Thus, the greater the unsaturated serum TBG (as measured in the amount of $T_3$ uptake by resin), the less protein-bound thyroxine is present in the plasma under most, but not all, conditions, so that the $T_3$ resin uptake result in hypo- or hyperthyroidism tends to parallel the PBI in most cases. The great difference between the two tests is that neither organic nor inorganic iodine contamination will affect the $T_3$ uptake. Note that the entire $T_3$ procedure is done in vitro, so no radioactivity is actually given to the patient himself. In the original $T_3$ method, the patient's red blood cells were used as $T_3$ acceptors. A drawback of the RBC method is that accuracy depends on the patient having relatively normal red cell quantities (hematocrit). Newer methods using synthetic resins are not dependent on hematocrit. As noted, the $T_3$ test by either the resin or RBC uptake method is affected in the same direction as the thyroxine tests in hypo- and hyperthyroidism, but is not falsely changed by iodine contamination. The $T_3$ is altered by most of the other medications and diseases which affect the PBI (e.g., Dilantin, pregnancy or estrogenic contraceptives, steroids, nephrotic syndrome, etc.). However, many of these conditions affect TBG quantity (TBG serum levels) rather than directly affecting serum thyroxine levels, and the $T_3$ results are thus altered in exactly the opposite way from the PBI. In addition, certain conditions such as severe acidosis (metabolic or respiratory), mongolism, and either heparin or Coumadin anticoagulant therapy have been reported to cause falsely high $T_3$ values, for unknown reasons. Occasionally, persons are found with congenitally high or low TBG levels.

Several modifications of the basic procedure are sold by commercial companies, and each modification has different areas where faulty technique would cause trouble. One source of confusion is that a commercial $T_3$ test which counts serum uptake gives exactly opposite results from one which counts resin uptake. The $T_3$ has been the subject of a growing number of clinical evaluations. Although some published reports are highly favorable, most indicate that accuracy is poor in hypothyroidism and that there is still a significant amount of overlap with normal values in mild hyperthyroidism. The main advantages are simplicity of performance, the fact that iodine contamination problems are eliminated, and the possibility of calculating the free thyroxine index in combination with a $T_4$ procedure.

    Free Thyroxine ($T_F$): As mentioned previously, circulating thyroxine is present in two fractions—over 99% protein-bound, and a very small quantity of free (unbound) thyroxine. The amount of free thyroxine present depends on several factors, the most important being the ratio of protein-bound thyroxine to the total amount of serum protein-binding capacity available (i. e. , the degree of saturation of TBG).  Assuming normal levels of TBG, the amount of protein-bound thyroxine then depends directly on the amount of thyroid hormone production.  In hyperthyroidism there is increased thyroxine production, increased protein-bound thyroxine, increased TBG saturation, and more free thyroxine (because TBG saturation is increased, less binding capacity remains).  Free thyroxine test results thus parallel the PBI in hypo- and hyperthyroidism or treatment with thyroid medication.  In addition, reports indicate that free thyroxine is normal in patients whose TBG levels are altered by drugs or congenital or physiologic mechanisms.  If the TBG is "artificially" lowered by one of these means, the TBG-bound thyroxine also decreases, in order to preserve its normal degree of saturation.  Free thyroxine is temporarily increased by the thyroxine released from TBG, the pituitary is stimulated to decrease thyroid-stimulating hormone somewhat, the thyroid releases less thyroxine, less thyroxine is now available for the decreased amount of TBG present, a normal TBG saturation is now achieved despite the decreased total TBG level, and the free thyroxine level returns to normal.  The PBI is decreased despite normal free thyroxine, because less thyroxine is released by the thyroid in order to compensate for decreased TBG levels.  In other words, with decreased TBG levels, the reserve serum thyroxine bound to TBG is partially sacrificed in order to maintain a normal free thyroxine.  The opposite happens if TBG levels are "artificially" increased, as occurs with the hyperestrogenism of pregnancy or contraceptive drugs.  Here the TBG is increased, PBI is increased as a compensatory mechanism to maintain normal TBG saturation, and the free thyroxine remains within normal limits.

Direct measurement of free thyroxine is currently available in only a few reference laboratories.  Use of the current test technique is further limited by the surprising fact that many patients seriously ill with a variety of diseases have decreased free thyroxine test results while the true serum free thyroxine level is normal.  The Free Thyroxine Index and "Corrected" T4 by isotope more accurately reflect the true status of the patient.

Free Thyroxine Index:  Free thyroxine is not affected by TBG abnormalities, since TBG acts mostly as a storage depot.  Clark and Horn popularized a mathematical estimate of free thyroxine status.  The estimate is calculated by multiplying the T3 and T4 results together.  This is based on the fact that whereas T3 and T4 results parallel each other in hypo- and hyperthyroidism, they go in opposite directions when TBG-related factors influence test results.  Multiplying T3 and T4 results together thus tends to cancel out the effects of TBG-related factors without affecting results in thyroid disease.  Although the method has generally proved reliable, there is difficulty in separating borderline or mild hypo- or hyperthyroid from normal range. Two tests are involved; thus there are additional chances for error in the final result. The new "Corrected" $T_4$ seems to be more accurate in borderline cases.

"Corrected" $T_4$ by Isotope: This is also called "Normalized" $T_4$, "ETR," and other trade names. A method was recently found to correct $T_4$ results for effects of TBG abnormality. Whereas the usual $T_4$ test system employs only TBG from normal serum, this new technique compensates for patient TBG variations by first reacting the patient's thyroxine with normal TBG and then with the patient's own TBG. The result is a thyroxine test which is not affected by inorganic iodine or by organic iodine and should also not be affected by diseases or medications which alter TBG. The major drawbacks to the PBI are thereby eliminated, and most of the diseases and medications which affect the PBI should no longer be a problem. The only qualification is the newness of the technique, the current lack of adequate evaluation of commercial test kits, and the possibility that factors as yet unrecognized might affect the test. It seems likely that the "Corrected" $T_4$ by isotope will replace most other tests for thyroid function screening, although the PBI may survive because it is much cheaper.

To briefly summarize chemical thyroid tests: the iodine-endpoint tests (PBI, BEI, $T_4$ by column) are in one way or another affected by iodine contamination and by conditions altering TBG; the $T_3$ and $T_4$ by isotope are affected only by TBG alterations; and the "Corrected" $T_4$ and Free Thyroxine Index are not affected by either iodine or TBG.

$T_3$ by Radioimmunoassay: This technique provides a fairly accurate and specific measurement of actual total serum $T_3$. Its greatest usefulness is in the diagnosis of "$T_3$ thyrotoxicosis" (to be discussed later), in which $T_3$ levels are elevated and $T_4$ is normal. Additionally, $T_3$ by radioimmunoassay is elevated whenever $T_4$ production is elevated. This procedure should not be confused with the standard $T_3$ test; the standard $T_3$ test estimates $T_3$ indirectly by measuring the number of free (available or unsaturated) binding sites for $T_3$ remaining on patient TBG. Radioimmunoassay measures $T_3$ directly by using antibody against $T_3$. $T_3$ by radioimmunoassay is affected by congenital or drug-induced TBG abnormalities. Another drawback is considerable technical difficulty and expense, but this may be diminished in the future.

Another group of tests estimates thyroid function by assessing the effects of thyroid hormone on body metabolism or reactions. These include the Achilles tendon reflex (a physical measurement), basal metabolic rate, and serum cholesterol.

Achilles Tendon Reflex: Thyroid hormone status affects the speed of muscle reflex. Equipment is available to measure contraction or relaxation time. Although a few investigators claim good results, the usual accuracy is 50-75% in hypothyroidism and 20-50% in hyperthyroidism. Diabetes mellitus, pernicious anemia and other neurologic disorders, and thiourea drugs prolong reflex time; estrogens and corticosteroids shorten it.

Basal Metabolic Rate (BMR): This supposedly measures body reaction as a whole to circulating thyroid hormone. Most methods are indirect, utilizing rate of oxygen uptake by means of breathing a measured amount of oxygen in a closed-circuit tank apparatus. If increased amounts of oxygen are breathed in, theoretically the patient has an abnormally high basal metabolic rate, and vice versa for decreased metabolism. Unfortunately, so many variables are involved that the test is most reliable only when the clinical situation is already so obvious that it is not really necessary. A truly basal state is difficult to achieve and maintain. Anxiety, obesity, adrenal dysfunction, and equipment malfunction are some of the other major obstacles to accurate results. The main use of BMR today is to follow the therapeutic effects of thyroid replacement drugs such as triiodothyronine which cannot be monitored by other thyroid tests.

Cholesterol is an indirect measurement of metabolic rate; this reflects a not-well-understood effect of thyroid hormone on cholesterol synthesis. Cholesterol is often elevated in myxedema and much less frequently is decreased in hyperthyroidism (in classic cases). Serum cholesterol is, however, a poor test of thyroid function for several reasons:

1. Many diseases influence cholesterol metabolism in various ways.
2. Changes from normal range tend to occur only in a far-advanced thyroid disease; much more so in hypothyroidism than in hyperthyroidism.
3. Cholesterol determination is one of the least accurate tests in the clinical laboratory. Also, the normal range itself is so wide that many persons could be abnormal and still have values which fall within the population normal.

Thus far, discussion has been limited to tests useful in the diagnosis of hypothyroidism and hyperthyroidism. There are several other procedures which are helpful in special situations.

Thyroid Scan: Thyroid uptake of radioactive isotopes such as $I^{131}$ may be counted by a special device which produces a visual over-all pattern of gland radioactivity. This allows visual localization of areas which may be hyperactive or hypoactive. The procedure is useful in two situations:

1. To show whether thyrotoxicosis is caused by diffuse hyperplasia or by a hyperfunctioning nodule ("hot nodule" or "toxic nodule").
2. To demonstrate hypofunction in a nodule, thus increasing suspicion of carcinoma ("cold nodule").

Most reports agree that a hyperfunctioning nodule is very rarely malignant. Single nonfunctioning nodules have a 10-20% incidence of malignancy; truly nonfunctioning nodules are much

more likely to be malignant than nodules which retain some function.
The difficulty is that normal tissue above or below a nonfunctioning
area may contribute some degree of apparent function to the nonfunctioning region.

Thyroid-Stimulating Hormone (TSH) Test:  In some patients
with myxedema, the question arises as to whether the etiology is
primary thyroid disease or malfunction secondary to pituitary deficiency.  This problem may be investigated by performing the RAI
before and after administration of an appropriate amount of TSH.  In
pituitary insufficiency, the thyroid usually will respond to TSH; if
hypofunction is primary disease of the thyroid, RAI uptake will not
be significantly improved.

The procedure may be very useful in patients who have been
on long-term thyroid hormone treatment and who must be re-evaluated as to whether the original diagnosis of hypothyroidism was correct.  The TSH test can be done while thyroid hormone is still being
administered, whereas it would take several weeks after cessation
of long-term therapy for the pituitary-thyroid relationship to reach
pretherapy equilibrium.

Another method of differentiating primary from secondary
myxedema is direct serum assay of TSH.  This can now be done in
various reference laboratories.  In primary myxedema, TSH levels
are elevated, since normal feedback control is reduced.

Thyroid Suppression Test:  This is frequently called "T3 suppression," although thyroid hormone could be used instead of T3.
Normal persons decrease RAI values to less than 50% of baseline
level after a standard dose of T3 daily for 1 week.  This is felt to be
a reliable test, and may be very useful in diagnosis of borderline
hyperthyroid patients.  Chemical thyroxine tests may be used instead of the RAI.  In conjunction with thyroid scan, the basic technique may be used to demonstrate that a nodule seen on original scan
is autonomous.  This is very helpful, since reports indicate that 50-
80% of toxic nodular goiter patients have normal RAI, and many have
normal thyroxine tests.  The procedure must be used with caution in
elderly persons, especially those with cardiac disease.

T3 Thyrotoxicosis is a relatively new entity found in association with Graves' disease or with toxic nodular goiter.  Standard thyroxine and T3 tests are normal.  The 24-hour RAI may be normal
(even low-normal) or increased.  T3 suppression tests are usually
abnormal and indicative of hyperthyroidism.  At present, the most
conclusive proof is obtained by quantitative T3 measurement using
radioimmunoassay (a different procedure from the standard T3 test).
This demonstrates elevated total T3 levels.  However, since TBG
abnormalities may affect T3 by radioimmunoassay (which measures
total serum T3), confirmation is advisable with the T3 suppression
test or some method of TBG assay.  Since TBG deficiency or decrease may falsely lower total serum T4 (in contrast to metabolically
active "free" T4) even more than effects on total serum T3, TBG

abnormality should be ruled out before attributing hyperthyroidism to $T_3$ hyperproduction rather than $T_4$.

Selection of Thyroid Tests: Each procedure measures one facet of thyroid hormone production, transport, or utilization; each has advantages and disadvantages, so that selection should simply involve choosing what information is needed in the particular situation. The best screening test for hypo- or hyperthyroidism is the new "Corrected" $T_4$ by isotope. However, if a patient has an obvious clinical hyperthyroidism, all of the thyroxine or radioisotope tests are equally good; since the question is not that of diagnosis but only of confirmation, only one test probably is sufficient. In obvious myxedema, any of the thyroxine tests is adequate, the $T_3$ is not quite as good, and the RAI is substantially less efficient. In a patient with hyperthyroid symptoms but definitely normal $T_4$, a thyroid scan followed by a $T_3$ suppression test may be worthwhile in order to rule out a subclinical toxic nodule. "$T_3$ thyrotoxicosis" might also be a possibility; if so, $T_3$ by radioimmunoassay is helpful. Except in special cases (such as thyroiditis), there is nothing to be gained by ordering more than one thyroxine test (PBI, BEI, $T_4$ by column or isotope) at the same time; all give the same information, differing only in the particular agents which interfere. There is hardly ever any need for BMR or serum cholesterol. The RAI is no longer needed for diagnosis of hyper- or hypothyroidism; normal values are changing, the test requires two patient visits plus the administration of radioisotopes, results are not reliable in mild hypothyroidism, technique is often poor, and various other factors alter test results. However, there are a few situations in which RAI may be useful. In "factitious" hyperthyroidism (due to deliberate ingestion of thyroid hormone or its incorporation into medication such as diet control pills), the RAI is low when thyroxine tests are elevated. In TSH stimulation or $T_3$ suppression tests, RAI is the standard procedure used, although a thyroxine test could probably be substituted.

In any case, good clinical judgment is even more important than laboratory results. If the clinical status of the patient does not agree with the laboratory values, the test results should be rechecked.

Hashimoto's Disease is a form of chronic thyroiditis characterized histologically by marked lymphocytic infiltration of the thyroid gland. Clinically, the disease is much more common in females, and the main symptom is the onset of thyroid enlargement. The general category of Hashimoto's disease has been divided into two subgroups—so-called lymphocytic thyroiditis and ordinary (adult) Hashimoto's. Lymphocytic thyroiditis is most frequent in children and young adults, and presents with a diffusely slowly enlarging thyroid gland, with or without other minor symptoms. Thyroid function tests include a PBI which is usually either elevated or high normal, and a BEI which remains normal. Many patients show a PBI-BEI discrepancy of more than 2.0 mcg. /100 ml. , whereas the normal limit is 1.0 mcg./100 ml. Other thyroid function tests are variable, although the RAI is often elevated early in the disease. Adult Hashimoto's disease is more frequent than lymphocytic thyroiditis; again, it is most common in females, but has a predilection for the 30-50-year-old age group. The goiter produced is often of relatively rapid onset; it is diffuse, although sometimes irregular. There may be pressure symptoms in the neck from the enlarged gland. As the disease progresses, hypothyroidism is frequent. Thyroid function test results usually are normal, except when hypothyroidism develops. There may be a PBI-BEI discrepancy over 1.0 mcg./100 ml., although not as frequently as in childhood lymphocytic thyroiditis. Thyroid scan often shows multiple areas of decreased isotope uptake. Exact diagnosis of Hashimoto's disease is important for several reasons: to differentiate the condition from thyroid carcinoma; because a diffusely enlarged thyroid raises the question of possible thyrotoxicosis; and because treatment with thyroid hormone gives excellent results, especially in childhood lymphocytic thyroiditis. Incidentally, adenomatous goiter is said to have a PBI-BEI discrepancy of 1-2 mcg./100 ml. in 10% of cases, and one report raises the possibility of a similar finding in rare cases of thyroid carcinoma.

Both subgroups of Hashimoto's disease are now considered to be either due to, or associated with, an autoimmune disorder against thyroid tissue. Autoantibodies against one or another element of thyroid tissue have been detected in most cases. In addition, there is an increased incidence of serologically detectable thyroid autoantibodies in the rheumatoid-collagen disease group, conditions themselves associated with disturbances in the body autoimmune mechanisms. Various systems have been devised for detection of circulating thyroid autoantibodies for aid in the diagnosis of Hashimoto's disease. The most readily available procedure is a rapid latex-agglutination slide test, called the TA test (thyroid antibody test). This primarily detects antibodies to thyroglobulin, and is similar in principle to the rheumatoid factor latex test (p. 264). Crude extract of thyroglobulin antigen is attached to an indicator (latex particles); significant titers of antithyroglobulin antibody in the serum attacks the antigen and thereby clumps the latex particles. The TA test has been reported to be reasonably sensitive and specific. However, as with most screening tests, false positives and false negatives occur, and must be expected. A small but significant percentage of patients with thyrotoxicosis, thyroid carcinoma, and the rheumatoid-collagen disease group have positive test results. Although there is an increased incidence of chronic thyroiditis histologically resembling Hashimoto's disease in thyrotoxicosis and thyroid carcinoma, some false positive TA tests occur without associated histologic thyroiditis, so that differentiation of these conditions by means of an autoantibody test cannot be made blindly. The TA test may also be positive in some cases of myxedema which cannot be established as being due to Hashimoto's disease. On the other hand, false negative TA tests have been reported in up to 30% of patients with acceptable Hashimoto's disease.

Another procedure, called the tanned red cell (TRC) test, is more sensitive to thyroid autoimmune disease. Most investigators find over 85% positive in Hashimoto's, with lesser percentages in other thyroid disorders. Titers in disease other than chronic thyroiditis tend to be low. The TRC technique is preferable to the TA test; since both tests are nonspecific, a negative TRC result would be stronger evidence against chronic thyroiditis.

Thyroiditis usually is classified as acute, subacute, and chronic. Except for Hashimoto's disease, the other varieties are not frequent, so will be mentioned only briefly. Acute thyroiditis usually is infectious in nature, and physical findings usually are those of localized infection. Thyroid function tests usually are normal. Subacute thyroiditis (De Quervain's, giant-cell, or granulomatous thyroiditis) is of unknown etiology, but possibly is viral or autoimmune in nature. Histologically, there are areas of thyroid acini degeneration surrounded by multinucleated giant cells. If the disease is localized, the only functional abnormality is possible focal hyperfunction on thyroid scan. If the disease is more widespread, RAI uptake is low, and the PBI is elevated (or high normal) due to release of thyroglobulin from damaged acini. There may be an increased PBI-BEI discrepancy. Thyroid autoantibodies occasionally may be detected, but are not common.

Finally, Riedel's struma is another type of chronic thyroiditis, consisting of extensive thyroid parenchymal fibrosis. In most cases, function tests are normal; in a few, results are hypothyroid.

In acute and subacute thyroiditis, nonspecific parameters of inflammation such as the erythrocyte sedimentation rate (ESR) usually are abnormal. In Hashimoto's disease, about 50% have an elevated ESR, more commonly in the childhood type. However, adenomatous goiter may also sometimes have an increased ESR.

Parathyroid Disease: Hyperparathyroidism is an uncommon disease, but nevertheless an important one, especially from the surgical standpoint. By far the most common manifestation is renal stones, but metabolic bone disease often is present, and peptic ulcer may be associated. The disease always enters into the differential diagnosis of hypercalcemia, because this is one of its most prominent laboratory signs. Typically, in addition to hypercalcemia, there is low serum phosphorus, elevated alkaline phosphatase and increased urine calcium (the Sulkowitch test is a commonly used semiquantitative urine method) due to the action of excessive parathyroid hormone. In the blood, there tends to be a reciprocal relationship between serum calcium and phosphorus, with low serum phosphorus giving high calcium in response, and vice versa. Parathyroid hormone prevents renal tubular reabsorption of phosphorus, thus allowing serum phosphorus to drain out into the urine, giving depressed blood levels. This is balanced by drawing calcium out of bone to raise serum calcium. Although the classic picture of primary hyperparathyroidism has been just described, in some cases one or more components may be lacking. Some patients have borderline or normal serum calcium, some have normal phosphorus, and a considerable number have normal alkaline phosphatase. In these cases other tests are needed for preoperative diagnosis.

One of the most frequently used is the phosphate reabsorption test. The patient drinks several glasses of water and then voids completely. One hour after voiding, a blood sample is obtained for phosphorus and creatinine. Exactly 2 hours after beginning the test the patient again voids completely and the urine volume and urine concentration of creatinine and phosphate are obtained. It is then possible to calculate the creatinine clearance and find the amount of phosphorus filtered per minute by the glomeruli. Comparing this with the actual amount of phosphate excreted per minute gives the amount reabsorbed by the tubules per minute or the tubular reabsorption of phosphate (TRP). A rough approximation is afforded by the formula:

$$\% \text{ TRP} = 1 - \left[ \frac{\text{Urine PO}_4 \text{ conc. X serum creatinine conc.}}{\text{Urine creatinine conc. X serum PO}_4 \text{ conc.}} \right] \text{X } 100$$

A low index value of less than 80% means diminished tubular reabsorption and thus suggests primary hyperparathyroidism. This test becomes increasingly unreliable when the creatinine clearance is low due to severe renal disease, and is definitely not reliable in the presence of renal insufficiency. Moreover, other causes of hypercalcemia such as sarcoidosis and myeloma have been reported to sometimes give a "positive" (reduced) TRP. Finally, the TRP has been reported normal in a significant number of primary hyperparathyroidism cases. Another test which may be useful is a "suppression test" utilizing large doses of adrenocortical steroids. After 1 week, the serum calcium level in most (but not all) cases of primary hyperparathyroidism is not affected, whereas the steroids will suppress elevated calcium levels due to most other etiologies. Again, exceptions occur, especially with metastatic carcinoma to bone.

Bone changes diagnostic of hyperparathyroid disease may be found radiologically in a significant minority of patients with primary hyperparathyroidism (one report quotes 20-25%, although this probably is higher than average experience). These are found most often in the phalanges, so that x-rays of the hands are often worth while. Patients with secondary hyperparathyroidism (chronic renal disease; malabsorption diseases) also may show these abnormalities. Other radiologic bone changes may be present (up to 45% of cases) but are not diagnostic.

The more common causes of hypercalcemia and metabolic bone disease, with their classic laboratory findings, are shown in Table 13. Here again, there may be variations in some of the val-

TABLE 13.—DIAGNOSIS OF CALCIUM-PHOSPHORUS DISEASES

| | Serum $Ca^{++}$ | Serum P | Alk. Phos. | Acidosis | Urine $Ca^{++}$ |
|---|---|---|---|---|---|
| Primary hyperparathyroidism | H | L | $H/N^{\#}$ | | H |
| Vitamin D excess | H | N/L | N/H | | H |
| Sarcoidosis | H | N | H | | H |
| Secondary hyperparathyroidism | L/N | H | H | + | H |
| Renal acidosis | L/N | N/L | H | + | H |
| Sprue | L/N | N/L | H | | L |
| Osteomalacia | L/N | L/N | H | | L |
| Paget's disease | N | N | H | | N/H |
| Metastatic neoplasm to bone* | N/H | N | N/H | | N/H |
| Hypoparathyroidism | L | H | N | | L |
| Osteoporosis | N | N | N | | N/H |
| Hyperthyroidism | N/H | N/H | N/H | | N/H |

(Table abbreviated for High, Normal, or Low; second letter, if present, means less common finding.)

*Depends on primary tumor and type of bone lesion produced. Metastatic carcinoma to bone is one of the most common etiologies for hypercalcemia, perhaps the most common.

# Alkaline phosphatase is high in textbook cases of primary hyperparathyroidism.

ues in patients. The clinical history, physical examination and other laboratory tests usually can separate out these other diseases. For example, in secondary hyperparathyroidism caused by chronic renal disease, there usually is anemia with an elevated BUN, which are absent in classic primary hyperparathyroidism. However, even in the primary disease, after long periods the kidney may be so damaged by calculi with superimposed infection or by renal tissue calcification that it is difficult to tell primary from secondary. Chest and bone roentgenograms often will reveal metastatic carcinoma lesions. Diagnosis of many of the other diseases is discussed elsewhere in the book. Laboratory error may produce apparent hypercalcemia, so the initial serum calcium elevation should be rechecked before extensive workups are begun.

Hypoparathyroidism is uncommon. Most cases used to occur

when the parathyroids were inadvertently removed during thyroid-
ectomy. Chemical hypocalcemia is rather frequent in hospitalized
patients but usually is not symptomatic. Decrease of serum albumin
by 1 Gm./100 ml. produces decrease in serum calcium of approximately 0.8 mg./100 ml. Uremia is frequently associated with hypocalcemia.

## REFERENCES

Achilles Reflex Time in the Diagnosis of Thyroid Dysfunction, Med.
    Letter Drugs & Therapeutics 9:43, 1967.
Anderson, J. R., et al.: Diagnostic tests for thyroid antibodies: A
    comparison of the precipitin and latex-fixation (Hyland TA) tests,
    J. Clin. Path. 15:462, 1962.
Bauer, R. E.: The present status of the diagnosis of hypothyroid-
    ism, Ann. Int. Med. 44:207, 1956.
Blahd, W. H. (ed.): Nuclear Medicine (2nd ed.; New York: Blakisto
    Company, 1972).
Caplan, R. H., and Kujack, R.: Thyroid uptake of radioiodine. A
    re-evaluation, J. A. M. A. 215:916, 1971.
David, N. J., et al.: The diagnostic spectrum of hypercalcemia,
    Am. J. Med. 33:88, 1962.
Davis, P. J.: Factors affecting the determination of the serum
    protein-bound iodine, Am. J. Med. 40:918, 1966.
Dowling, J. T., et al.: Abnormal iodoproteins in the blood of eu-
    metabolic goitrous adults, J. Clin. Endocrinol. 21:1390, 1961.
Hamolsky, M. W., et al.: The plasma protein-thyroid hormone
    complex in man. III. Further studies on the use of the in vitro
    red blood cell uptake of $I^{131}$-L-triiodothyronine as a diagnostic
    test of thyroid function, J. Clin. Endocrinol. 19:103, 1959.
Leboeuf, G., and Bongiovanni, A. M.: Thyroiditis in Childhood, in
    Levine, S. Z. (ed.): Advances in Pediatrics (Chicago: Year Book
    Medical Publishers, Inc., 1964), Vol. XIII, p. 183.
Magliotti, M. F., et al.: The effect of disease and drugs on the
    twenty-four hour $I^{131}$ thyroid uptake, Am. J. Roentgenol. 81:54,
    1959.
McConahey, W. M., et al.: Comparison of certain laboratory tests
    in the diagnosis of Hashimoto's thyroiditis, J. Clin. Endocrinol.
    21:879, 1961.
Meachim, G., and Young, M. H.: DeQuervain's subacute granu-
    lomatous thyroiditis: Histological identification and incidence, J.
    Clin. Path. 16:189, 1963.
Murphy, B. E. P.: In vitro tests of thyroid function, Seminars
    Nuclear Med. 1:301, 1971.
Myers, W. P. L., et al.: Endocrine syndromes associated with
    nonendocrine neoplasms, M. Clin. North America 50:763, 1966.
Nelson, J. C., et al.: The normal thyroidal uptake of iodine,
    California Med. 112:11, 1970.

Nelson, J. C. , et al. : Serum TSH levels and the thyroidal response
to TSH stimulation in patients with thyroid disease, Ann. Int. Med.
76:47, 1972.
Rose, N. R. , and Witebsky, E. : Thyroid Autoantibodies in Thyroid
Disease, in Levine, R. , and Luft, R. (eds.): Advances in Meta-
bolic Disorders (New York: Academic Press, 1968), Vol. 5,
p. 231.
Saxena, K. M. , and Crawford, J. D. : Juvenile lymphocytic thy-
roiditis, Pediatrics 30:917, 1962.
Sisson, J. C. : Principles of, and pitfalls in, thyroid function tests,
J. Nuclear Med. 6:853, 1965.
Sterling, K. , et al. : T-3 thyrotoxicosis, J. A. M. A. 213:571, 1970.
Strott, C. A. , and Nugent, C. A. : Laboratory tests in the diagnosis
of hyperparathyroidism in hypercalcemic patients, Ann. Int. Med.
68:188, 1968.
Volpe, R. , et al. : Thyroid function in subacute thyroiditis, J. Clin.
Endocrinol. 18:65, 1958.
Werner, S. C. (ed.): The Thyroid (3rd ed. ; New York: Hoeber Med-
ical Division, Harper & Row, Publishers, 1971).
Yeager, G. H. , et al. : Thyroiditis: A review and presentation of
forty pathologically proven cases of chronic thyroiditis, South.
M. J. 50:1005, 1957.

# CHAPTER 29

# Adrenal Function

The adrenal glands produce several important hormones. A summary of these hormones, their actions, and their major metabolites is shown in Figure 15. Histologically, the adrenal cortex is divided into three areas. A narrow outer (subcapsular) region is known as the zona glomerulosa. It is thought to produce aldosterone. The cortex middle zone, called the zona fasciculata, mainly elaborates 17-hydroxycortisone, also known as hydrocortisone or cortisol. It is the principal zone. A thin inner zone, called the zona reticularis, manufactures compounds with androgenic or estrogenic effects. Pathways of synthesis for adrenal hormones are outlined in Figure 16. The adrenal medulla produces epinephrine and norepinephrine. Excess or deficiency of these hormones leads to well-recognized diseases. Diagnosis is made by demonstrating excess or deficiency of the substance in question, either the hormone itself or its metabolites. In diseases of the adrenal cortex, three steroid tests form the backbone of laboratory diagnosis—17-hydroxycorticosteroids, 17-ketosteroids, and 17-ketogenic steroids. Before discussing the use of these steroid tests in various syndromes, it might be useful to consider what actually is being measured.

## 17-Hydroxycorticosteroids (17-OH-CS)

These are $C_{21}$ compounds which possess a dihydroxyacetone group on carbon number 17 of the steroid nucleus (Fig. 17). In the blood, the principal 17-OH-CS is hydrocortisone. In urine, the predominating 17-OH-CS are tetrahydro metabolites (breakdown products) of hydrocortisone and cortisone. Therefore, measurement of 17-OH-CS can be used to estimate the level of cortisone and hydrocortisone production. Estrogen therapy (including oral contracep-

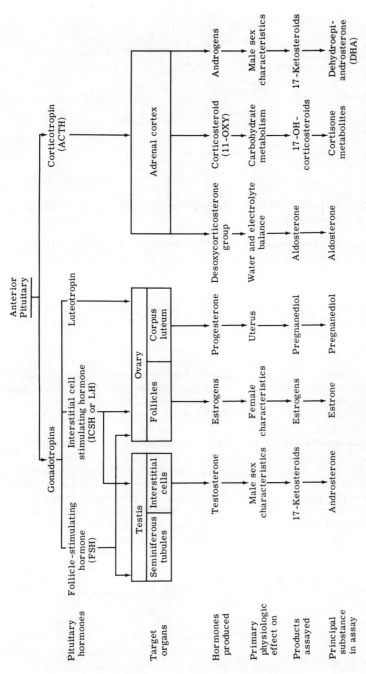

Fig. 15.—Derivation of principal urinary steroids. (From Handbook of Specialized Diagnostic Laboratory Tests [7th ed.; Van Nuys, Calif.: BioScience Laboratories, 1966] , p. 5.)

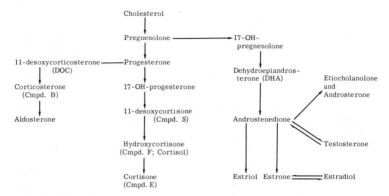

Fig. 16.—Adrenal cortex steroid synthesis. (Several alternate pathways are omitted.)

tives) will elevate plasma 17-OH-CS, although degradation of these compounds is delayed and urine 17-OH-CS are decreased.

### 17-Ketosteroids (17-KS)

These are $C_{19}$ compounds with a ketone group on carbon number 17 of the steroid nucleus (see Fig. 17). They are measured in urine only. Most of the 17-KS are derived from androgens, although lesser amounts come from early steroid precursors and a small percentage from hydrocortisone breakdown products. The principal urinary 17-KS is a compound known as dehydroisoandrosterone (dehydroepiandrosterone; DHA). This is formed in the adrenal and has a weak androgenic effect. DHA is not a metabolite of cortisone or hydrocortisone, and therefore 17-KS cannot be expected to mirror or predict levels of hydrocortisone production.

In adrenogenital or virilization syndromes, high levels of 17-KS usually mean congenital adrenal hyperplasia in babies and adrenal tumor in older children and adults. In both cases, steroid synthesis is abnormally shifted away from cortisone formation toward androgen production. High levels are occasionally found in testicular tumors, if the tumor produces androgens greatly in excess of normal testicular output. In Cushing's disease, 17-KS production is variable, but adrenal hyperplasia is often associated with mild-to-moderate elevation, while adrenal carcinoma frequently produces moderate or marked urinary values. In adrenal tumor, most of the increase is due to DHA.

Low levels of 17-KS are not very important because of normal fluctuation and the degree of inaccuracy in assay. Low levels of 17-KS are usually due to a decrease in DHA. This may be caused by many factors, but the most important is stress of any type (such as trauma, burns, chronic disease, etc.). Therefore, normal 17-KS levels are indirectly a sign of health.

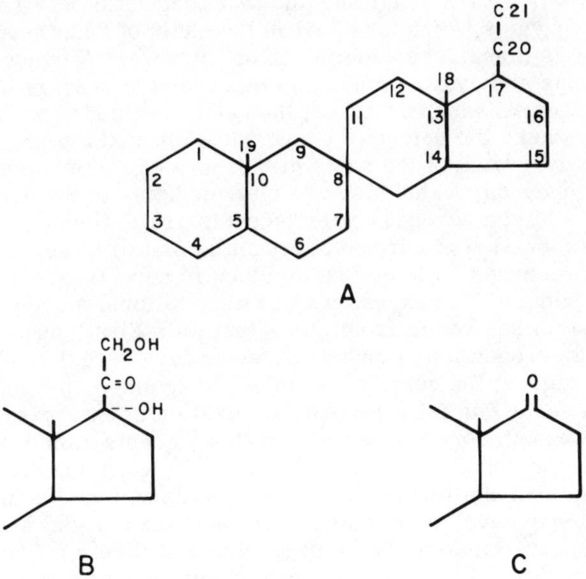

Fig. 17.—Adrenocortical steroid nomenclature. A, basic 17-hydroxycorticosteroid nucleus with standard numerical nomenclature of the carbon atoms. B, configuration of hydrocortisone at the C-17 carbon atom. C, configuration of the 17-ketosteroids at the C-17 carbon atom.

## 17-Ketogenic Steroids

These are $C_{21}$ compounds which can be oxidized to 17-ketosteroids. The ketogenic steroids thus constitute the difference between 17-KS determinations done before and after oxidation. The 17-ketogenic compounds include the 17-OH-CS group and also pregnanetriol. Pregnanetriol is a metabolite of 17-OH progesterone (a precursor of cortisone). Since pregnanetriol elevation occurs only in a very few conditions (the adrenogenital syndrome) in which 17-OH-CS are not also elevated, in most situations a urinary 17-ketogenic steroid determination could be used (if desired) instead of urinary 17-OH-CS. Whereas the metabolite of 17-OH-progesterone (pregnanetriol) is included in 17-ketogenic assays, the metabolite of progesterone (pregnanediol) is not a 17-ketogenic steroid.

A list of compounds which may interfere with 17-OH-CS or 17-KS (and ketogenic) determinations is found on page 434.

I. The Adrenogenital Syndrome

This is a rare syndrome due to a congenital defect in one of several enzymes which take part in the chain of reactions whereby cortisone is manufactured from its precursors. Although formation of cortisone and hydrocortisone is blocked, the precursors of these steroids are still manufactured; the actual compound produced depends on where the defective enzyme has blocked the normal synthesis pathway. Most of the early precursors of cortisone are estrogenic compounds, which also are intermediates in the production of androgens by the adrenal cortex (see Fig. 16). Normally, the quantitative production of adrenal androgen is small; however, if the steroid precursors pile up (due to block in normal formation of cortisone), some of this excess may be used to form more androgens.

Two things result from this situation. First, due to abnormally high production of androgen, secondary sexual characteristics are affected. If the condition is manifest in utero, pseudohermaphroditism results in females (masculinization of external genitalia) and macrogenitosomia praecox in males (accentuation of male genitalia). If the condition does not become clinically manifest until after birth, virilism (masculinization) results in females and precocious puberty develops in males. Second, the adrenal glands themselves increase in size due to hyperplasia of the steroid-producing adrenal cortex. This results because normal pituitary production of ACTH (the adrenal cortex stimulating hormone) is controlled by the amount of cortisone and hydrocortisone produced by the adrenal. If more cortisone is produced than the body needs, this inhibits the pituitary and decreases ACTH production; if the body has less cortisone than it needs, the pituitary produces more ACTH. In congenital adrenal hyperplasia, cortisone production is partially or completely blocked, the pituitary produces more and more ACTH in attempts to increase cortisone production, and the adrenal cortex tissue becomes hyperplastic under continually increased ACTH stimulation.

This condition is diagnosed by the finding of increased 17-ketosteroids in the urine. 17-ketosteroids are composed mainly of the metabolites or breakdown products of androgens. In most cases, urinary pregnanetriol (a metabolite of 17-OH-progesterone) is also elevated.

II. The Virilization Syndrome

This rare syndrome occurs in older children and in adults. It is manifested by virilism in females and by excessive masculinization in males. It may be due to idiopathic adrenal cortex hyperplasia, adrenal cortex adenoma, or cortex carcinoma. Tumor is more common than hyperplasia in these cases. Virilism in a female child or an adult leads to hirsutism, clitoral enlargement, deepening of the voice, masculine contour, and breast atrophy. The syndrome may be simulated in females by idiopathic hirsutism, arrhenoblastoma of the ovary, and possibly by the Stein-Leventhal syndrome. Urinary 17-ketosteroids are elevated with normal or decreased 17-OH-corticosteroids when the adrenal is involved. Ovarian arrhenoblastoma gives normal or only slightly elevated urine 17-ketosteroids, since androgen is produced in smaller quantities but is more potent, thus giving clinical symptoms without greatly increased quantities. In prepubertal males, the symptoms are those of precocious puberty; in adult males, excessive masculinization is difficult to recognize. A similar picture may be associated with certain testicular tumors.

## III.  Cushing's Syndrome

About 50-60% of cases with the syndrome are due to simple hyperplasia of the adrenal cortex; most are idiopathic, but a few are secondary to pituitary basophil tumors. About 30-40% are caused by cortex adenomas, with cortex carcinomas accounting for 10% or less. Very uncommonly, the syndrome may be produced by nonadrenal tumors, mainly small-cell undifferentiated ("oat-cell") lung carcinoma. The highest incidence of the syndrome is found in adults, with females affected four times more than males. Major symptoms and signs include body trunk obesity, "buffalo hump" fat deposit on the back of the neck, abdominal striae, osteoporosis, and a tendency to diabetes, easy bruising, and hypertension. Laboratory findings include hyperglycemia (either fasting or 2-hour postprandial) in about 50%, hypokalemia with alkalosis in about 35%, and lymphopenia with mild leukocytosis. Serum sodium may be elevated or normal. Total circulating eosinophils are decreased. Red blood cell counts and hemoglobin are often increased, sometimes to polycythemic levels.

Laboratory diagnosis of Cushing's syndrome requires demonstration of consistently elevated 17-OH-corticosteroid secretion. Assay of 17-OH-CS in blood is still technically rather difficult so that this test is not widely available. Assay in urine is not easy, but is more so than for blood, and can be obtained in most sizable laboratories. A single random 17-OH-CS in either plasma or urine is not very reliable, although a definitely elevated value would increase suspicion of adrenal hypersecretion. In plasma, stress or estrogen effect of pregnancy may produce elevated random levels, and mild degrees of Cushing's syndrome may have normal 17-OH-CS. Urine is somewhat more helpful than plasma as a single test. About 10-15% of Cushing's syndrome patients are said to have consistently normal urine values, while some patients with obesity or hyperthyroidism have consistently increased urine 17-OH-CS levels. If plasma 17-OH-CS determinations are available, a better screening test for Cushing's syndrome than a single determination consists of two plasma specimens, one at 8 A.M. and the other at 5 P.M. Normally, there is a diurnal variation in plasma levels (not urine lev-

els), with the afternoon specimen being less than 50% of the morning value. In Cushing's syndrome, this variation is absent in 90%
or more patients. Unfortunately, significant decrease in plasma
diurnal variation is not specific for Cushing's syndrome, since it
has been demonstrated in occasional patients with a wide variety of
conditions.

The most accurate simple screening procedure is said to be a
rapid dexamethasone suppression test. Oral administration of 1 mg.
of dexamethasone at 11 P.M. suppresses pituitary ACTH production,
so that the normal 8 A.M. peak of plasma cortisol fails to develop.
Normal and obese persons produce 8 A.M. plasma cortisol values
less than 50% of baseline levels (some require suppression to 5 $\mu$g./
100 ml. or less). Over 95% of Cushing's syndrome patients are said
to exhibit abnormal test responses, with less than 5% false positive
results. Stress may negate the suppressive effects from small
amounts of dexamethasone, so that a barbiturate is usually given
with the test dose. Estrogens or very serious illness may produce
false positive tests (failure to suppress normally). Additional evidence to support abnormal screening test results may be obtained by
using the standard dexamethasone suppression test.

Confirmation of the diagnosis depends mainly on tests which
involve either stimulation or suppression of adrenal hormone production. It is often possible with the same tests to differentiate between
the various etiologies of primary hyperadrenalism. Normally, increased pituitary ACTH production increases adrenal corticosteroid
release. Increased plasma corticosteroid levels normally inhibit
pituitary release of ACTH and therefore suppress further adrenal
steroid production. Adrenal tumors, as a rule, produce their hormones without being much affected by suppression tests; on the other
hand, they tend to give little response to stimulation, as though they
behave independently of the usual hormone control mechanism. Also, if urinary 17-ketosteroids are markedly increased (over twice
normal), this strongly suggests carcinoma; adenoma is most often
associated with normal or even low values, while hyperplasia produces mildly or moderately elevated levels. However, hyperplasia
and carcinoma values overlap, and ketosteroid levels may be normal with either hyperplasia or carcinoma.

The dexamethasone suppression test probably is the most widely used confirmatory procedure. Dexamethasone (Decadron) is a synthetic steroid with cortisone-type actions but is approximately thirty
times more potent than cortisone, so that amounts too small for laboratory measurement may be given to suppress pituitary ACTH production. If low doses (2 mg./day) are used, normal adrenals will show
significantly decreased urine 17-hydroxycorticosteroid values while
those with Cushing's syndrome from any etiology will not. If larger
doses (8 mg./day) are used, those with cortical hyperplasia will usually show significantly depressed urine 17-OH-CS, but hormone-
producing adenomas or carcinoma will be relatively unaffected.

A second way to accomplish the same thing is to use metyrapone, available commercially as Metopirone. This blocks the production of cortisone, so that the pituitary releases more ACTH in order to try to increase adrenal cortisone production. Although cortisone is not manufactured, the very close precursors of cortisone are; they pile up and are excreted in the urine. Since they are included in 17-hydroxycorticosteroid measurements, response to metyrapone is a sharp increase in urine 17-hydroxycorticosteroids in both normal adrenals and those with hyperplasia; tumors show little change.

A third method is direct stimulation by ACTH. Cortex hyperplasia and some cases of adenoma show increased blood 17-hydroxycorticosteroids. Carcinoma and some adenomas do not respond. Results apparently are more variable in cortex hyperplasia than with the suppression tests, and various conditions other than Cushing's syndrome have been reported to occasionally give abnormal responses. Interestingly enough, nonadrenal neoplasms which cause Cushing's syndrome produce exactly the same patterns in the various tests as does primary carcinoma of the adrenal.

## IV. Primary Aldosteronism

Primary aldosteronism (Conn's syndrome) is another syndrome caused by adrenocortical hyperfunction—this time by oversecretion of aldosterone, the chief electrolyte-regulating hormone of the adrenal. This works mainly in the kidney, where it causes retention of sodium, leading to secondary loss of potassium. Edema is absent. Symptoms include hypertension, weakness, and polyuria. Hypokalemia is the most prominent laboratory finding; there usually is mild alkalosis and low urine specific gravity. Hypernatremia is found in classic cases, but a sizable minority of patients have high normal or normal serum sodium. 17-OH-CS and 17-KS excretion are normal. Hemoglobin and WBC are also normal. Other diseases which may give hypokalemia and hypertension include Cushing's syndrome, essential hypertension combined with mercurial or thiazide diuretic therapy, and malignant hypertension.

Diagnosis of primary aldosteronism may be suggested by failure to raise serum potassium on regular diet plus 100 mEq. of potassium a day (in addition, urine potassium excretion should increase during potassium loading, assuming normal salt intake of 5-8 Gm./ day). A more definitive test requires demonstration of increased urinary aldosterone in a 24-hour specimen. Currently, this involves a complicated isotope or chromatographic procedure which is very difficult and takes several days to perform. At present, only large medical centers or reference laboratories offer the test. Aldosterone may also be increased in certain other conditions ("secondary aldosteronism"):

1. Hyponatremia or low salt intake.
2. Potassium loading.

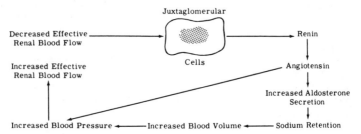

Fig. 18.—Renal pressor system.

3. Generalized edema (cirrhosis, nephrotic syndrome, congestive heart failure).
4. Malignant hypertension.
5. Renal ischemia of any etiology (including renal artery stenosis).
6. Pregnancy or estrogen-containing medications.

Current explanations for the effects of these conditions on aldosterone point toward decreased effective renal blood flow (Fig. 18). This triggers certain pressure-sensitive glomerular afferent arteriole cells called the juxtaglomerular apparatus into compensatory release of an enzyme called renin. Renin sets up a chain reaction leading to formation of a vasoconstrictor substance which in turn leads to release of adrenal aldosterone.

The importance of secondary aldosteronism is that some of these situations also are associated with hypertension (either as cause or treatment). Of these, nephrosis has normal blood pressure and serum potassium. Cirrhosis and malignant hypertension may have normal or decreased potassium. Malignant hypertension usually has papilledema, which is rare in aldosteronism, and a normal or low serum sodium. In cirrhosis with hypokalemia, serum sodium generally is low normal or decreased, blood pressure usually is not elevated, and ascites or other signs of liver disease usually are present.

Treatment of hypertension by diuretics or sodium restriction will increase aldosterone secretion. Since the body may be sodium-deficient with serum sodium still within normal range, it is advisable to give patients a high-salt diet or salt supplements for several days before collecting specimens for aldosterone. As a further check, the 24-hour urine aldosterone specimen should be assayed for sodium. Finding sodium values of less than 40 mEq./L. suggests decreased sodium secretion, implying a sodium deficit and therefore a falsely increased aldosterone. In occasional individuals, aldosterone hypersecretion may fluctuate, so that a single normal determination does not completely rule out the diagnosis.

Some patients with primary aldosteronism have normal serum potassium. Since hypertension from several different etiologies

may be associated with increased urine aldosterone and normal serum potassium, this may create diagnostic difficulty. The most
specific test for primary aldosteronism is a combination of increased urine aldosterone and decreased plasma renin. Decreased
renin alone is not sufficient, since nearly 25% of hypertensive patients demonstrate decreased plasma renin without having Conn's
syndrome. Low salt diet and upright posture are manipulations
which stimulate renin production in normal individuals and thus help
to separate the decreased renin of Conn's syndrome from a temporary decrease of some other etiology. Certain precautions are essential in collecting and processing the blood specimen (p. 452).
    Plasma renin is technically a difficult test. Radioisotope im-
munoassay has improved simplicity and accuracy over the old bio-
assay methods, but present-day commercial kits are economically
suitable only for large numbers of specimens. Therefore, only
university or reference laboratories offer the test. Certain factors
influence plasma renin values. Sodium depletion, upright posture,
various diuretics, estrogens, and many of the antihypertensive drugs
tend to increase renin secretion. Renovascular hypertension and
some cases of malignant hypertension do likewise. Decreased renin
occurs in 25% of persons with hypertension, besides patients with
primary aldosteronism or Cushing's syndrome and those undergoing
therapy with L-dopa, methyldopa (Aldomet), or guanethidine. Primary aldosteronism has increased aldosterone excretion, which
many of these other conditions lack; and, in addition, use of stimuli
which increase renin production yield renin values still below normal
in Conn's syndrome while forcing renin values into normal range or
above in the other listed conditions.

## V. Addison's Disease

    This condition is adrenocortical insufficiency from any cause.
Tuberculosis used to be the most frequent etiology, but now is second to idiopathic atrophy. Steroid therapy, if long-term, causes
cortex atrophy from disuse, and if steroids are abruptly withdrawn
symptoms will develop rapidly. Other cases are due to infection,
idiopathic hemorrhage, or replacement by metastatic carcinoma.
The most frequent metastatic tumor is from the lung, and it is interesting that there often can be nearly complete replacement without any symptoms. Weakness and fatigability are early manifestations of Addison's disease, often brought on by infection or stress.
Other signs and symptoms of the classic syndrome are weight loss,
hypotension of varying degree, a small heart, pigmentation of the
skin, and sometimes mild hypoglycemia. Laboratory studies show
low serum sodium and chloride with elevated potassium. There
may be a normocytic normochromic mild anemia, and relative lymphocytosis with decreased neutrophils. The diagnosis may be suspected on clinical grounds and the finding of increased sodium and

chloride in the urine despite low serum levels. Total circulating eosinophils usually are close to normal, although not always so.

A definitive diagnosis is possible using ACTH stimulation. A 24-hour urine specimen is taken the day before the test. Twenty-five units of ACTH in 500 cc. saline is given intravenously during 8 hours while another 24-hour urine specimen is obtained. In normal persons, there will be at least a 2-4 fold increase in urine 17-OH-corticosteroids. In Addison's disease, practically no response is found. If pituitary deficiency is suspected, the test should be repeated the next day, in which case there will be a gradual, although relatively small, response. If exogenous steroids have been given over long periods, especially in large doses, the test period may have to be prolonged up to 7 days. If maintenance steroids are necessary during the test period, small doses of dexamethasone should be used to avoid measuring the treatment steroid along with endogenous production. If steroid measurements are not available, the Thorn test is a reasonably satisfactory substitute, although not as accurate. First, a count of total circulating eosinophils is done. Then the patient is given 25 units of ACTH, either intravenously in the same way as the ACTH test described above or in the form of long-acting ACTH gel given intramuscularly. Eight hours after ACTH is started, another total circulating eosinophil count is made. Normally, cortisone causes depression of eosinophil production. Therefore, a normal response to the test ACTH stimulation would be a drop of total circulating eosinophils of more than 50% (from baseline values). A drop of less than 50% is considered suspicious for adrenal insufficiency. False positive responses (less than 50% drop) may occur in any condition which itself produces eosinophilia (such as acute episodes of allergy).

One technical note: for adrenal suppression or stimulation tests in general, many authorities recommend direct plasma 17-OH-corticosteroid determination in preference to the more indirect urine metabolite measurements. However, what the physician orders may depend on what laboratory procedures are available in his area. Also, it usually is advisable to obtain a creatinine value on urine samples submitted for steroid assay. Since creatinine has a fairly stable excretion rate, finding values less than normal would suggest inadequate specimen collection. This precaution is, in fact, advisable any time a 24-hour urine sample is collected for quantitative chemical analysis.

Adrenal Medulla Dysfunction

The only syndrome in this category is produced by pheochromocytomas. Pheochromocytoma is a tumor of the adrenal medulla which often secretes epinephrine or norepinephrine. This causes hypertension, which may be continuous or intermittent. Although rare, pheochromocytoma is one of the few curable causes of hyper-

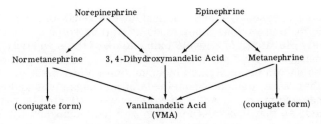

Fig. 19.—Catecholamine metabolism.

tension, and thus should be tested for in any patient with hypertension of either sudden or recent onset.   This is especially true for
young or middle-aged persons.   The original tests for pheochromocytomas were pharmacologic, based on the fact that epinephrine
effects could be neutralized by adrenergic blocking drugs such as
Regitine.   After basal blood pressure has been established, 5 mg.
of Regitine are given intravenously and the blood pressure is checked
every 30 seconds.   The test is positive if systolic blood pressure
decreases more than 35 mm. or diastolic levels decrease 25 mm.
or more and remain decreased 3-4 minutes.   Laboratory tests have
proved much more reliable than the pharmacologic procedures,
which have an appreciable percentage of false positives and negatives.   The catecholamines epinephrine and norepinephrine are excreted by the kidney, about 3-6% free (unchanged) and the remainder
as various metabolites (Fig. 19).   Of these metabolic products, the
major portion is vanilmandelic acid (VMA), and the remainder
(about 20-40%) are compounds known as metanephrines.   Therefore,
one can measure either urinary catecholamines, metanephrines, or
VMA.   Advantages of VMA are that there is less fluctuation between
night and day specimen levels, the amounts excreted are greater
than those of its precursors, and certain ("screening") methods are
easier to do in the laboratory than catecholamines or metanephrines.
The advantage of catecholamines is that when elevations occur they
are as a rule more marked than the VMA elevations.   The advantage
of metanephrines is increased reliability over some of the VMA procedures.   However, all three tests give nearly equal results.   A
small but significant percentage of cases are missed by any of the
three tests, especially if the tumor secretes intermittently.   Occasionally, one test will be positive when another is normal.   Some
claim that metanephrines are slightly better in this respect than the
others.   Catecholamine production may be increased after severe
exercise (although mild or moderate degrees have no appreciable
effect) and uncommonly by emotional stress.   Other diseases which
may increase catecholamine production (and thereby the excretion
of either free catecholamines or their metabolites) are thyrotoxicosis, Cushing's disease, myocardial infarction, hemolytic anemia,

and occasional cases of lymphoma and severe renal disease. In addition, coffee and various other foods as well as some drugs may give falsely elevated VMA levels using some of the standard ("screening") techniques. An abnormal result with the "screening" VMA techniques should be confirmed by some other VMA method. Although other VMA methods or methods of metanephrines and catecholamines are more reliable, they too may be affected by certain substances, so that it is best to check with individual laboratories for details on substances which affect their particular test method. Fasting blood sugar is elevated in about 50% of pheochromocytoma.

Cushing's disease and primary aldosteronism are two conditions which often produce hypertension. As noted on page 148, unilateral renal disease (rarely bilateral renal artery stenosis) may also be a cause. As described earlier, pheochromocytoma is another etiology. These diseases are classified as secondary hypertension, in contrast to primary idiopathic (essential) hypertension. Although these particular diseases which cause secondary hypertension form a relatively small minority of hypertension cases, they are important because they are surgically curable. The patient usually is protected against the bad effects of hypertension by early diagnosis and cure. Those patients who must be especially investigated are those who are young (under age 50), who develop symptoms over a short period, or who have a sudden worsening of the hypertension after previous mild stable blood pressure elevation.

## REFERENCES

Amery, A., and Conway, J.: A critical review of diagnostic tests for pheochromocytoma, Am. Heart J. 73:129, 1967.

The Adrenal, Clinician I (Chicago: G. D. Searle & Co., 1971).

Bongiovanni, A. M., and Root, A. W.: The adrenogenital syndrome, New England J. Med. 268:1283, 1342, 1391, 1963.

Channick, B. J., et al.: Suppressed plasma renin activity in hypertension, Arch. Int. Med. 123:131, 1969.

Conn, J. W., et al.: Preoperative diagnosis of primary aldosteronism, Arch. Int. Med. 123:113, 1969.

Conn, J. W.: Aldosteronism in hypertensive disease, M. Times 98:116, 1970.

Greendyke, R. M.: Adrenal hemorrhage, Am. J. Clin. Path. 43:210, 1965.

Gunnells, J. C., Jr., et al.: Plasma renin activity in healthy subjects and patients with hypertension, Arch. Int. Med. 119:232, 1967.

Kaplan, N. M.: Primary Aldosteronism, in Astwood, E. B. (ed.): Clinical Endocrinology II (New York: Grune & Stratton, Inc., 1968), p. 467.

Laragh, J. H., and Kelly, W. G.: Aldosterone: Its Biochemistry
and Physiology, in Levine, R., and Luft, R. (eds.): Advances in
Metabolic Disorders (New York: Academic Press, Inc., 1964),
Vol. 1, p. 217.
Lauler, D. P.: When to hospitalize for adrenal insufficiency, Hosp.
Practice 3:35, 1968.
Lauler, D. P.: When to hospitalize for primary aldosteronism,
Hosp. Practice 4:48, 1969.
Liddle, G. W., et al.: Nonpituitary neoplasms and Cushing's syn-
drome, Arch. Int. Med. 111:471, 1963.
Liddle, G. W., and Shute, A. M.: Cushing's Syndrome as a Clinical
Entity, in Stollerman, G. H. (ed.): Advances in Internal Medicine
(Chicago: Year Book Medical Publishers, Inc., 1969), Vol. 15,
p. 155.
Nelson, D. H.: Determining plasma and urinary corticosteroids,
Postgrad. Med. 46:135, 1969.
Nichols, T., et al.: Steroid laboratory tests in the diagnosis of
Cushing's syndrome, Am. J. Med. 45:116, 1968.
Pertsemlidis, D., et al.: Pheochromocytoma: 1. Specificity of
laboratory diagnostic tests. 2. Safeguards during operative re-
moval, Ann. Surg. 169:376, 1969.
Rose, L. I., et al.: The 48-hour adrenocorticotropin infusion test
for adrenocortical insufficiency, Ann. Int. Med. 73:49, 1970.
Ross, E. J., et al.: Cushing's syndrome; diagnostic criteria,
Quart. J. Med. 35:149, 1966.
Sawin, C. T.: Measurement of plasma cortisol in diagnosis of
Cushing's syndrome, Ann. Int. Med. 68:624, 1968.
Sheps, S. G., et al.: Current experience in the diagnosis of pheo-
chromocytoma, Circulation 34:473, 1966.
Spark, R. F., and Melby, J. C.: Hypertension and low plasma
renin activity: Presumptive evidence for mineralocorticoid ex-
cess, Ann. Int. Med. 75:831, 1971.
Zimmerman, B.: Pituitary and adrenal function in relation to sur-
gery, S. Clin. North America 45:299, 1965.

# CHAPTER 30

# Pituitary Function Tests, Miscellaneous Hormone Tests, and Tests in Obstetrics

### Tests of Pituitary Function

The most common areas of pituitary dysfunction are growth hormone deficiency of childhood, pituitary insufficiency in adults, and acromegaly in adults.

Pituitary insufficiency in adults is most commonly due to postpartum hemorrhage (Sheehan's syndrome). Gonadal failure is usually the first deficiency to appear; it is followed some time later by myxedema. Diagnosis can be made, using indirect methods, by proving normal adrenal 17-ketosteroid response to ACTH stimulation or normal thyroid hormone response to TSH. The metyrapone (Metopirone) test (p. 359) can also be used. Growth hormone secretion deficiency may now be measured directly via radioimmunoassay, which in some cases is more sensitive than indirect tests. Lowest basal plasma levels are found in the morning after awakening but before arising. Specimens must be drawn when the patient is fasting at this time. Values are elevated by exercise of any type, various foods, and estrogens. Because the basal normal range overlaps with hypopituitarism values, stimulation tests are used for definitive diagnosis. These procedures depend on hypoglycemia as a stimulus to growth hormone production. Hypoglycemia may be produced directly, using insulin, or indirectly, using the amino acid arginine. Tolbutamide and glucagon have also been suggested. Pituitary insufficiency cannot be documented on the basis of one test alone, since about 20% of normal persons fail to respond either to insulin or to arginine.

Acromegaly is produced in adults by increase of growth hormone, usually from an eosinophilic adenoma of the pituitary. About two thirds of these patients are females. Signs and symptoms include bitemporal headaches, disturbances of the visual field, optic atrophy, hand and face physical changes, and decreased carbohydrate tolerance. About 65-75% of patients display sella turcica enlargement on skull x-rays. Growth hormone assay usually reveals levels above the upper limit of 5 ng./ml. The standard method of confirming the diagnosis is a suppression test using glucose. Normal persons nearly always respond with a decrease in growth hormone levels to less than 50% of baseline levels, while acromegalic patients in theory have autonomous tumors and should show little if any effect of hyperglycemia. One recent study, however, noted relatively normal suppression in a significant percentage of acromegalics.

The metyrapone test (Metopirone; SU-4885; Liddle test) may be used as a test of pituitary hypofunction. Sometimes the pituitary does not function normally, but is still able to put out the small quantities of ACTH needed to maintain adrenal cortisone output at normal or nearly normal levels under nonstressful basal conditions. To demonstrate this, one first shows that the adrenal can respond normally to ACTH, then does the metyrapone test and shows that the adrenal does not put out significantly greater amounts of 17-OH-CS (the pituitary is not able to respond to the block in cortisone production by putting out more ACTH).

Miscellaneous Hormone Tests

Plasma testosterone may be useful in a variety of conditions relating to hypogonadism, virilization, and hirsutism. In males, hypogonadism due to Klinefelter's syndrome, deficiency of interstitial cell stimulating hormone, or primary gonadal failure have subnormal values. Patients with cirrhosis frequently have depressed levels. In females, Stein-Leventhal (polycystic ovary) syndrome is usually associated with elevated plasma testosterone when virilization is present. Idiopathic hirsutism patients may have elevated values, but at least 40% are normal. Estrogen decreases testosterone levels. Arrhenoblastomas frequently secrete testosterone. Virilization due to adrenal cortex etiology (adrenogenital syndrome) is usually accompanied by increased urine 17-ketosteroids, but reports differ on how frequently plasma testosterone is elevated.

Pregnancy tests are based on the fact that the placenta secretes chorionic gonadotropin, a hormone which has a luteinizing action on ovarian follicles, but whose actual function is not definitely established. It appears in detectable titer between the 28th and 32nd days after the beginning of the last menstrual period, reaching a level of about 500 international units of gonadotropic activity. A peak is reached about the 63rd day but ranging between the 50th and 80th days, with values reaching 200,000 I.U., then slowly falls to levels of between 2,000 and 10,000 I.U. This level is maintained for the remainder of pregnancy except for a brief rise and fall in the third trimester.

    The first practical biologic test for pregnancy was the Ascheim-
Zondek test, published in 1928. Urine was injected into immature female mice and a positive test was indicated by corpus luteum development in the ovaries. This took 4-5 days to perform. Clinical accuracy is reported as up to 98%. A few false positives and negatives
occur. The next widely used procedure was the Friedman test, which
was similar except that female rabbits were used and the test took
3 days. Other variations on these procedures were used, but it was
not until the frog tests were described that a significant advance occurred. Using male frogs, urine or serum is injected and the animal catheterized 1-2 hours later. The presence of spermatozoa
gives a positive test. The frog test has approximately a 95% reliability, although some report even better. False negative and false
positive results do occur, although they are uncommon. Phenothiazine drugs (e. g. , Thorazine) give a considerable number of
false positives. The test is almost always positive at the 40th day
of pregnancy, although sometimes sooner. All these biologic tests
share the problems which go with using animals. In the past few
years, it was discovered that antibodies to human chorionic gonadotropin could be produced by injecting the gonadotropin into animals.
This raised the possibility of developing an immunologic pregnancy
test using antigen-antibody reactions.
    Both tube tests and slide tests are now available. In general,
the tube tests require 2 hours to perform, but tend to be a little
more accurate. The slide tests take 2-3 minutes. A few procedures
based on chemical techniques are being marketed. There is significant variation in accuracy and sensitivity among all these tests
(p. 454). In general, most immunologic tests are over 95% accurate. Each becomes positive between the 35th and 40th days (counting from the first day of the last menstrual period), sometimes
sooner, and is almost always positive by the 41st day. Proteinuria
(over 25 mg./100 ml.) causes false positive results (p. 454) in many
of the commercial slide tests; certain psychiatric drugs (such as
Thorazine) give false positives in a few of the commercial procedures. In the third trimester, and occasionally even in the second,
false negative results with any of the immunologic tests may be obtained in some patients, due to the much lower gonadotropin levels
at this time. Occasional false positive results from some of the
pregnancy tests have been reported in postmenopausal women; presumably this is due to increased luteinizing hormone, which cross-
reacts with current antibody preparations to chorionic gonadotropin.
    Pregnancy tests are useful in certain situations other than
early diagnosis of normal pregnancy. In possible abortion, a dying
trophoblast is usually associated with low levels of chorionic gonadotropin and predicts present or inevitable abortion. However, normal levels are found in some cases where the embryo dies but the
trophoblast carries on. In ectopic pregnancy, the tests are positive
only about half the time, so a negative test definitely does not rule

out this diagnosis. Hydatidiform mole and chorionepithelioma are associated with increased production of chorionic gonadotropin. When such levels are present at a time when low or negative values are expected, it suggests the diagnosis, especially if a rising titer is found. Quantitative dilution tests have to be run to confirm this. "False positives" may occur in normal multiple pregnancy such as twins.

## Tests in Obstetrics

Urinary estriol levels may help predict impending fetal damage or death resulting from placental insufficiency. Estriol is an estrogenic compound; after the second month of pregnancy it is produced in steadily increasing quantities by the placenta. The procedure is to obtain weekly serial determinations after 30 weeks' gestation in high-risk patients, or as an immediate test if fetal distress occurs; 24-hour urine collections are obtained, since excretion fluctuates during the day. A marked decline from previous values, especially if sustained, is considered significant evidence of placental malfunction. Coupled with clinical evidence of fetal distress, or in a high-risk patient, cesarean section may be indicated. Those considered high risk are diabetics, hypertensives, and those with a history of stillbirths. The test is not valid in liver damage, such as occurs with Rh erythroblastosis or eclampsia, because the liver also produces estriol. Urinary tract infection and certain drugs such as steroids and Mandelamine affect the test results. The test at present is chromatographic, so it is not done in most routine laboratories.

Since estriol comprises about 95% of urinary estrogens in pregnancy, total estrogens (much easier technically) could be substituted for estriol. Results using total estrogens are a little more variable than estriol patterns.

Tests are described elsewhere which are useful in other obstetrical conditions such as eclampsia (p. 134), urinary tract infection (p. 170), and hemolytic disease of the newborn (p. 104).

Placenta localization: Vaginal bleeding in the third trimester of pregnancy is most frequently caused by placenta previa. In this condition the placenta is located near the cervical opening instead of in its usual position near the upper end of the uterus. Placenta previa location is therefore a hazard to normal delivery and might necessitate caesarean section. Radioisotope scanning and ultrasound "B mode" scanning are now being used for placental localization. Ultrasound "B mode" (not yet widely available) has the advantage that no radioactivity is needed; however, the fetal dose by radioisotope scan is very small—much smaller than what the fetus would receive from ordinary x-ray pelvimetry studies.

Fetal maturity tests: Tests are also available for monitoring fetal maturity via amniocentesis. Bilirubin levels in erythroblastosis

is discussed in Chapter 10 (p. 104 ).  Amniotic creatinine, cell stain
with Nile blue sulfate,  fat droplet evaluation, and osmolality, alone
or in combination, have been tried with satisfactory but not outstand-
ing results.  A new test, the lecithin/sphingomyelin (L/S) ratio, may
well replace all previous techniques.  Lecithin is a phospholipid
which is a major component of alveolar surfactant.  Surfactant is a
substance which lowers the surface tension of the alveolar lining,
stabilizes the alveoli in expiration, and helps prevent atelectasis.
Surfactant deficiency causes neonatal respiratory distress syndrome
(hyaline membrane disease).  In amniotic fluid, sphingomyelin normally exceeds lecithin before the 26th week; thereafter, lecithin
concentration is slightly predominant until approximately the 35th
week, when lecithin swiftly rises to more than twice sphingomyelin
levels.  After lecithin becomes twice sphingomyelin, there is no
longer any danger of hyaline membrane disease.  The L/S ratio thus
becomes a test for fetal maturity.  Certain precautions must be
taken.  Contamination by maternal vaginal secretions or bleeding
into the amniotic fluid may cause a false increase in lecithin.  The
amniotic fluid specimen must be cooled immediately and kept frozen
if not tested promptly, in order to avoid destruction of lecithin by
certain enzymes in amniotic fluid.

## REFERENCES

Albert, A. , and Northcutt, R. C.:  Pituitary gonadotropin assays,
    Postgrad. Med. 46:96, 1969.
Andrews, B. F.:  Amniotic fluid studies to determine fetal maturity,
    Pediat. Clin. North America 17:49, 1970.
Behrman, S. J.:  The complete fertility workup, Hosp. Practice
    1:50, 1966.
Christy, N. P.:  Pituitary Insufficiency, in Astwood, E. B. (ed.):
    Clinical Endocrinology (New York: Grune & Stratton, Inc., 1960),
    p. 53.
Daughaday, W. H.:  Growth hormone assay in acromegaly, gigantism,
    dwarfism, and hypopituitarism, Postgrad. Med. 46:84, 1969.
Davis, M. E. , and Fugo, N. W.:  Diagnosis and treatment of men-
    strual disorders, M. Clin. North America 45:3, 1961.
Doe, R. P. , and Gold, E. M.:  The metyrapone test for pituitary
    function, Postgrad. Med. 46:157, 1969.
Gluck, L.:  Pulmonary surfactant and neonatal respiratory distress,
    Hosp. Practice 6:45, 1971.
Gordon, D. A. , et al.:  Acromegaly: A review of 100 cases, Canad.
    M. A. J. 87:1106, 1962.
Hobson, B. M.:  Pregnancy diagnosis, J. Reprod. Fert. 12:33, 1966.
Jubiz, W. , et al.:  Single-dose metyrapone test, Arch. Int. Med.
    125:472, 1970.
Kahn, C. B. , et al.:  Laboratory assessment of diabetic pregnancy:
    A brief review, Diabetes 21:31, 1972.

Kerber, I. J., et al.: Immunologic tests for pregnancy, Obst. & Gynec. 36:37, 1970.

Krieger, D. T.: The hypothalamus and neuroendocrine pathology, Hosp. Practice 6:127, 1971.

Lamb, E.: Immunologic pregnancy tests, Obst. & Gynec. 39:665, 1972.

Lawrence, A. M.: Glucagon in medicine: New ideas from an old hormone, M. Clin. North America 54:183, 1970.

Lawrence, A. M., et al.: Growth hormone dynamics in acromegaly, J. Clin. Endocrinol. 31:239, 1970.

Lipsett, M. B., et al.: Physiologic basis of disorders of androgen metabolism, Ann. Int. Med. 68:1327, 1968.

McCullagh, E. P., and Brandon, J. M.: Acromegaly, in Astwood, E. B. (ed.): Clinical Endocrinology I (New York: Grune & Stratton, Inc., 1960), p. 36.

Mitchell, M. L., et al.: Detection of growth-hormone deficiency—The glucagon stimulation test, New England J. Med. 282:539, 1970.

O'Leary, J. A., and Bezjian, A. A.: Amniotic fluid fetal maturity score, Obst. & Gynec. 38:375, 1971.

Ontjes, D. A.: Tests of anterior pituitary function, Metabolism 21:159, 1972.

Scarpelli, E. M.: Pulmonary surfactant system, Clin. Notes on Resp. Dis. 9:3, 1970.

Spellacy, W. N., et al.: Human growth hormone levels in normal subjects receiving an oral contraceptive, J. A. M. A. 202:451, 1967.

Weingold, A. B.: Monitoring the fetal environment, Postgrad. Med. 48:232 (Sept.); 201 (Oct.), 1970.

# CHAPTER 31

# Tests for Syphilis

Clinical syphilis usually is subdivided into primary, secondary, latent, and tertiary stages. The primary stage begins after an average 3-6 weeks' incubation and is manifested by the development of a primary-stage lesion, or chancre, near the site of infection. The time of appearance is variable; the lesion often is inconspicuous and overlooked, especially in the female. The chancre usually heals and, in classic cases, skin and sometimes mucous membrane lesions develop about 4-6 weeks after appearance of the chancre, marking the secondary stage. After a few days or weeks, the secondary stage lesions disappear, and the patient enters the latent stage. This lasts, on the average, 3-5 years. During this time, about half the untreated patients apparently become spontaneously cured, or, at least, do not develop further evidence of infection. About 25% remain in a latent ("late latent") status; the remaining 25% develop tertiary-stage sequelae such as neurologic, cardiovascular, or ocular syphilis.

Diagnostic procedures in syphilis include darkfield examination, immunologic tests, and cerebrospinal fluid examination, depending on the clinical situation.

## DARKFIELD EXAMINATION

Darkfield examination should be performed on all primary and any suitable secondary lesions. Darkfield may be the only way to make an early diagnosis, since immunologic test antibodies often do not appear until late in the primary stage. The technique of obtaining the specimen without contamination by blood or surface bacteria is very important. The lesion should be cleansed thoroughly with water or normal saline and a sterile gauze pad. No soap or antiseptics are used. Care must be taken not to produce bleeding, since

TABLE 14.—TYPES OF IMMUNOLOGIC SYPHILIS TESTS

| Specific | Crossreacting | Fortuitous |
|----------|---------------|------------|
| TPI | RPCF | STS |
| FTA | | |

RBC will obscure the organisms. After having been blotted dry, the lesion will accumulate a clear serous exudate in a few minutes. If it does not, it may be abraded gently with gauze, but not enough to cause bleeding. The serous fluid exudate is taken off in a pipet or capillary tube for examination with a darkfield microscope. The causative organism, Treponema pallidum, has a characteristic morphology and motility under darkfield, but experience is necessary for interpretation, since nonpathogenic varieties of spirochetes may be found normally in the genital areas.

## IMMUNOLOGIC TESTS FOR SYPHILIS

Immunologic tests for syphilis depend on the fact that diseases caused by infectious organisms are characterized by development of antibodies toward that organism. These antibodies can be specific or nonspecific (Table 14), the nonspecific group either of cross-reacting type (sharing a common antigen with another organism) or fortuitous type (provoked by some nonspecific portion of the organism).

The first practical serologic test for syphilis (STS) was a complement-fixation technique invented by Wassermann. He used extract from a syphilitic liver. Subsequently, it was found that the main ingredient of the substance he used actually had nothing to do with syphilitic infection and was present in other tissues besides liver. It is a phospholipid which is now commercially prepared from beef heart and therefore called cardiolipin. The present-day STS reagent is a mixture of purified lipoproteins including cardiolipin, cholesterol, and lecithin. Apparently, an antibody called reagin is produced in syphilis which will react with this cardiolipin-lipoprotein complex. Why reagin is produced is not entirely understood; it is not a specific antibody to T. pallidum. There is a lipoidal substance in spirochetes, and it is possible that it is similar enough to the cardiolipin-lipoprotein complex that antibodies produced against it may also fortuitously react with cardiolipin.

There are two basic types of STS procedures to detect reagin:

1. Complement-Fixation (CF) Reaction: This was the procedure used by Wassermann. The original technique has been superseded by the Kolmer modification. There are several defects in this system. The patient's serum may be anticomplementary (contain substances which bind, and thus inactivate, complement). The CF test is a two-stage procedure, and the second stage of the re-

action has to incubate overnight.  Complement and sheep RBC are among the reagents needed, and these may be of poor quality.  Contamination of glassware may give anticomplementary results.

2.  Flocculation Reaction:  In this system, the patient's serum is heated; for unknown reasons, heating seems to enhance the reaction.  Then a suspension of cardiolipin antigen particles is added to the serum and mixed.  If positive (reactive), the serum reagin antibody present will combine with the antigen, producing a microscopic clumping or flocculation of the antigen particles.  The reaction is graded according to degree of clumping.  It was found that the preliminary heating step could be eliminated if certain chemicals were added to the antigen, and this modification is called the rapid plasma reagin (RPR) test.

Not all serums from known syphilitics gave positive reactions to these tests.  It was discovered that the number of positives could be increased by altering the ratio of antigen ingredients.  However, usually when the percentage of positive results increased significantly, more false positives were reported.  The various modifications in common use are listed in Table 15.

A peculiarity of the STS exists when antibiotic treatment is given.  If treated early in the disease, the STS will revert to negative.  However, the longer the disease has been present before treatment, the longer the STS takes to become negative; in many cases, it will never become negative even with adequate treatment (this is called "Wassermann fastness").

Another problem developed when some patients were found to give definitely positive STS but just as definitely did not have syphilis or any exposure to it.  These are called biologic false positive reactions (BFP).  The main known causes for BFP can be classified under three headings:

1.  Acute BFP—due to many viral or bacterial infections, and to many febrile reactions such as hypersensitivity or vaccination.  These usually give low-grade or moderate (1-2+) STS reactions and return to normal within a few weeks.

2.  Chronic BFP—due to chronic systemic illness such as the rheumatoid-collagen disease group, malaria, or chronic tuberculosis.

---

## TABLE 15.—STS PROCEDURES

| CF Tests | Flocculation Tests | |
|---|---|---|
| Kolmer (modified Wassermann) | VDRL | |
| | RPR | Most widely used |
| | Kahn | |
| | Hinton | |
| | Kline | |
| | Mazzini | |

3. Nonsyphilitic treponemal diseases such as yaws or pinta.

To further add to the confusion, some of these patients may have syphilis in addition to one of the diseases known to give BFP reactions. Because of this, everyone hoped for a way to use T. pallidum organisms themselves as antigen rather than depend on the nonspecific reagin system.

Syphilitic spirochetes can be cultured in rabbits. Eventually, a test was devised by Nelson called the Treponema pallidum immobilization or TPI test. This basically consists of incubating live syphilitic spirochetes with the patient's serum. If specific anti-syphilitic antibody is present, it will attack the spirochetes and immobilize them, causing them to stop moving when viewed under the microscope. This involves an antibody which is different from reagin and which is specific against pathogenic Treponema spirochetes. Besides T. pallidum, other Treponema spirochetal diseases such as yaws may thus give positive reactions. The main disadvantages of this test are that it means working with live spirochetes, necessitates an animal colony, is difficult to perform accurately and is expensive. Routine laboratories cannot do it using present techniques. The TPI behaves toward treatment like the STS. If treated early, the TPI will revert to negative; if treated late, it may remain permanently reactive.

The TPI is done using the Nichol strain of pathogenic spirochetes. It has been discovered that a certain nonpathogenic Treponema spirochete called the Reiter strain can be cultured more easily and cheaply on artificial media. Antigen prepared from this organism was adapted to a complement-fixation technique and the result was the Reiter protein complement fixation (RPCF).

The Reiter antibody is different from the Treponema immobilizing antibody of the TPI. Apparently, both the nonpathologic Reiter and the pathologic Nichol spirochete share a common protein antigen, and it is this protein which is used in the RPCF. In addition, the Nichol organism has a specific antigen which results in the immobilizing antibody response of the TPI. Several investigators have found the RPCF to be almost as sensitive and specific as the TPI, although others have been definitely less enthusiastic about sensitivity in late syphilis. The Reiter antibody also appears at a different time than does the TPI antibody. The main disadvantages of the RPCF are those inherent in all CF tests; namely, variation in reagents and technique plus the 2 days required.

Fluorescent techniques have been a relatively recent addition to laboratory methods. A procedure has been adapted for the detection of syphilis, using the Nichol spirochetes. Instead of working with living organisms, the spirochetes are dead. The patient's serum is incubated on a slide with the organisms; afterward is added a preparation of antibodies produced by animals against human globulins. These animal antihuman-globulin antibodies were previously tagged with a fluorescein dye. Since human antibodies against syphilis are gamma globulins, the fluorescein-tagged animal antibodies against human globulin will combine with any antibodies against syphilis present in the patient's serum. If the patient's antibody has combined previously with the spirochetes, the fluorescent anti-globulin material will attach to the patient's antibody on the spiro-chetes, and the spirochetes will be fluorescent when viewed with an ultraviolet microscope.

Unfortunately, fluorescent work is not as simple as the de-scription given above or the recent literature would imply. Many technical problems remain. These tests at present are not suitable for mass production screening, although they are less time-consum-ing than the RPCF and easier than the TPI. Many substances will give varying degrees of natural fluorescence, and it is sometimes difficult to decide whether a preparation is actually positive or not. There may be nonspecific antigen-antibody binding of cross-reaction type, as well as specific reaction. When the animal antihuman-globulin antibody is conjugated with fluorescein, not all the fluores-cein binds to the antibody, and the free fluorescein remaining may stain various proteins, including the spirochetes, nonspecifically, when the tagged mixture is added to the patient's serum.

A very promising recent modification is called the FTA ab-sorption test (FTA-ABS). Here the nonspecific cross-reacting anti-bodies are absorbed out of the patient's serum onto Reiter Trepone-ma antigen. Antibody to T. pallidum is not absorbed out by this technique, so that the absorbed serum can then be run through the regular FTA procedure.

The sensitivity and specificity of these tests should be dis-cussed next. Sensitivity may be defined as the ability to detect syphilis, or the percentage of positive (reactive) test results in pa-tients with syphilis. Specificity refers to the ability of the test to be reactive only in syphilis, or the percentage of positive results in persons who do not have syphilis ("false positive" reactions). Stud-ies have been done sending duplicate samples to various laboratories from known syphilitic patients in various stages of their disease and also from normal persons. Besides this, many reports have ap-peared from laboratories all over the world comparing one test with another in various clinical stages of syphilis, in nonsyphilitic dis-eases, and in apparently normal persons. These are summarized in Table 16.

Note the considerable variation in results. Several factors must be involved besides the inherent sensitivity and specificity of the individual tests themselves.

1. Antibiotic treatment may cause some previously reactive syphilitic cases to become nonreactive.

2. Some persons may have unsuspected subclinical syphilis.

3. True BFP reactions, either acute or chronic.

4. Most important, there is obvious variation in laboratory technique and ability. Some laboratories introduce their own modi-fications into standard techniques.

TABLE 16.—COMPARISON OF SEROLOGIC TESTS FOR SYPHILIS

Approximate Percentage Reported Reactive

|  | STS | RPCF | TPI | FTA-ABS |
|---|---|---|---|---|
| Primary | 48-96 (50-70) | 50-83 (55-65) | 26-68 (35-65) | 80-87 (85-86) |
| Secondary | 98-100 | 85-97 | 67-99 (80-95) | 99-100 |
| Latent | 75-100 | 86-95 | 84-100 (90-95) | 95-96 |
| Tertiary | 55-95 (60-75) | 44-90 (70-80) | 78-100 (90-91) | 95-100 (97) |
| Congenital | 66-95 (70) | 82-100 (90) | 82-93 | 99-100 |
| Normal | 0.5-10.0 (1.0) | 0.0-10.0 (2.5) | 0.0-3.0 (2.0) | 0.0-1.0 (0.8) |
| Nonsyphilitic disease* | 5-45 (5.0) | 3-27 (9.0) | 2.8-8.0 (6.0) | 0.6-14+ (1.5) |
| Biologic false positive diseases++ | 25-45 | (4.0) | (2.5) | 0-16+ (1.5) |

N. B.: Numbers in parentheses indicate either the percentage most frequently reported or figures extracted from a large Public Health interlaboratory cooperative study (SERA study).

*Miscellaneous nonspirochetal diseases with no history or clinical evidence of syphilis.

+FTA-ABS reactive, TPI nonreactive (see text, p. 378).

++Nonspirochetal diseases known to produce a high incidence of BFP reactions in the STS.

The time of antibody appearance differs for the various antibodies. In general, the FTA-ABS test becomes positive in significant numbers of cases in the middle or end of the primary stage, followed by the RPCF, then the STS, and, finally, the TPI. All these procedures are usually positive in the secondary stage, and also probably the early latent stage.

In tertiary (late) syphilis, there is a well-documented tendency for the STS to revert spontaneously to negative, even if the patient is untreated. This is reported to occur in a substantial minority of cases. The RPCF may do likewise, but only in a smaller minority of patients. The TPI in untreated tertiary syphilis is said to be usually positive (assuming good technique, etc.), but false negatives do occur—at least 5% and more likely 10%. The FTA-ABS is reported to be even more sensitive than the TPI in tertiary syphilis, although occasional false negatives may occur even with the FTA-ABS.

At this point it might be useful to summarize those tests for syphilis which currently are most widely used.

STS: The STS is cheap, easy to do, and suitable for mass production testing. Its sensitivity and specificity are adequate, and positivity develops reasonably early in the disease. Reagents are well standardized and reproducibility is good. Disadvantages are the problem of BPF reactions, relatively poor sensitivity in primary syphilis, and the tendency in late syphilis for spontaneous reversion to negative.

TPI: Most reports agree that, up to the present, the TPI was the most reliable and most specific test available; it still is the one against which all the others are measured. There are several cautions to be observed with TPI specimens. Visibly hemolyzed blood is unsatisfactory. Antibiotic treatment should be stopped at least 2 weeks prior to drawing the sample, and all antibiotic information should be recorded on the request slip. This is especially true for penicillin, no matter how small the amount given. The TPI is a difficult test to perform, and results will vary somewhat depending on the particular laboratory, but also to some extent in the same laboratory. Therefore, some false positives or negatives will occur, strictly on a technical basis, although hopefully a good laboratory can keep these to a minimum. This means that if clinical judgment does not agree with the TPI results, a careful re-evaluation of the problem is necessary, but eventually a repeat TPI may be needed.

FTA: The fluorescent antibody techniques are still being investigated and modified. At present, the FTA-ABS seems well established. It is reported to have relatively good sensitivity in primary syphilis (except in early cases) and to have even better sensitivity in late syphilis than the TPI. It is said to be at least as specific as the TPI; possibly even better. Nevertheless, surveys report up to 5-10% variation between laboratories, and weak reactions are still a problem. Therefore, its reported sensitivity and specificity cannot yet be considered established beyond a doubt under all conditions and in all laboratories. For example, several reports list a disturbingly high incidence of positive FTA-ABS reactions in patients who were STS-positive but TPI-negative. Some of these were eventually diagnosed as syphilitic. Most of the remainder were weakly reactive or 1+; recommendation now is that such specimens should be repeated and the 1+ reclassified as "borderline" if it becomes negative when repeated. Occasional false positive FTA-ABS have been reported in persons with hyperglobulinemia of varying etiology. No laboratory test is free from the possibility of technical error, and the FTA-ABS is no exception. The FTA-ABS has currently replaced all other treponemal tests, and the TPI is becoming very difficult to obtain.

The best selection of tests for syphilis depends on the clinical situation.

1. If the patient has definite early clinical syphilis, an STS should be done to help confirm the diagnosis and also to note the effect of treatment on the STS in case diagnosis is required subsequently for possible reinfection.

2. If the patient has possible or equivocal syphilis, or late syphilis, an STS should be done. If the initial STS is positive, the FTA-ABS should be done as a confirmatory test. If the confirmatory test is negative, the next step depends on the clinical situation. If syphilis is a strong possibility, it probably would be a good idea to repeat the confirmatory test 1 or 2 months later. If the initial STS is negative, it may be that nothing further is needed. However, if syphilis is a strong possibility (especially tertiary syphilis), it is probably a good idea to get a confirmatory test anyway, since these are more sensitive than the STS in late syphilis.

3. If a routine screening STS is found to be positive in a person with no history or clinical evidence of syphilis, a confirmatory test should be done. If the confirmatory test is negative, the patient should be screened for diseases known to cause a high incidence of BFP reactions. In this respect, a weakly positive STS may be due only to an acute BFP etiology, and the STS should be negative in 2-3 months. If the confirmatory test is positive, past or present syphilis is a strong probability. Nevertheless, since false positive (and also false negative) reactions may occur occasionally even in the "confirmatory" tests, in certain cases it may be necessary to repeat the confirmatory test.

## CONGENITAL AND CENTRAL NERVOUS SYSTEM SYPHILIS

Congenital syphilis often gives a confusing serologic picture. Syphilitic infants usually have a positive STS. Sometimes, however, these infants have negative serologies at birth, and these may remain negative up to 3 months before the titer begins rising. On the other hand, if the mother has a positive STS, even though she was adequately treated, many infants will have a positive STS due to passive transfer of maternal antibodies through the placenta. The same is true for the TPI or FTA. If the mother has been adequately treated, the infant's positive serology will decline to negative by approximately 3-4 months and no treatment is necessary. The TPI may be positive for as long as 7 months.

Central nervous system syphilis may also require serologic tests for diagnosis. The standard serologic tests for syphilis such as the VDRL are usually, but not always, positive in the blood when they are positive in the CSF. A lack of relationship is most often found in the tertiary stage, when the blood VDRL sometimes reverts to normal. Conversely, the CSF is very often negative when the peripheral blood VDRL is positive, since CNS syphilis usually is a tertiary form developing symptoms only after years of infection, and in many cases of syphilis the CNS is not clinically involved at all. Despite lack of clinical CNS symptoms, actual CNS involvement is apparently fairly common and often begins as early as the secondary stage, although the clinical symptoms, if they develop, do not show up until the tertiary stage years later. Many people never develop any clinical evidence of CNS infection. The best criteria of disease activity are elevated cell count and CSF protein. The serology indicates disease which has been present for a certain length of time, without necessarily being currently active. The CSF serology (STS) usually is negative in those patients with so-called biologic false positive blood STS reactions.

The three most important forms of CNS lues are general paresis, tabes dorsalis, and vascular neurosyphilis. In general paresis, the CSF serology almost always is positive in untreated cases. In tabes dorsalis, the CSF serology is said to be usually positive in early untreated cases, but up to 50% of late or so-called burnt-out cases may be negative. In vascular neurosyphilis, approximately 50% are positive. Sometimes the blood or CSF may have a negative STS but a positive TPI, since once the TPI or FTA are positive they usually remain reactive if not treated early. If the CSF has a positive TPI, the blood TPI or FTA is almost always positive. However, 15-25% of patients with definite CNS syphilis have been reported to have a negative spinal fluid TPI. The TPI or FTA usually are not done on spinal fluid, since there is no problem of BFP reactions in the spinal fluid STS, and the blood TPI or FTA are positive in most cases of CNS syphilis.

## REFERENCES

Anderson, R. I., and Kent, J. F.: Evaluation of the Treponema pallidum immobilization test of serum and cerebrospinal fluid, Am. J. Clin. Path. 32:233, 1959.

Atwood, W. G., et al.: The TPI and FTA-ABS tests in treated late syphilis, J. A. M. A. 203:549, 1968.

Berner, J. E., et al.: Evaluation of the Reiter protein complement-fixation (RPCF) test for syphilis, Cleveland Clin. Quart. 27:162, 1960.

Bradford, L. L., et al.: Fluorescent treponemal absorption and Treponema pallidum immobilization tests in syphilitic patients and biologic false positive reactors, Am. J. Clin. Path. 47:525, 1967.

Carr, R. D., et al.: The biological false positive phenomenon in elderly men, Arch. Dermat. 93:393, 1966.

Eng, J., and Wereide, K.: The TPI test in untreated syphilis, Brit. J. Ven. Dis. 38:223, 1962.

Goldman, J. N., and Lantz, M. A.: FTA-ABS and VDRL slide test reactivity in a population of nuns, J. A. M. A. 217:53, 1971.

Harner, R. E., et al.: The FTA-ABS test in late syphilis, J. A. M. A. 203:545, 1968.
Kampmeier, R. H.: The late manifestations of syphilis: Skeletal, visceral, and cardiovascular, M. Clin. North America 48:667, 1964.
Kolmer, J. A.: Clinical Diagnosis by Laboratory Examinations (3d ed.; New York: Appleton-Century-Crofts, Inc., 1961), p. 434.
Magath, T. B.: The serologic problem of syphilis, even today, Am. J. Clin. Path. 34:338, 1960.
Miller, J. L., et al.: Significance of the Treponema pallidum immobilization test on spinal fluid, J. A. M. A. 160:1394, 1956.
Moore, M. B., and Knox, J. M.: Sensitivity and specificity in syphilis serology: Clinical implications, South. M. J. 58:963, 1965.
Nicholas, L., and Beerman, H.: Present day serodiagnosis of syphilis: Review of some of the literature, Am. J. M. Sc. 249:466, 1965.
Sequeira, P. J. L.: An examination of the treponemal Wassermann reaction and Reiter complement-fixation test, Brit. J. Ven. Dis. 35:139, 1959.
Serology Evaluation Research Assembly (SERA), U. S. Public Health Service Publication no. 650, 1957.
Smith, J. L., et al.: Seronegative ocular and neurosyphilis, Am. J. Ophth. 59:753, 1965.
Sparling, P. F.: Diagnosis and treatment of syphilis, New England J. Med. 284:642, 1971.
Syphilis and Other Venereal Diseases (Symposium), M. Clin. North America, Vol. 48, No. 3, May, 1964.

# CHAPTER 32

# Laboratory Aspects of Cancer

Unfortunately, there is no laboratory test to detect all cancer. There are, however, certain circumstances in which the laboratory may be of assistance.

Renal carcinoma often causes microscopic hematuria, and bladder carcinoma likewise; this may be the only clue to the diagnosis. In addition, hypernephroma, on occasion, is a well-recognized cause of fever of unknown origin. The reported incidence of fever in renal cell carcinoma varies from 11 to 33%. It has rarely but repeatedly been associated with secondary polycythemia (about 3% of cases), although a large minority has anemia, and the majority do not show hemoglobin abnormality.

In renal cell carcinoma (hypernephroma), symptoms and urinary findings vary according to the location, size, and aggressiveness of the tumor. Hematuria is the most frequent finding, either gross or microscopic, being detected at some time in 75-80% of cases. Flank pain is much less commonly present, and a palpable abdominal mass usually suggests relatively large size. Proteinuria may sometimes be found. The intravenous pyelogram (IVP) is the most useful screening test for renal cell carcinoma, and, if carefully done, will also detect many cases of carcinoma in the renal pelvis and ureters. Once a space-occupying lesion is identified in the kidney, the question often arises as to its nature. Drip-infusion tomography seems at present to be one of the best methods to distinguish a solid renal tumor from a renal cyst. Selective renal angiography is equally effective, and could be performed if tomography were inconclusive. No technique is infallible, however, since, uncommonly, a tumor may become exceptionally cystic due to internal necrosis. Urine cytology has relatively little value at present in the diagnosis of renal cell carcinoma. Metastatic car-

cinoma or malignant lymphoma in the kidney usually does not produce significant clinical or urinary findings.

Prostatic carcinoma often may be detected chemically because
normal prostatic tissue is rich in the enzyme acid phosphatase, and
adenocarcinomas arising from this area often retain the ability to
produce this enzyme. Generally speaking, the presence of elevated
serum acid phosphatase means that a prostatic carcinoma has me-
tastasized. However, 10-15% give elevated values without demonstrable metastasis. About 25% with metastases, but no skeletal invasion, show abnormal values, and between 50 and 80% with bone
involvement. Most prostatic skeletal metastases are osteoblastic
in nature, and, therefore, alkaline phosphatase shows elevation in
up to 90% of cases, depending on extent of involvement. One difficulty results from the fact that various widely used chemical methods vary in their specificity for prostatic acid phosphatase. Platelets are rich in nonprostatic acid phosphatase and certain other conditions might conceivably result in elevated serum levels if a relatively nonspecific method is used. Another difficulty which sometimes arises comes from the fact that acid and alkaline phosphatase
are very similar enzymes, differing mainly in their optimum pH.
Therefore, when alkaline phosphatase is very high for any reason,
some of the enzymes may react at a lower pH than normally, giving
so-called spillage into the acid phosphatase range. Fortunately, in
situations where prostatic acid phosphatase is needed, the likelihood
of coexistent sources of nonprostatic acid phosphatase is small. A
differential procedure has been advocated based on the finding that
L-tartrate will inhibit prostatic phosphatases, so that when there is
doubt about the origin of elevated acid phosphatase, the test may be
repeated with the tartrate inhibition procedure. After tartrate, elevated values suggest a nonprostatic origin. There is dispute concerning the accuracy of this technique. Elevated values of prostatic
phosphatase may be produced by prostatic infarcts as well as carcinoma.

Certain acid phosphatase procedures have recently been marketed with claims of specificity for prostatic phosphatase. Unfortunately, these may also produce false high values when alkaline
phosphatase is markedly elevated.

Tumors of the Gastrointestinal Tract (tumors of the lower GI
tract were discussed in Chapter 26): Screening tests include rectal
examination and examination of the stool for occult blood. Tumor
anywhere in the GI tract, benign or malignant, frequently results in
blood found in the stool, sometimes gross, although much more often
occult. The most frequent malignancies are from colon and rectum,
stomach, and the head of the pancreas. Many people advocate sigmoidoscopy as a routine screening test for rectal and sigmoid colon
carcinoma in all people over age 40.

In carcinoma of the stomach, under the best conditions, x-ray
examination is said to be about 90% accurate in demonstrating gas-

tric carcinoma.   Unfortunately, this still leaves open the question
as to the nature of the lesion demonstrated.   Some type of efficient
screening test for gastric malignancy needs to be developed in order to make early diagnosis possible, since 5-year survival rates
usually are less than 20%.   This refers both to demonstration of
early lesions and to obtaining proof of malignancy once a lesion is
found.   Gastric aspiration for free acid (after histamine) may be
helpful; achlorhydria would considerably increase suspicion of carcinoma.   Cytology of gastric washings is useful.   However, gastric
cytology is not as successful as results from specimens of uterine
or even of pulmonary neoplasia, since small gastric tumors may not
shed many neoplastic cells, and interpretation of gastric Papanicolaou
("Pap") smears in general is more difficult.   Gastric aspiration
specimens for cytology should be placed in ice immediately in order
to preserve the cells.

Newer methods include the use of tetracycline and acridine
orange fluorescent techniques.   Tetracycline is given orally for
several days, followed by gastric lavage and examination of the
sediment under ultraviolet light.   Tumor tissue seems to selectively
take up the tetracycline, and, since tetracycline is naturally fluorescent, the tumor cells will appear fluorescent under the ultraviolet
microscope.   The usefulness of this technique is still not conclusively
established.   The same may be said of the acridine orange stain,
which is applied to smears of gastric contents and which stains actively proliferating cells intensely under ultraviolet light.

Carcinoids are relatively uncommon tumors found mainly in
the GI tract, although a minority are located in the lungs.   The appendix is the most frequent site of origin; these are almost always
benign.   Carcinoids are next most frequent in the terminal ileum or
rectum.   Tumor in these locations frequently is malignant.   When
metastases are extensive, a characteristic syndrome is often produced.   This is due to the production of the vasoconstrictor serotonin by liver metastases.   The diagnosis can be made by testing for
abnormal levels of the chief metabolic breakdown product of serotonin, 5-hydroxyindoleacetic acid (5-HIAA), in the urine.   Although
usually elevated, sometimes the level fluctuates, and repeat determinations may be needed if a normal result is obtained in the presence of characteristic symptoms.   Surprisingly, malignant rectal
carcinoids rarely produce this syndrome.   Certain foods may elevate urinary 5-HIAA (p. 434).

Pancreatic carcinoma sometimes may be suspected by recent
onset of diabetes in a patient with jaundice.

Islet cell tumors of the pancreas often produce insulin, either
intermittently or frequently.   Certain criteria have been accepted
for presumptive diagnosis, known as "Whipple's triad."   A glucose
tolerance test may be done to rule out other causes of hypoglycemia;
this should last for 5 hours, preceded by a fasting period of 8-12
hours.   A tolbutamide tolerance test is more reliable.   Eighty to 90%

of spontaneous hypoglycemia is due to causes other than islet cell
tumors, about 70% being due to so-called functional hypoglycemia.

Carcinoma of the Breast: Until 1960, diagnosis of mammary
carcinoma depended on discovery of a breast mass by physical examination, followed by a biopsy of the lesion. It has been said that,
with experience, carcinoma as small as 1 cm. may be regularly detected by palpation. More recently, x-ray study of the breast (mammography) has begun to receive considerable attention. Several
favorable reports have been published, and several mass screening
surveys have been attempted. To date, available information on the
status of mammography includes the following:

1. Breast carcinoma can be seen by mammography in some
   cases in which it is not palpable.
2. Screening surveys utilizing mammography are reporting
   detection of 2-3 times the normally expected rate of breast
   carcinoma.
3. Proper technique is of the utmost importance; this calls
   for special training and conscientious technicians.
4. Mammography is definitely not infallible. The average
   good radiologist will probably miss a malignant diagnosis
   in about 20% of cases, and call a benign lesion malignant
   in about 10%. Biopsy is still essential for all breast
   lesions.
5. Mammography is best in the postmenopausal or large
   breast where fatty tissue predominates. In these circumstances, probably 80-90% of malignant tumors can be diagnosed correctly, whereas the figure decreases to 55%
   under age 45.
6. Mammography is useful to indicate the site for biopsy when
   several breast masses are present, and has shown that the
   incidence of a carcinoma in the opposite breast from previous malignancy is 7.5-10%, while the incidence of simultaneous bilateral breast carcinoma is nearly 3%.
7. At present, mammography is not an ideal screening procedure, because only a rather limited number of satisfactory studies can be performed daily under present conditions in the average radiologic office.

Carcinoma of the Uterus (Cervix and Endometrium): The mainstay of screening for uterine carcinoma is the Papanicolaou ("Pap")
smear. For Pap examination of the cervix, material is best obtained directly from the cervix by some type of scraping technique.
For endometrium, vaginal secretions in the posterior fornix provide much better information than cervical or endocervical specimens. Vaginal irrigation smears are reported to be 50-75% as accurate as the cervical scrape for detection of cervical carcinoma.
Suspicious or definitely positive Pap smears should be followed up
with a biopsy of the site indicated, in order to confirm the diagnosis
and determine the extent and character of the neoplasm. For cer-

vix, a conization procedure, or at least a four-quadrant biopsy, is
the method of choice.  For the endometrium, dilatation and curet-
tage (D & C) should be done.

Carcinoma of the Lung: Chest x-ray has been the usual means
of detecting lung cancer.  Unfortunately, best results are obtained
from the less common peripheral lesions rather than the more usual
bronchogenic carcinomas arising from major bronchi.  In general,
chest x-rays are not an efficient means of early diagnosis, and this
is especially true for the miniature films used in mass survey-type
work.  If a patient over age 40 has symptoms such as chronic cough,
hemoptysis, or recurrent pneumonia, sputum samples should be
collected for cytology.  These should be obtained once daily (before
breakfast) for 3 days.  The material should be from a "deep cough";
saliva is not adequate.  If adequate sputum cannot be obtained, aerosol induction may be helpful.  If the specimen cannot be taken to the
lab immediately, it should be collected in a fixative such as 70% alcohol.  Twenty-four-hour collections are not advised, due to cell disintegration.  A good specimen is the key to success in pulmonary
cytology, because interpretation is more difficult than with uterine
material.

Pheochromocytoma: This is a tumor of the adrenal medulla
which often secretes epinephrine or norepinephrine.  This causes
hypertension, which may be continuous or intermittent.  Pheochromocytoma has an association with medullary carcinoma of the thyroid
(p. 429).  Tests include catecholamines, VMA, or metanephrines;
all are discussed in Chapter 29 (p. 363).

Zollinger-Ellison syndrome is caused by a non-beta islet tumor of the pancreas.  About 60% are malignant.  Occasionally, the
tumor may occur in the wall of the duodenum.  The three major
components of the syndrome are intractable peptic ulcer, severe
chronic diarrhea (40% of cases, with potassium loss especially
prominent), and multiple peptic ulcers (12%) or ulcer in unusual
locations (usually the jejunum; jejunal ulcer comprises 25% of
cases).  About 20-25% have adenomas in other endocrine organs.
About 50% have a single duodenal ulcer.  Diagnosis is based on
demonstration of elevated serum gastrin and basal gastric hypersecretion and hyperacidity; some consider these an integral part of
the syndrome.  Basal (1-hour) acid secretion greater than 10 mEq.
HCl/hour is strongly suspicious of Zollinger-Ellison.  Histamine
stimulation fails to double basal values.  Blood gastrin assay is now
available in a few reference laboratories and should be more widely
used in future to confirm diagnosis and postoperatively to assess
complete removal of all tumors.

Liver Cancer: Tumor in the liver is most often metastatic.
The liver is more frequently subject to metastases than any other
organ; 25-50% of all (metastasizing) cancers reach the liver.  The
GI tract (including the pancreas), breast, kidney, lung, melanomas,
and sarcomas are especially apt to produce hepatic metastases.

Tests for detection include alkaline phosphatase, liver scan, and liver biopsy (Chapter 19). Primary liver cell carcinoma (hepatoma) is more common in cirrhosis. On liver scan, it typically appears as a large, dominant, space-occupying lesion. The fetoprotein test (p. 222) is often positive. Liver biopsy is essential to verify a diagnosis of cancer in the liver, since nonneoplastic diseases may produce abnormalities identical to those of neoplasia in any of the tests mentioned (except possibly the fetoprotein test).

Multiple Myeloma: This is a disease of malignant plasma cells. They invade the bones and bone marrow some time during the course of the disease, but, surprisingly, only very seldom appear in the peripheral blood. Bone marrow aspiration usually is positive by the time symptoms develop, but sometimes may take longer to become diagnostic. There usually are over 20% plasma cells in the myeloma bone marrow. If less than this, many have to be immature if a diagnosis is to be possible, because other diseases can sometimes give up to 20% marrow plasma cells, most of them mature forms. Anemia develops at some time during the disease; this is generally moderate in degree and of normocytic-normochromic type. The erythrocyte sedimentation rate (ESR) is usually moderately to markedly elevated. By far the most common symptom in myeloma is bone pain, most often in the spine. X-ray films show two types of bone lesions; about 25% have diffuse osteoporosis and 50% or more show "punched out" osteolytic lesions, most commonly in skull, vertebral spine, and pelvis. There may be both osteolytic lesions and osteoporosis. Alkaline phosphatase usually is normal except when fractures due to the bone lesions develop. Twenty to 35% of myeloma cases have hypercalcemia. Serum protein electrophoretic pattern and Bence Jones protein have been discussed elsewhere. About half of those with Bence Jones eventually develop kidney damage because of their disease.

Neuroblastoma: This is one of the most frequent tumors of childhood, during which it comprises the most frequent abdominal neoplasm except for Wilms' tumor of infancy. Neuroblastoma usually presents as an abdominal mass, and frequently the only method of diagnosis is abdominal exploration with biopsy. Treatment by combined radiation and chemotherapy is beginning to produce worthwhile results, so that diagnosis has become more than just of academic interest. Urine VMA has been found elevated in over 90% of patients, although some elevations were not present initially. Homovanillic acid (HVA), a metabolic product of the catecholamine precursor dopamine, is reported to be abnormal in about 80% of patients. VMA and HVA positive results combined include nearly 100% of patients. Bone marrow aspiration has been reported positive in up to 50% of cases. Therefore, bone marrow aspiration should be done in all cases, since the finding of marrow metastases rules out surgery alone as a curative procedure.

Metastatic Carcinoma to Bone: Any carcinoma, lymphoma, or sarcoma may metastasize to bone, although those primary in certain organs do so much more frequently than others. Breast, prostate, lung, kidney, and thyroid are the most common carcinomas. Once in bone they may cause local destruction which is manifested on x-ray by osteolytic lesions. In some cases there is osseous reaction with the formation of new bone or osteoid, and this appears on x-ray films as osteoblastic lesions. Prostate carcinoma is usually osteoblastic; breast and lung are more commonly osteolytic, but a significant number are osteoblastic. The others are usually osteolytic only.

About half the carcinomas metastatic to bone replace or at least injure bone marrow to such an extent as to give hematologic symptoms. The degree of actual replacement often is relatively small in relation to the total amount of bone marrow, so that some sort of toxic influence of the cancer on the blood-forming elements has been postulated. Whatever the mechanism, about half the patients with metastatic carcinoma to bone have anemia when first seen (that is, a hemoglobin at least 2 Gm./100 ml. less than the lower limit of normal). When the hemoglobin is less than 8 Gm./100 ml., nucleated red cells and immature white cells may appear in the peripheral blood, and thrombocytopenia may be present. By this time there is often extensive marrow replacement.

Because of bone destruction and local attempts at repair, the serum alkaline phosphatase is often elevated. Roughly one third of patients with metastatic carcinomas to bone from lung, kidney, or thyroid have elevated alkaline phosphatase on first examination; for breast carcinoma this may be true in up to 50% of cases, while, for the prostate, reports vary from 70 to 90%.

If an x-ray skeletal survey is taken, bone lesions will be seen in approximately 50% of cases with actual bone metastases. More are not detected on first examination because lesions must be over 1.5 cm. to show on x-ray films, because parts of the bone are obscured by overlying structures, and because the tumor spread may be concealed by new bone formation. Almost any bone may be affected, but the vertebral column is by far the most common and is involved most of the time whether seen on x-ray film or not.

Bone scanning for metastases has been done using radioactive isotopes of elements which take part in bone metabolism. Currently, strontium-85 is the most widely used. Bone scanning will detect foci of metastatic tumor considerably in advance of x-ray lesions. The main difficulty is the fact that strontium remains in bone for a long time, and the patient gets a relatively large dose of radiation. Current Atomic Energy Commission rules limit use of $Sr^{85}$ to patients who have known cancer. New isotopes are becoming available.

Bone marrow aspiration will show tumor cells in a certain number of patients with metastatic carcinoma to bone. Reports do not agree whether there is any difference in positive yield between

the sternum and iliac crest.   Between 7 and 40% of the patients with
tumor in the bone have been said to have a positive bone marrow.
This varies with the site of primary tumor, whether the marrow was
done early or late in the disease, and whether random aspiration or
aspiration from x-ray lesions was performed.   The true incidence
of positive marrows is probably about 15%.   Prostatic carcinoma
has the highest rate of yield, since this tumor metastasizes to bone
the most frequently, mostly to the vertebral column and pelvic bones.

The question often arises as to the value of bone marrow aspiration in suspected metastatic carcinoma to bone.   In this regard,
the following statements seem valid:

1.   It usually is difficult or often impossible to determine
either the exact type or the origin of tumor cells from
marrow aspiration.

2.   If localized bone lesions exist on x-ray and it is for some
reason essential to determine their nature, a direct bone
biopsy of these lesions using a special needle is much better than random marrow aspiration or even aspiration of
the lesion area.   In this way, a histologic tissue pattern
may be obtained.

3.   If a patient has a normal alkaline phosphatase, no anemia,
and no bone lesions on skeletal survey x-ray (and in addition, a negative acid phosphatase in cases of prostatic
carcinoma), the chances of obtaining a positive bone marrow aspiration are less than 5%.   Therefore, these studies
should be done first before considering a bone marrow.

4.   If a patient has known carcinoma or definite evidence of
carcinoma and has x-ray lesions of bone, there is usually no practical value in getting chemical studies or bone
marrow aspiration apart from academic interest, except
in certain special cases.   These cases mainly concern
situations in which anemia or thrombocytopenia may be
caused by a disease which the patient has in addition to
the carcinoma.

Tumors of the Central Nervous System:   There is no chemical
laboratory test to detect neoplasia in the central nervous system.
Brain tumors, however, may show changes in the cerebrospinal
fluid.   About 70% have increased pressure, and the same percentage
show increased protein, depending to some extent on the size and
location of the lesion.   The cell count is usually normal, but up to
30% may have slight-to-moderate increase.   The best procedures
for detection of brain tumors (not including spinal cord or cerebel-
lum) are brain scan and an arteriogram.   The brain scan utilizes
any of several radioisotopes which seem to concentrate in tumor tissues rather than normal brain tissue.   This produces an area of increased radioactivity corresponding to the tumor.   The accuracy of
this technique is reported as 80-90% (although not all types of tumors
give equally good results), and there is little technical difficulty or

morbidity. However, infarcts and hemorrhage may also give increased intracerebral radioactive pickup and may have similar patterns to a tumor. Arteriograms depend on contrast media injection into arteries leading to the tumor (usually the common carotid artery). Tumor masses push aside and displace blood vessels, and this distortion or shift in normal vascular pattern can be seen on an x-ray film taken quickly after injection. The accuracy of this procedure can be as good as the brain scan, but requires much more expert interpretation, and is somewhat more dependent on the size and location of the lesion. For pituitary lesions, special x-ray views of the sella turcica are needed, attempting to demonstrate alterations secondary to the expanding tumor mass. Brain scan may demonstrate a pituitary or parapituitary tumor, but accuracy is probably 50% or less.

Miscellaneous Tests in Cancer: Metastatic tumors to bone will produce hematologic symptoms if sufficient marrow replacement occurs. This must be distinguished from the anemia of neoplasia, which appears in a considerable number of cases without direct marrow involvement and whose mechanism may be hemolytic, toxic depression of marrow production, or of completely unknown etiology. Generally speaking, one always suspicious sign of extensive marrow replacement is the presence of thrombocytopenia in a patient with known cancer. Another is the appearance of nucleated red cells in the peripheral blood, sometimes with slightly more immature white cells in addition. This does not occur in multiple myeloma, even though this disease often produces discrete bone lesions on x-ray and the malignant plasma cells may replace much of the bone marrow.

Serum lactic dehydrogenase (LDH) is sometimes elevated in extensive carcinomatosis, often without any obvious reason. This is especially true in lymphoma, where it has been reported abnormal in up to 50% of cases. LDH is especially useful in diagnosis of effusion due to malignancy. If LDH of these fluids is appreciably higher than serum LDH and hemolysis is not present, then suspicion of malignancy is high. Absence of hemolysis, however, is essential for accurate LDH determinations; this may be difficult to ensure, since effusions caused by carcinoma are often bloody.

## REFERENCES

Bell, M.: Newer chemical diagnostic tests (neuroblastoma symposium), J. A. M. A. 205:105, 1968.

Blahd, W. H. (ed.): Nuclear Medicine (2d ed.; New York: McGraw-Hill Book Company, Inc., 1971).

Brown, D. H.: The urinary excretion of vanilmandelic acid (VMA) and homovanillic acid (HVA) in children with retinoblastoma, Am. J. Ophth. 62:239, 1966.

Clark, R. C., et al.: Reproducibility of the technique of mammo-
graphy (Egan) for cancer of the breast, Am. J. Surg. 109:127,
1965.
Clifton, J. A., et al.: Bone marrow and carcinoma of the prostate,
Am. J. M. Sc. 224:121, 1952.
Cooley, R. N.: Diagnostic accuracy of radiologic studies of biliary
tract, small intestine, and colon, Am. J. M. Sc. 246:610, 1963.
Delta, B. G., and Pinkel, D.: Bone marrow aspiration in children
with malignant tumors, J. Pediat. 64:542, 1964.
Gershon-Cohen, J.: Mammography, thermography, and xerography,
CA 17:108, 1967.
Gilbertson, V. A.: X-ray examination of the chest—Unsatisfactory
method of detection of early lung cancer in asymptomatic individ-
uals, J. A. M. A. 188:1082, 1964.
Grabstald, H.: Renal cell cancer (parts I, II and III), New York J.
Med. 64:2539, 2658, 2771, 1964.
Grann, V., et al.: Comparative study of bone marrow aspiration
and biopsy in patients with neoplastic disease, Cancer 19:1898,
1966.
Haverback, B. J., Stubrin, M. I., and Majcher, S. J.: Serotonin
and Related Substances, in Disease-a-Month (Chicago: Year Book
Medical Publishers, Inc., April, 1966).
Jaffe, B. M.: Diagnosis of occult Zollinger-Ellison tumors by
gastrin radioimmunoassay, Cancer 29:694, 1972.
Kantor, S., et al.: Carcinoid tumors of the gastrointestinal tract,
Am. Surgeon 27:448, 1961.
Lauby, V. W., et al.: Value and risk of biopsy of pulmonary lesions
by needle aspiration, J. Thoracic & Cardiovas. Surg. 49:159,
1965.
Lipsett, M. B., et al.: Humoral syndromes associated with non-
endocrine tumors, Ann. Int. Med. 61:733, 1964.
Martin, J. R., and Johnson, L.: Multiple myelomatosis: A review
based on 68 patients, Canad. M. A. J. 76:605, 1957.
Nathanson, L., and Fishman, W. H.: New observations on the Regan
isoenzyme of alkaline phosphatase in cancer patients, Cancer
27:1388, 1971.
Ochsner, A., Sr., et al.: Gastric carcinoma, Am. Surgeon 27:333,
1961.
Osserman, E. F.: Plasma-cell myeloma. II. Clinical aspects,
New England J. Med. 261:952, 1006, 1959.
Ozgelen, F. N., et al.: Cytology in lung cancer, J. Thoracic &
Cardiovas. Surg. 49:221, 1965.
Pillers, E. M. K., et al.: The bone marrow in malignant disease,
Brit. J. Cancer 10:458, 1956.
Pool, J. L.: Diagnosis and Treatment of Lung Cancer, in Banyai,
A. L., and Gordon, B. L. (eds.): Advances in Cardiopulmonary
Diseases (Chicago: Year Book Medical Publishers, Inc., 1963),
Vol. I, p. 121.

Ptak, T. , and Kirsner, J. B. : The Zollinger-Ellison Syndrome,
Polyendocrine Adenomatosis, and Other Endocrine Associations
with Peptic Ulcer, in Stollerman, G. H. , et al. (eds.): Advances
in Internal Medicine (Chicago:  Year Book Medical Publishers,
Inc. , 1970), Vol. 16, p. 213.

Rao, N. V. , et al. : Needle biopsy of parietal pleura in 124 cases,
Arch. Int. Med. 115:34, 1965.

Schwartz, M. K. , et al. : Comparative value of phosphatases and
other serum enzymes in following patients with prostatic carcinoma, Cancer 16:583, 1963.

Schwartz, M. K. : Biochemical procedures in different forms of
cancer, M. Clin. North America 55:613, 1971.

Scott, W. G. : Mammography and the training program of the American College of Radiology, Am. J. Roentgenol. 99:1022, 1967.

Sherlock, P. , and Kim, Y. S. : Unusual gastrointestinal manifestations of cancer and newer techniques in the diagnosis of gastrointestinal cancer, M. Clin. North America 50:747, 1966.

So-Bosita, J. L. , et al. : Endometrial jet washer, Obst. & Gynec.
36:287, 1970.

Tickton, H. E. , and Trujillo, N. P. : Enzymes in Neoplastic and
Surgical Diseases, in Coodley, E. L. (ed.): Diagnostic Enzymology (Philadelphia:  Lea & Febiger, 1970), p. 205.

Zollinger, R. M. : Ulcerogenic tumor of the pancreas, Am.
Surgeon 29:751, 1963.

# CHAPTER 33

# Congenital Diseases

Congenital disease will be considered as any clinical condition resulting from a genetically determined abnormality. Such a category provides a wide variety of unrelated disorders. Although a great many syndromes and diseases are known, only those for which adequate laboratory diagnostic tests are available will be included.

## I. HEMATOLOGIC DISEASES

These include principally the hemoglobinopathies (p. 37), red cell glucose-6-phosphate dehydrogenase deficiency (p. 43), and the hemophilias (p. 74), and were discussed in the appropriate sections on hematology. The Philadelphia chromosome abnormality found in chronic myelogenous leukemia was noted in reviewing that disease (p. 62).

## II. DISEASES OF CARBOHYDRATE METABOLISM

1. Renal Glucosuria: This is a disorder of the renal tubule glucose transport mechanism, mentioned on page 326.
2. Lactosuria: A surprising number of infants, more commonly premature, show neonatal intolerance to lactose, clinically manifested by gastrointestinal upsets. Urinary lactose is increased and can be detected by one of the copper sulfate reducing sugar urine methods; glucose oxidase enzyme paper tests are negative. Specific chemical tests may then be done if desired to positively identify the substance as lactose. Benign lactosuria in adults is apparently not uncommon in the last trimester of pregnancy and the puerperium.

3. Galactosemia: This is based on congenital inability to utilize galactose and thus differs from lactosuria, which represents a temporary inability to hydrolyze lactose, a major precursor of galactose. Normally, galactose is metabolized to galactose-1-phosphate and thence, through several intermediate steps, to glucose-1-phosphate. In galactosemia, there is a deficiency of the enzyme galactose-1-phosphate uridyl transferase which mediates the conversion of galactose-1-phosphate to the next step in the sequence toward glucose-1-phosphate. The defect is transmitted by a recessive gene, and the enzyme affected is located in red blood cells.

Galactosemia usually is not clinically evident at birth, but symptoms commence within a few days after beginning a milk diet. Vomiting, diarrhea, and "failure to thrive" are common. Physiologic jaundice may seem to persist, or jaundice may develop later with hepatomegaly. Splenomegaly occurs in only about 10-30% of cases. Eye signs, consisting of lens cataracts, develop after several weeks in about 50%. Mental retardation is a frequent sequel without treatment. The disease is treatable with a lactose-free diet, if begun early enough.

There are multiple laboratory abnormalities. Urinalysis shows proteinuria and galactosuria. Galactose in the urine may be detected by a positive copper sulfate reducing test combined with a negative glucose oxidase method; urine chromatography or specific chemical tests are available for more precise identification. Currently, this is the way most of these patients have been detected. However, galactosuria depends on lactose ingestion, and may be absent if the infant refuses milk or persistently vomits. There is also abnormal amino acid urinary excretion, and this can be detected by urine paper chromatography, although little is added to the diagnosis by such information. Positive urine galactose results must be confirmed by some type of blood galactose determination, since occasional normal newborns have transient galactosuria. Serum chromatography for galactose is a valuable aid in confirmation of the diagnosis, and there are new screening tests available by which the galactose-1-phosphate uridyl transferase in RBC may be measured semiquantitatively. These enzymatic screening tests measure a red cell enzyme which is relatively unstable; therefore, it would be better to request serum chromatography if the specimen must be sent to a distant laboratory.

Hepatomegaly is a frequent finding, although the liver is not always palpable. Jaundice may or may not be present. Liver function tests should be interpreted with caution, since normal values are different from adults; nevertheless, the SGOT is said to be often considerably elevated. Liver biopsy has been used in certain problem cases; the histologic changes are suggestive but not conclusive, and consist of early fatty metamorphosis, with a type of cirrhosis pattern often developing after about 3 months of age.

The galactose tolerance test used to be the most widely used method for confirmation of galactosemia. However, there is considerable danger of hypoglycemia and hypokalemia during the test, and it has been replaced by chromatography and red cell enzyme assay.

4. Disaccharide Malabsorption: Occasionally this is a cause of chronic diarrhea or vomiting in newborns or infants. This probably is not common, especially compared to the frequency of diarrhea and vomiting in infants, but it is beginning to receive more attention. Certain enzymes are present in small intestine mucosal cells which aid absorption of various carbohydrates by preliminary hydrolyzation. Affected patients have varying degrees of specific enzyme deficiency, and thus cannot properly absorb the substance that depends on that enzyme. Clinically, the most common problems are with the disaccharides sucrose and lactose. Lactose is present in milk, while sucrose is a common source of carbohydrate supplement. A presumptive diagnosis can be made by careful substitution of foods, at least for lactose and sucrose. Of course, cessation of symptoms does not necessarily mean that intolerance was the real etiology. Of some help as a screening procedure is the fact that when excessive amounts of these carbohydrates reach the large intestine, bacterial fermentation often will turn the stool from a normally neutral to a strongly acid pH. In addition, a test (such as Clinitest) for reducing substances has also been advocated. Strongly acidic stool pH may be found in certain other conditions associated with diarrhea, especially steatorrhea. To make a definitive diagnosis at present requires either specific carbohydrate tolerance tests or small intestine biopsy for enzyme assay.

5. Glycogen Storage Disease: This abnormality contains a spectrum of syndromes resulting from defective synthesis or utilization of glycogen. Clinical manifestations depend on the organ or tissue primarily affected and the specific enzyme involved. The disease in one or another of its clinical syndromes may affect the liver, heart, or skeletal muscle. The most common is von Gierke's disease, which clinically involves primarily the liver. Hepatomegaly usually is the only sign during the first few months of life, except for poor body growth. Liver function tests usually are within normal limits. There usually is a fasting hypoglycemia, but a diabetic type of glucose tolerance test. Mild anemia is frequent. Liver biopsy shows increased hepatic cell glycogen, but, to demonstrate glycogen, the specimen should be fixed in absolute alcohol rather than the usual fixatives. Certain pediatric research centers have techniques for pinpointing the specific enzyme responsible in the various forms of glycogen storage disease.

### III.  DISEASES OF LIPID STORAGE

1. Histiocytosis-X: This term was coined to include three

closely related diseases of unknown etiology, all three characterized
by proliferation of histiocytic cells, but with one of the three associated with lipid storage.  Letterer-Siwe disease is a rapidly progressive fatal condition seen mostly in early childhood and infancy.  There
is widespread involvement of visceral and reticuloendothelial organs
by atypical histiocytes, with accompanying anemia and thrombocytopenia.  Bone marrow aspiration or, occasionally, lymph node biopsy
is the usual diagnostic procedure.  Eosinophilic granuloma is the
benign member of the triad.  It is seen most often in later childhood,
and most commonly presents as isolated bone lesions.  These usually are single but may be multiple.  The lungs may occasionally be
involved.  The lesion is composed of histiocytes with many eosinophils and is diagnosed by direct biopsy.  Hand-Schüller-Christian
disease is somewhat intermediate between the other two in terms of
chronicity and histology.  Bone lesions, often multiple, are the major abnormalities.  Soft tissue and reticuloendothelial organs sometimes may be affected.  There may be very few systemic symptoms
or there may be anemia, leukopenia, and thrombocytopenia.  The
lesions are composed of histiocytes containing large amounts of
cholesterol in the cytoplasm and accompanied by fibrous tissue and
varying numbers of eosinophils.  Diagnosis usually is by direct biopsy of a lesion.

2. Gaucher's disease:  This is a disorder in which the glyco-
lipid cerebroside compound kerasin is phagocytized by the reticuloendothelial system.  There seem to be two subgroups of this disorder—a fatal disease of relatively short duration in infancy accompanied by mental retardation, and a more slowly progressive
disease of older children and young adults without mental retardation.  Splenomegaly is the most characteristic finding, but the liver
and occasionally the lymph nodes also may become enlarged.  The
most characteristic x-ray findings are aseptic necrosis of the femoral heads and widening of the femoral marrow cavities; although
typical, these findings may be absent.  Anemia is frequent, and
there may be leukopenia and thrombocytopenia due to hypersplenism.
The serum acid phosphatase usually is elevated if chemical methods
are used which are not reasonably specific for prostatic acid phosphatase.  There are several widely used chemical methods, and
while none is absolutely specific for prostatic acid phosphatase,
some are considerably more so than others.  Definitive diagnosis
is most easily made by bone marrow aspiration.  Wright-stained
bone marrow smears often show the characteristic Gaucher cells,
which are large mononuclear phagocytes whose cytoplasm is filled
with a peculiar linear or fibrillar material.  Splenic puncture is
even better than bone marrow aspiration, but is a more complicated procedure.  Biopsy of the spleen, and sometimes the liver,
can yield the diagnosis on histologic section with special stains—or,
better, tissue analysis for lipids—but should be reserved for special
problem cases.

3. Niemann-Pick disease: This is similar clinically and pathologically to the fatal early childhood form of Gaucher's disease, except that the abnormal lipid involved is a phospholipid sphingomyelin. Diagnosis is established by bone marrow aspiration, although the cells are not as characteristic as those of Gaucher's disease. Spleen or liver biopsy with histologic special stains or tissue lipid analysis are probably the most definitive studies.

There are several diseases in the lipid storage category; a complete list is given on page 455. Definitive diagnosis can now be obtained by enzyme analysis of the patient's white blood cells or by tissue culture of fibroblasts obtained from the patient's skin. In addition, in most of these diseases it is possible to perform specific glycosphingolipid analysis from liver biopsy specimens. It is recommended that a university medical center specializing in such problems or the Neurological Diseases branch of the National Institutes of Health be contacted for details on how to proceed with any patient suspected of a lipid storage disease. It is highly preferable that the patient be sent directly to the center, for biopsy or required specimen collection, in order to avoid unnecessary and costly delays and to prevent damage to the specimen in transport.

### IV.  DEFECTS IN AMINO ACID METABOLISM
### (AMINOACIDOPATHIES)

A.    Primary (Metabolic) Aminoacidopathies

1. Phenylketonuria (PKU): This condition is due to deficiency of a liver enzyme needed to convert the amino acid phenylalanine to tyrosine. With its major utilization pathway blocked, phenylalanine accumulates in the blood and leads to early onset of progressive mental deficiency. This disease is one of the more common causes of hereditary mental deficiency, and one of the few whose bad effects can be prevented by early treatment of the infant. At birth, the infant usually has normal serum levels of phenylalanine (less than 2 mg./100 ml.) due to maternal enzyme activity, although some cases of mental damage in utero occur. After birth, and after beginning a diet containing phenylalanine (such as milk), serum levels begin to gradually rise. After they reach the 12-15 mg./100 ml. level, utilization of phenylalanine by other metabolic pathways has reached such an extent that a characteristic substance known as phenylpyruvic acid begins to appear in the urine. This becomes detectable by urine screening tests (ferric chloride or Phenistix) at some time between 3 and 6 weeks of age. Since some degree of damage may have been done by that time, it is desirable to make an earlier diagnosis.

The most widely used screening test for elevated serum phenylalanine is the Guthrie test. This is a bacterial inhibition procedure. A certain substance which competes with phenylalanine in Bacillus

subtilis metabolism is incorporated into culture media; this essentially provides a phenylalanine-deficient culture medium.  B. subtilis
spores are seeded into this medium, but, in order to produce significant bacterial growth, a quantity of phenylalanine equivalent to more
than normal blood levels must be furnished.  Next, a sample of the
patient's blood is added, and the presence of abnormal quantities of
serum phenylalanine is reflected by bacterial growth in the area
where the specimen was applied.  The Guthrie test, if properly done,
is adequately sensitive and accurate, and will reliably detect definitely abnormal levels of serum phenylalanine (4 mg./100 ml. or
over).  The Guthrie test also fulfills the requirements for an acceptable screening method.  There are, however, two main drawbacks to the use of this procedure.  First, the standard practice is
to obtain a blood specimen from an infant before discharge from the
hospital.  Unfortunately, in the majority of patients, it takes 2 to 4
days on a high-protein (milk) diet before the serum phenylalanine
reaches the definitely abnormal level of 4 mg./100 ml.  Therefore,
if the blood specimen is obtained before 4 full days on a milk diet
are completed and definitely if obtained before 3 full days, a certain
very significant percentage of PKU patients will be missed.  Second,
there are other possible causes of elevated neonatal serum phenylalanine such as liver disease, galactosemia, or late development of
certain enzyme systems.  In fact, some reports state that the majority of initially positive Guthrie tests are not due to PKU.  In some of
these "false positive" cases, harm could be done by prolonged PKU
treatment (low phenylalanine diet).  Therefore, an abnormal Guthrie
test should be followed up by more detailed investigation, including,
as a minimum, both the serum phenylalanine and tyrosine levels
(the typical PKU develops a serum phenylalanine of greater than
15 mg./100 ml. with a serum tyrosine of less than 5 mg./100 ml.
The tests may have to be repeated in 1-2 weeks if values have not
reached these levels).

    2.  Alkaptonuria (Ochronosis):  The typical manifestations of
this uncommon disease are the triad of arthritis, black pigmentation of cartilage (ochronosis), and excretion of homogentisic acid in
the urine.  Arthritis usually begins in middle age and typically involves the spine and the large joints.  Black pigmentation of cartilage
is most apparent in the ears, but may be noticed in cartilage elsewhere, or even may appear in tendons.  The intervertebral disks
often become heavily calcified and thus provide a characteristic
x-ray picture.  The disease is caused by abnormal accumulation of
homogentisic acid, an intermediate metabolic product of tyrosine,
caused by a deficiency of the liver enzyme homogentisic acid oxidase
which mediates its further breakdown.  Most of the homogentisic
acid is excreted in the urine, but enough slowly accumulates in cartilage and surrounding tissues to cause the characteristic changes
previously described.  Diagnosis is accomplished by demonstration
of homogentisic acid in the urine.  Addition of 10% sodium hydroxide

turns the urine black or gray-black. A false positive urine sugar
test is produced by copper reduction methods such as Benedict's or
Clinitest.

3. Other Primary Aminoacidopathies: These are several, varied, and rare. They are mostly diagnosed through paper chromatography of urine (or serum), looking for abnormal quantities of the
particular amino acid involved whose metabolic pathway has been
blocked. The most widely known diseases (apart from phenylketonuria and alkaptonuria) are maple syrup disease and histidinemia.
The most common is homocystinuria.

B. Secondary Aminoacidopathies

These are associated with a renal defect, usually of reabsorption, rather than a primary defect in the metabolic pathway of the
amino acid in question. The serum levels are normal. The most
common cause is a systemic disease such as Wilson's disease, lead
poisoning, or the Fanconi syndrome. In such cases, several amino
acids usually are found in the urine. Aminoaciduria may occur normally in the first week of life, especially in premature infants. A
much smaller number of patients have a more specific amino acid
renal defect with one or more specific amino acids excreted; the
most common of these diseases is cystinuria. Patients with cystinuria develop cystine renal calculi. Cystine crystals may be identified in acidified urine, providing the diagnosis. Otherwise, combined urine and serum paper chromatography are the diagnostic
methods of choice.

## V. DISORDERS OF CONNECTIVE TISSUE

Hurler's Syndrome (Gargoylism): There actually are several
subtypes of Hurler's, or Hurler-like syndromes, but the classic
case includes many of the following: short stature or dwarfism,
moderate lumbar kyphosis, saddle nose, clouding of the ocular cor-
neas, deafness, joint stiffness, hepatosplenomegaly, and abnormalities of heart valves. There often are varying degrees of mental
deficiency, but some patients have normal intelligence. The biochemical defect consists of abnormal tissue storage by connective
tissue cells of certain mucopolysaccharides, chondroitin sulfate B
and heparitin sulfate. There also is markedly increased urinary
excretion of the substances, which are not detectable in normal persons except uncommonly during the first week of life. Rapid screening tests have been devised for demonstration of mucopolysaccharides or chondroitin sulfuric acid in the urine. However, these have
been developed relatively recently, and probably are not widely
available as yet.

There are other disorders involving primarily connective tissue; a complete list is presented on page 456. The most characteristic laboratory finding is elevated urine mucopolysaccharides.

Differentiation can be made by chemical identification of the individual
substance excreted, plus inheritance patterns and clinical signs.
Tissue cell culture may prove to be the basic method of the future;
fetal cells from amniocentesis have been used by one investigator.
Some of these conditions display metachromatic granules in lymphocytes and occasionally in segmented neutrophils. Certain of these
diseases are frequently included among the chondrodystrophies,
since basic connective tissue defects frequently lead to cartilage
abnormalities.

## VI.  CHROMOSOMAL ABNORMALITIES

There are several conditions, some relatively common and
some rare, that result either from abnormal numbers of chromosomes, defects in size or configuration of certain specific single
chromosomes, or abnormal composition of the chromosome group
which determines sexual characteristics. Laboratory diagnosis, at
present, takes two forms. First, chromosome charts may be prepared on any individual by culturing certain body cells, such as
white blood cells from peripheral blood or bone marrow, introducing
a chemical such as colchicine, which kills the cells at a specific
stage in mitosis when the chromosomes become organized and separated, and then photographing and separating the individual chromosomes into specific groups according to similarity in size and
configuration. The most widely used system is the Denver classification. The 46 human chromosomes are composed of 22 chromosome pairs and, in addition, 2 unpaired chromosomes, the sex
chromosomes (XX in the female and XY in the male). In preparing
a Denver chromosome chart (karyotype) the 22 different paired
chromosomes are separated into seven groups, each containing 2
or more individually identified and numbered chromosomes. For
example, the first group contains chromosomes 1-3, the seventh
group chromosomes 21-22. In addition, there is an eighth group
for the 2 unpaired sex chromosomes. Chromosome culture takes a
substantial amount of experience and care in preparation and interpretation.

The second, and more widely used, technique provides certain
useful information about the composition of the sex chromosome
group. It was discovered by Barr that the nuclei of various body
cells contained a certain stainable sex chromatin mass (Barr body)
that appeared for each X chromosome more than one that the cell
possessed. Therefore, a normal male (XY) cell has no Barr body
because there is only one X chromosome, a normal female (XX) has
one Barr body, and a person with the abnormal configuration XXX
would have two Barr bodies. The most convenient method for Barr
body detection at present is called the buccal smear. It is obtained
by scraping the oral mucosa, smearing the epithelial cells thus collected onto a glass slide in a monolayer, and, after immediate

chemical fixation, staining with certain special stains. Comparison of the results with the secondary sex characteristics and genitalia of the patient allows presumptive diagnosis of certain sex chromosome abnormalities. The results may be confirmed, if necessary, by chromosome karyotyping.

Buccal smears should not be obtained during the first week of life or during adrenal corticosteroid or estrogen therapy, because these situations falsely lower the incidence of sex chromatin Barr bodies. Certain artifacts may be confused with the nuclear Barr bodies. Poor slide preparations may obscure the sex chromatin mass and lead to false negative appearances. Even normally, only about 40-60% of normal female cells contain an identifiable Barr body. The buccal smear is not capable, by itself, of demonstrating the true genetic sex; it is only an indication of the number of female (X) chromosomes present.

1. Klinefelter's Syndrome: In this condition, the patient looks outwardly like a male, but the sex chromosome makeup is XXY instead of XY. The external genitalia are usually normal, except for small testes. There is a tendency toward androgen deficiency and thus for gynecomastia and decreased body hair, but this may be slight or not evident. There also is a tendency toward mental deficiency, but many have perfectly normal intelligence. Patients with Klinefelter's syndrome are almost always sterile. Testicular biopsy used to be the main diagnostic method, with histologic specimens showing marked atrophy of the seminiferous tubules. At present, a buccal smear is the procedure of choice; it shows a "normal female" configuration with one Barr body (due to the two XX chromosomes). In the presence of unmistakably male genitalia, this usually is sufficient for clinical diagnosis. Chromosome karyotyping may be necessary to confirm doubtful cases.

2. Turner's Syndrome (Ovarian Agenesis): This is the most frequent chromosomal sexual abnormality in females, as Klinefelter's is for males. In Turner's syndrome, there is a deletion of one female (X) chromosome, so that the patient has only 45 chromosomes instead of 46, and only 1 female sex chromosome instead of 2. Typically, this leads to a female with relatively short stature but with normal body proportions. There is deficient development of secondary sex characteristics and small genitalia, although body hair usually is female in distribution. Some of these persons have associated anomalies such as webbing of the neck, coarctation of the aorta, and short fingers. These patients do not menstruate, and actually lack ovaries. Diagnosis may be made in most cases by buccal smear; this should be "sex chromatin negative," since Barr bodies appear only when the female sex chromosomes number more than one. If the buccal smear is "chromatin positive," a chromosome karyotype should be ordered, because some cases of Turner's syndrome have mixtures of normal cells and defective cells ("mosaicism").

3. Mongolism (Down's Syndrome): This is a relatively frequent disorder associated with two different chromosome abnormalities. The majority of patients have an extra chromosome in the number 21-22 chromosome group (therefore producing three chromosomes in this group instead of two, a situation known as "trisomy 21"). These patients have a total of 47 chromosomes. Their chromosome abnormality has nothing to do with the sex chromosomes, which are normal. This type of mongolism apparently is spontaneous, not inherited (that is, there is no family history of mongolism, and the parents have very little risk that they will have another similar child). Other patients with mongolism have an extra 21-type chromosome, but it is attached to one of the other chromosomes, most often in the 13-15 group (called the D group in some nomenclatures). This type of arrangement is called "translocation." It means that one of the parents had a normal total number of chromosomes, but one of the pair of number 21 chromosomes was attached to one of the number 15 chromosomes. The other number 21 and the other number 15 chromosome were normal. The cluster behaves in meiosis as though it were a number 15 chromosome. If the abnormal chromosome cluster is passed to the children, two situations could arise: a mongoloid child which received both the translocated 15-21 chromosome plus the normal number 21 chromosome, or a carrier who received the translocated 15-21 chromosome but did not receive the other (normal) number 21 chromosome.

Clinically, an infant or child with mongolism usually presents some combination of the following: prominent epicanthal folds at the medial aspect of the eyes, mental retardation or deficiency, broad hands and feet, and a single long transverse crease on the palm instead of several shorter transverse creases. Other frequent but still less common associated abnormalities are umbilical hernia, webbing of the toes, and certain types of congenital heart disease. There also is an increaséd incidence of acute leukemia.

Diagnosis usually can be made clinically, but chromosome karyotyping is a valuable means of confirmation and of diagnosis in equivocal cases. It probably is advisable to get chromosome karyotyping in most cases of mongolism, because the type of chromosome pattern gives an indication of the prognosis for future children.

4. Other Disorders Associated with Chromosomal Abnormalities: A wide variety of syndromes, usually composed of multiple congenital deformities and anomalies, are now found due to specific chromosomal abnormalities. The most common of these involve trisomy in the 13-15 (D) group and in the 16-18 (E) group. Some patients with habitual abortion have abnormal karyotypes. Various tumors have yielded abnormal chromosome patterns, but no one type of tumor has produced any consistent pattern (except for chronic myelogenous leukemia).

5. Commonly Accepted Indications for the Buccal Smear Procedure: These include the following:

1. Cases with ambiguous or abnormal genitalia.
2. Cases of male or female infertility without other known cause.
3. Persons with symptoms suggestive of Turner's syndrome or Klinefelter's syndrome, such as primary amenorrhea.

Indications for chromosome karyotyping include selected cases of those outlined above, for confirmation or initial diagnosis, and:

1. Mongoloid infants; also possible carriers.
2. Mentally defective persons.
3. Persons with multiple congenital anomalies.

## VII.  DISEASES OF SKELETAL MUSCLE

Several well-known disorders affecting skeletal muscle either are not congenital or do not as yet have any conspicuously useful laboratory test.  Among these are myasthenia gravis, a disorder affecting muscle electrical impulse conduction at the neuromuscular junction, whose diagnosis is most often made by pharmacologic tests such as response to edrophonium chloride.  A second group of disorders has the primary defect located in the central nervous system rather than in skeletal muscle itself.  These comprise various neurologic diseases which secondarily result in symptoms of muscle weakness.  A third, and very uncommon group, includes the myotonias, characterized by difficulty or inability to voluntarily cease contraction of certain muscles.

The muscular dystrophies comprise still another group, but one in which the clinical laboratory may be of assistance.  The muscular dystrophies usually are divided into three main subgroups—pseudohypertrophic (Duchenne) type; fascioscapulohumeral (Landouzy-Dejerine) type; and limb-girdle (Erb) type.  Pseudohypertrophic dystrophy affects only males, and may be either familial or sporadic. In the familial type, clinically unaffected females carry the gene.  In either type, the patient is clinically normal for the first few months of life; symptoms develop usually between 1 and 6 years of age.  The most frequent symptoms are lower extremity and pelvic muscle weakness.  There is spotty but progressive muscle fiber dissolution, with excessive deposition or replacement by fat and fibrous tissue. The latter process leads to the most characteristic physical finding of the disease—pseudohypertrophy of the calf muscles.  The usefulness of laboratory tests is based on the fact that certain enzymes are found in relatively high concentration in normal skeletal muscle. These include creatine phosphokinase, aldolase, SGOT, and LDH, as well as others.  Despite external pseudohypertrophy, the dystrophic muscles actually undergo individual fiber dissolution and loss of skeletal muscle substance; this is accompanied by release of these enzymes into the blood stream.  SGOT, LDH, and aldolase are found together in many tissues.  Pulmonary infarction, myocardial infarction, and acute liver cell damage as well as other conditions cause elevated serum levels of these enzymes. Aldolase follows a pattern similar to SGOT in liver disease, and to LDH otherwise. Creatine phosphokinase (CPK) is found in significant concentration only in brain, heart muscle, and skeletal muscle.

CPK and aldolase are considered the two most helpful tests in Duchenne's muscular dystrophy. They are elevated very early in the disease, well before clinical symptoms become manifest, and the elevations usually are over 10 times normal, at least for CPK. This marked elevation persists as symptoms develop. Eventually, after replacement of muscle substance has become chronic and extensive, the aldolase often becomes normal and the CPK may be either normal or only mildly elevated (less than 5 times normal). In the hereditary type of Duchenne's dystrophy, borderline or elevated CPK has been reported in variable numbers of carrier females; in one study, up to 80%. Aldolase is much less frequently abnormal. SGOT and LDH tend to parallel CPK and aldolase, but at a much lower level. Therefore, these enzymes frequently are normal in the later stages of the disease, when the more sensitive tests are still considerably abnormal, and are not of much use in detecting carriers. Muscle biopsy used to be the mainstay of diagnosis, but now probably should not be necessary except in unusual cases.

Fascioscapulohumeral dystrophy begins most often in adolescents and adults; the facial muscles are usually the first to become involved, and the upper part of the body is most affected. The disease is slowly progressive, but relatively benign. Serum enzymes, including CPK and aldolase, frequently are normal. Limb-girdle dystrophy seems to have a somewhat intermediate position between the other two types of dystrophy; it combines the areas of involvement of the other two, but usually without pseudohypertrophy. It is seen most frequently in adolescents and young adults. There is considerable variation in clinical aspects among individuals. Serum enzyme values are also variable; they are more likely to be abnormal in younger patients.

Other muscular disorders in which the serum enzymes may be elevated are trauma, dermatomyositis, and polymyositis. The levels of elevation are said to be considerably below those seen in early cases of Duchenne's dystrophy. Neurologic disease does not show elevated levels, even when marked secondary muscular atrophy occurs.

## VIII.  DISEASES OF MINERAL METABOLISM

1. Wilson's Disease (Hepatolenticular Degeneration): This most often becomes manifest between 7 and 15 years of age. Symptoms most often include dystonia (abnormal muscular rigidity) and tremor of the fingers, due to involvement of the basal ganglia (lentiform nuclei) of the brain. Dysarthria, mental disturbances, and a

flapping type of upper extremity intention tremor are frequent developments. Pafients with Wilson's disease almost invariably have developed a postnecrotic type of liver cirrhosis by the time clinical symptoms are manifest; uncommonly, the initial symptoms are those of hepatic failure. Wilson's disease is characterized by inability of the liver to manufacture normal quantities of an alpha-2-globulin named ceruloplasmin, which is the plasma transport agent for copper. For reasons not entirely understood, excessive copper is deposited in various tissues, producing eventual damage. Damage to the basal ganglia of the brain and to the liver were mentioned earlier; the kidney is also affected, leading to aminoaciduria, and copper is deposited in the cornea, producing a discolored zone called the Kayser-Fleischer ring.

The triad of typical basal ganglia symptoms, Kayser-Fleischer ring, and hepatic cirrhosis are diagnostic. However, the Kayser-Fleischer ring is seen in only about half the patients, and even in some of these slit lamp examination may be required for its identification.

Laboratory studies may be of value in diagnosis, especially in the preclinical or early stages. Plasma ceruloplasmin is always low (except in a few late cases), is low from birth, and is considered the best screening test for Wilson's disease. However, normal newborn infants apparently may have decreased ceruloplasmin levels, and it is not considered a reliable test (except to rule out Wilson's disease if normal) until about 3 months of age. Certain other diseases may be associated with low plasma ceruloplasmin; these include the nephrotic syndrome, malabsorption syndromes such as sprue, and infrequently a few other conditions. Another useful test, especially for confirmation, is liver biopsy. The characteristic findings are early or established postnecrotic type cirrhosis plus demonstration of increased hepatic copper content by special stains (or tissue analysis, if available). For histologic staining of copper, fixation of the biopsy specimen in alcohol rather than the routine fixatives is recommended. Here again, it is advisable to wait 6-12 weeks after birth.

Other laboratory abnormalities which may be present are a characteristically low serum uric acid, rather frequent hypercalcemia and low serum phosphorus, aminoaciduria including many amino acids, and sometimes glucosuria without hyperglycemia.

2. Hemochromatosis: This is an uncommon disease, predominantly affecting males, which is produced by excessive deposition of iron in various tissues, especially the liver. There is dispute as to whether hemochromatosis is due to an inborn error of metabolism or is a variant of nutritional cirrhosis in which iron deposition in body tissues is, for some reason, more pronounced. Most authors seem to favor the first hypothesis, so the disease is included in this chapter. At any rate, cirrhosis (usually Laennec's type) is always present when symptoms begin. Onset usually is be-

tween 40 and 60 years of age. Cirrhosis, diabetes mellitus, and bronze skin pigmentation form the classic triad of hemochromatosis, although diabetes may not be manifest in 20-50% (at least, not clinically manifest when the patient is first seen), and skin pigmentation is absent in over 15%, depending on the stage of the disease. Hypogonadism and a history of alcoholism or poor nutrition are frequent.

Laboratory findings include those of diabetes mellitus, discussed in Chapter 27. Liver function tests are those expected in portal cirrhosis; in some cases there are minimal abnormalities. The body iron abnormality is expressed in a high serum iron coupled with a decreased total iron-binding capacity (i. e., marked saturation of the TIBC). In addition, hemosiderin very often can be demonstrated in the urinary sediment by iron stains. Liver biopsy shows cirrhosis plus marked parenchymal deposition of iron.

Diagnosis is made more difficult because various other conditions may produce some of these laboratory changes. Hemosiderosis due to multiple blood transfusions over long periods can mimic idiopathic hemochromatosis closely, but the history of transfusions usually is available. A diabetic type of oral glucose tolerance test is not uncommon in nonhemochromatotic cirrhosis, and there may be increased skin pigmentation. Hemolytic anemia may give similar serum iron and TIBC values, and is found occasionally in association with cirrhosis. Even liver biopsy may not always yield unequivocal results, because many patients with cirrhosis have increased hepatic iron deposition, and some of these may have enough to make a clearcut decision either difficult or impossible.

## IX. ABNORMALITIES OF GLANDULAR SECRETION

Cystic fibrosis (mucoviscidosis, or fibrocystic disease of the pancreas) is a hereditary condition which affects the exocrine glands of the body. It is best explained at present as a recessive gene whose full expression depends on a homozygous genetic status. The disease is rare in Negroes. Both mucus-producing and nonmucus-producing exocrine glands are affected. The mucous glands produce abnormally viscid secretions which may inspissate, plug the glands, and generate obstructive complications. In the lungs, this may lead to recurrent bronchopneumonia, the most frequent and most dangerous symptom of cystic fibrosis. Next most common is complete or partial destruction of the exocrine portions of the pancreas, leading to various degrees of malabsorption, steatorrhea, digestive disturbances, and malnutrition. This manifestation varies in severity, and about 15% of patients have only a minimal disorder or even a normal pancreatic exocrine function. Less common findings are those of biliary cirrhosis, most often focal, due to obstruction of bile ductules, and intestinal obstruction by inspissated meconium (meconium ileus), found in 10-15% of newborns with cystic fibrosis.

Nonmucus-producing exocrine glands such as the sweat glands do not ordinarily cause symptoms. However, they are also affected, because the sodium and chloride concentration in sweat is higher than normal in patients with cystic fibrosis, even though the volume of sweat is not abnormally increased. Therefore, unusually high quantities of sodium and chloride are lost in sweat, and this fact is utilized for diagnosis. Screening tests have been devised (silver nitrate or Schwachman test) which depend on the incorporation of silver nitrate into agar plates or special paper. The patient's hand is carefully washed and dried, since previously dried sweat will leave a concentrated chloride residue and give a false positive result. After an extended period, or after exercise to increase secretions, the palm or fingers are placed on the test surface. Excess chlorides will combine with the silver nitrate to form visible silver chloride. For definitive diagnosis, sweat is collected by means of a plastic bag arrangement or some other method such as iontophoresis, and the specimen is subjected to quantitative electrolyte analysis. A sweat chloride content greater than 60 mEq./L. is considered definitely abnormal. For diagnostic sweat collection, it is recommended that the hand not be used, because the concentration of electrolytes in the palm is significantly greater than elsewhere. Also, the quantity of sweat collected for analysis is important; volumes less than 50 mg. are not considered reliable.

Clinically normal heterozygotes and relatives of patients with cystic fibrosis have been reported to give abnormal sweat electrolytes in 5-20% of cases, although some investigators dispute these findings.

## X.  ENZYME ABNORMALITIES

Congenital Cholinesterase Deficiency: Cholinesterase is an enzyme best known for its role in regulation of nerve impulse transmission via breakdown of acetylcholine at the nerve synapse and neuromuscular junction. Two categories of cholinesterase are distinguished: acetylcholinesterase ("true cholinesterase"), found in RBC and nerve tissue; and serum cholinesterase ("pseudocholinesterase"). Cholinesterase deficiency became important when it was noted that such patients were predisposed to develop prolonged periods of apnea after administration of succinylcholine, a competitor to acetylcholine. Serum cholinesterase is thought to have greatest effect in degradation of succinylcholine. Serum cholinesterase deficiency may be congenital or acquired; the congenital type is uncommon but is responsible for most of the cases of prolonged apnea. The patient with congenital deficiency seems to have an abnormal ("atypical") cholinesterase, of which several genetic variants have been reported. Serum cholinesterase assay is the best screening test for cholinesterase deficiency. If abnormally low values are found, it is necessary to perform inhibition procedures with dibucaine and fluoride in order to distinguish congenital deficiency ("a-typical" cholinesterase) from acquired deficiency of normal enzyme. Deficiency of normal enzyme may cause prolonged succinylcholine apnea, but not predictably and usually only in very severe deficiency. Acute and chronic liver disease is the most frequent etiology for acquired deficiency.  Hypoalbuminemia is frequently associated in hepatic or nonhepatic etiologies.  A considerable number of drugs lower serum cholinesterase levels (p. 437) and thus might potentiate the action of succinylcholine.

Cholinesterase is also decreased in organic phosphate poisoning (p. 242); this affects both red cell and plasma enzyme levels. Screening tests have been devised using "dip-and-read" paper strips. These are probably satisfactory to rule out phosphate insecticide poisoning, but are not accurate in diagnosis of potential for succinylcholine apnea.

Alpha-1 Antitrypsin Deficiency:  This deficiency has been associated with two different diseases:  pulmonary emphysema in adults (relatively common) and cirrhosis in children (rare).  This type of emphysema is characteristically (although not invariably) more severe in the lower lobes.  A substantial number of those with homozygous antitrypsin deficiency are affected; reports differ on whether heterozygotes have increased predisposition to emphysema or to pulmonary disease.  The most useful screening test at present is serum protein electrophoresis; alpha-1 globulin peak is absent or nearly absent in homozygotes.  More definitive diagnosis, as well as separation of severe from intermediate degrees of deficiency, may be accomplished by quantitation of alpha-1 antitrypsin using methods such as immunodiffusion.  Estrogen therapy (birth control pills) may elevate alpha-1 antitrypsin levels.

## REFERENCES

Anderson, C. M., and Freeman, M.: Sweat test results in normal persons of different ages compared with families with fibrocystic disease of the pancreas, Arch. Dis. Childhood 35:581, 1960.

August, G. P.: Diagnosis of disorders of sexual maturation, Pediat. Clin. North America 18:313, 1971.

Bartholomew, C. G., and Dahlin, D. C.: Intestinal polyposis and mucocutaneous pigmentation (Peutz-Jeghers syndrome), Minnesota Med. 41:949, 1958.

Basford, R. L., and Henry, J. B.: Lactose intolerance in the adult, Postgrad. Med. 41:A-70, 1967.

Bell, R. S.: The radiographic manifestations of alpha-1 antitrypsin deficiency, Radiology 95:19, 1970.

Berry, H. K., et al.: Phenylketonuria, in Disease-a-Month (Chicago: Year Book Medical Publishers, Inc., December, 1966).

Burkhart, J. M., et al.: The chondrodystrophies, Mayo Clin. Proc. 40:481, 1965.

Carpenter, G. G., et al.: Phenylalaninemia, Pediat. Clin. North America 15:313, 1968.

Carter, C. H., et al.: Classification of inborn errors of metabolism associated with mental retardation, J. Florida M. A. 54:1147, 1967.

Crouch, W. H., Jr., and Evanhoe, C. M.: Inborn errors of metabolism, Pediat. Clin. North America 14:269, 1967.

Dmowski, W. P., and Greenblatt, R. B.: Abnormal sexual differentiation, Am. Fam. Phys. 3:73, 1971.

Dubin, I. N.: Idiopathic hemochromatosis and transfusion siderosis: A review, Am. J. Clin. Path. 25:514, 1955.

Eggen, R. R.: Chromosome Diagnostics in Clinical Medicine (Springfield, Ill.: Charles C Thomas, Publisher, 1964).

Ferguson-Smith, M. A.: Chromosomal abnormalities. II: Sex chromosome defects, Hosp. Practice 5:88, 1970.

Gatti, R. A., and Good, R. A.: The immunological deficiency diseases, M. Clin. North America 54:281, 1970.

Good, R. A.: Disorders of the immune system, Hosp. Practice 2:39, 1967.

Gordon, R. S., et al.: Protein-Losing Gastroenteropathy, in Disease-a-Month (Chicago: Year Book Medical Publishers, Inc., August, 1966).

Guthrie, R.: Guthrie test and repeated examinations (Questions and Answers), J. A. M. A. 197:303, 1966.

Haemmerli, U. P., and Kistler, H.: Disaccharide Malabsorption, in Disease-a-Month (Chicago: Year Book Medical Publishers, Inc., July, 1966).

Hirschhorn, K.: Chromosomal abnormalities I: Autosomal defects, Hosp. Practice 5:39, 1970.

Lichtenstein, L.: Histiocytosis X, A. M. A. Arch. Path. 56:84, 1953.

MacDonald, R. A.: Hemochromatosis, Postgrad. Med. 41:56, 1967.

Melicow, M. M., and Uson, A. C.: A periodic table of sexual anomalies, J. Urol. 91:402, 1964.

Mone, J. C., and Mathe, W. E.: Qualitative and quantitative defects of pseudocholinesterase activity, Anaesthesia 22:55, 1967.

Nyhan, W. L., and Tocci, P.: Aminoaciduria, in DeGraff, A. C., and Creger, W. P. (eds.): Annual Review of Medicine (Palo Alto, Calif.: Annual Reviews, Inc., 1966), Vol. 17, p. 133.

O'Brien, W. M., et al.: Biochemical, pathologic, and clinical aspects of alkaptonuria, ochronosis, and ochronotic arthropathy, Am. J. Med. 34:813, 1963.

Osoba, D.: Thymic function, immunologic deficiency, and autoimmunity, M. Clin. North America 56:319, 1972.

Sharp, H. L.: Alpha-1 antitrypsin deficiency, Hosp. Practice 6:83, 1971.

Shwachman, H.: The sweat test, Pediatrics 30:167, 1962.

Smith, D. W.: Dysmorphology (teratology), J. Pediat. 69:1150, 1966.

Snyderman, S. E.: Diagnosis of metabolic disease, Pediat. Clin. North America 18:199, 1971.

Stanbury, J. B., et al.: The Metabolic Basis of Inherited Disease (3d ed.; New York: McGraw-Hill Book Company, 1972).

Viamonte, M., Jr., et al.: Angiographic findings in a patient with tuberous sclerosis, Am. J. Roentgenol. 98:723, 1966.

Waisman, H. A.: Some newer inborn errors of metabolism, Pediat. Clin. North America 13:469, 1966.

Welsh, J. D.: Isolated lactose deficiency in humans: Report on 100 patients, Medicine 49:257, 1970.

Zundel, W. S., and Tyler, F. H.: The muscular dystrophies, New England J. Med. 273:537, 596, 1965.

# CHAPTER 34

# Special Category Tests

This chapter includes tests which should be mentioned for special reasons but which seemed better left out of the main text for the sake of succinctness. Some are too new, and original reports need independent confirmation; some have generated highly favorable evaluations that have not been confirmed by the experience of others; some are older tests which are being replaced but occupy a prominent place in the older medical literature; and others are rarely used procedures which might be useful in very unusual circumstances. The tests are listed by the chapters in which they could have been placed.

## CHAPTER 2. FACTOR-DEFICIENCY ANEMIA

Formiminoglutamic acid (FIGLU) is a compound which is derived from the amino acid histidine, and which requires active folic acid (tetrahydrofolic acid) for normal metabolism to glutamic acid. In significant folic acid deficiency, FIGLU cannot be properly utilized, and is excreted into the urine in abnormal quantities. Vitamin $B_{12}$ deficiency will also influence FIGLU metabolism to some extent, because $B_{12}$ is necessary for the conversion of folic acid to metabolically active tetrahydrofolic acid. Urine assay for FIGLU has proved rather difficult, and several techniques are available. Some of these have poor sensitivity, others are not sufficiently specific, and others are technically difficult. In order to circumvent some of the problems of sensitivity and specificity, a loading dose of oral histidine (15 Gm. in three divided doses in 12 hours) with a 24-hour urine collection for FIGLU has proved helpful. Challenge with a loading dose of histidine augments FIGLU excretion in folic acid deficient states. FIGLU excretion after histidine loading is reported to be a reasonably accurate parameter of folic acid deficiency. FIGLU measurement is not widely available. Histidine may produce a reticulocyte response in megaloblastic anemia. Collection of urine must be done using a container with acid as a preservative. Many diseases produce elevated FIGLU excretion, so that false positive results will be common. Treatment of megaloblastic anemia returns FIGLU to normal.

Methylmalonic acid (MMA) excretion has been proposed as a specific test for B12 deficiency. However, the assay is difficult and not always reliable; patients with mild serum B12 decrease and mild megaloblastosis may still have normal MMA values; and some patients with folic acid deficiency anemia are reported to have elevated urine MMA because of coexisting B12 deficiency. Treatment of B12 deficiency restores MMA to normal.

With availability of serum B12 and folic acid assay, there seems little use for FIGLU or MMA determination.

References:

Chanarin, I. , et al. : Urinary excretion of histidine derivatives in megaloblastic anemia and other conditions and a comparison with the folic acid clearance test, J. Clin. Path. 15:269, 1962.

Chanarin, I. : The Megaloblastic Anaemias (Oxford, England: Blackwell Scientific Publications, 1969).

## CHAPTER 4.  DEPLETION ANEMIA

Paroxysmal cold hemoglobinuria is a rare but famous cause of hemolytic anemia. The most frequent etiology is syphilis. Cold temperatures trigger episodes of intravascular hemolysis, producing hemoglobinuria. The Donath-Landsteiner test detects cold-acting antibodies responsible for this hemolysis.

### Sickle Hemoglobin Tests

The Sickledex test is becoming widely used. It seems to be based on deoxygenation of sickle hemoglobin, which then becomes insoluble and precipitates in certain media. The test is said to be reliable, with certain drawbacks which should be appreciated. False negative results may be obtained in patients whose hemoglobin is less than 10 Gm. /100 ml. (or hematocrit 30%) unless extra blood is used. Reagents may deteriorate and inactivate. Dysglobulinemia (Waldenstrom's, myeloma, cryoglobulinemia) may interfere. Infants less than 6 months old may react negatively, because fetal hemoglobin is not yet completely transferred to adult hemoglobin. Certain rare non-S sickling hemoglobins will be positive.

The Murayama test has been proposed recently as a specific screening test for Hgb S. This is based on differential solubility of S hemoglobin at different temperatures. The only other non-S hemoglobin thus far reported positive is C (Harlem), which is rare and which also sickles in other sickling tests, but migrates with Hgb C on electrophoresis. However, the Murayama test is too cumbersome in its present form to use in most laboratories.

References:

Nalbandian, R. M., et al.: Sickledex test for hemoglobin S; A critique, J. A. M. A. 218:1679, 1971.

Nalbandian, R. M., et al.: Molecular basis for the specific test for hemoglobin S (Murayama test), Ann. Clin. Lab. Sc. 1:26, 1971.

## CHAPTER 7.  BLOOD COAGULATION

Tests for Fibrinolysin

The following tests are in limited use and merit some attention:

1. "Split products" tests ("Fi" test, etc.): Antifibrinogen antibodies attack not only fibrinogen but also certain of the fragments ("split products") cleaved from fibrinogen or fibrin by either primary or secondary fibrinolysin. Disseminated intravascular coagulation (DIC) is associated with intravascular fibrin clots and compensatory secondary fibrinolysin production. Fibrinogen is, by definition, absent from serum. Split products from fibrinolysins remain in serum after clotting of plasma by thrombin. Some investigators feel serum split products testing is useful in DIC; others report that the sensitivity of the test is poor.

2. Staphylococcal clumping: Staphylococci contain a substance which, under proper conditions, will agglutinate the organisms in the presence of fibrinogen or fibrin split products. The test is not widely used; it is reported to have sensitivity equal to or slightly greater than the "Fi" test.

3. Ethanol gelation: It is postulated that certain concentrations of ethyl alcohol allow breakup of abnormal complexes formed by fibrinogen and fibrin monomer, with subsequent gel formation by the fibrin monomer. With certain modifications, the procedure has been praised by some but reported to have inadequate sensitivity by others.

References:

Breen, F. A., and Tullis, J. L.: Ethanol gelation: A rapid screening test for intravascular coagulation, Ann. Int. Med. 69:1197, 1968.

Marder, V. J., et al.: Detection of serum fibrinogen and fibrin degradation products, Am. J. Med. 51:71, 1971.

## CHAPTER 10.  IMMUNOHEMATOLOGIC REACTIONS

The Witebsky test is a test for ABO hemolytic disease of the newborn.  The test is positive in about half the cases.  In this procedure, fetal red cells from the cord blood are placed into adult (blood group) AB serum.  Agglutination of the fetal RBC is a positive test.  This used to be considered one of the best tests for ABO hemolytic disease of the newborn despite the fact that its mechanism is unexplained.  The test is not indicated if the baby is blood group O or the mother is group AB.

## CHAPTER 11.  BLOOD TRANSFUSIONS

Central venous pressure (CVP) is frequently used as an estimate of blood volume status.  There are, however, circumstances in which CVP does not accurately reflect the relation between blood quantity and vascular capacity; these include pulmonary hypertension (emphysema, embolization, mitral stenosis), left ventricular failure, and technical factors of catheter placement and maintenance.

References:

> Bigger, J. T. , Jr. , et al. :  Management of cardiac problems in the intensive care unit, M. Clin. North America 55:1183, 1971.
> Gump, F. E. :  Physiological measurements and their interpretation, M. Clin. North America 55:1141, 1971.

## CHAPTER 16.  VIRAL, RICKETTSIAL, AND MISCELLANEOUS INFECTIOUS DISEASES

Streptococcus MG is a test for the mycoplasma-induced antibodies of primary atypical pneumonia.  The test is based on the unusual reactivity of these antibodies for material from this strain of the streptococcal organism.  The majority of investigators feel that the test is not as sensitive as cold agglutinins.  The "strep MG" test is positive in less than 40% of cases, although reports range from 10 to 80%.

A new antigen ("Milan antigen") has been reported in association with short-incubation hepatitis A in the same manner that Australia antigen is associated with long-incubation hepatitis B.  Verification by others is needed.

Reference:

> Del Prete, S. , et al. :  Epidemic hepatitis—Associated antigen (Milan antigen), Am. J. Dis. Child. 123:326, 1972.

## CHAPTER 19.  LIVER FUNCTION TESTS

Cephalin flocculation test (ceph. floc.):  In acute and
chronic liver cell necrosis or inflammation, abnormal globulins are often produced.  Depending on their nature, they may
be precipitated by certain substances such as zinc sulfate or
buffered thymol, or be detected by excessive attachment to
certain surfaces such as colloidal gold or cephalin-cholesterol
particles.  Zinc sulfate turbidity tests have been demonstrated
to be nearly specific for gamma globulin.  The thymol turbidity test responds either to changes in gamma globulin or to
lipoproteins migrating in the beta globulin area.  The cephalin
flocculation test is more complex and responds to either of
two stimuli.  Gamma globulin will precipitate the cephalin
emulsion, but is normally prevented from doing so by certain
stabilizing factors, probably in the alpha-1 globulin area.  In
acute hepatic parenchymal cell injury, the stabilizing factors
vanish from serum in 24-48 hours, allowing normal amounts
of gamma globulin present to give a positive ceph. floc. reaction.  On the other hand, excessively large amounts of
gamma globulin may be sufficient to overcome normal amounts
of stabilizing factor present and likewise give a positive test.
However, the ceph. floc. does not seem to depend primarily
on hypergammaglobulinemia, since certain types of globulins
have a peculiar reactivity out of proportion to their actual
quantity.

The technique of the ceph. floc. consists of incubating
the patient's serum with a cephalin-cholesterol emulsion in
the dark for 24 hours.  Any resulting flocculation or precipitation is graded 1 to 4 plus.  Normal serums are negative,
but 1+ is regarded as within normal range and only 2+ or over
is considered significant, in order to rule out error in visually estimating very weak reactions.  As noted earlier, the test
is usually positive in acute hepatocellular injury from any
cause, except when very mild.  The stabilizing factor remains
absent until hepatocellular healing is well established, but following relatively mild or brief episodes, the ceph. floc. may be
elevated only a few days.  The test cannot show the degree of
damage or the amount of tissue affected.  It usually is normal in
certain diseases such as obstructive jaundice without superimposed
infection, chronic passive congestion (as opposed to acute types),
small-to-moderate degrees of metastatic carcinoma, and solitary
liver abscess.  However, occasionally some of these conditions may
have a positive result, especially with extensive metastasis and
jaundice.  Since there must be active cell necrosis to get a positive
test (unless abnormal globulins are present), there usually are negative results in fatty liver, inactive cirrhosis, often in moderately
active cirrhosis, or in healing stages of acute diseases.  Positive

results may be found in a certain percentage of cases in primarily nonhepatic diseases, as mentioned earlier, although some of these may also have liver involvement. These include collagen diseases, infectious mononucleosis, SBE, viral pneumonia, malaria, pernicious anemia, and a few others.

Both the SGOT and SGPT, if they show elevation, do so before the ceph. floc. becomes abnormal, but they all return to normal ranges considerably in advance of the ceph. floc. Therefore, the ceph. floc. sometimes will be abnormal in the presence of normal enzyme studies, due either to a minimal amount of hepatocellular damage or from obtaining the tests after the enzymes had returned to normal. In general, the ceph. floc. is less sensitive than the SGOT, but is elevated longer and is more specific for hepatic cell acute destruction. It may be helpful to assess activity of cirrhosis and as a parameter of therapy in hepatitis.

The ceph. floc. is probably of most use as a means to confirm acute liver cell damage in a patient when the SGOT is normal or only minimally elevated. There usually is little use in getting a ceph. floc. if the SGOT is elevated. With the advent of enzyme tests, such as SGOT, which are more sensitive for hepatocellular injury, the ceph. floc. is not as important as it once was. The ceph. floc. is not reliable in the neonatal period, and before the age of 6 months may sometimes be normal even with extensive acute liver cell damage.

The zinc sulfate test demonstrates elevations of gamma globulin, but serum protein electrophoresis can do this more informatively.

The thymol turbidity test roughly correlates with the results of the ceph. floc. It seems less sensitive than the ceph. floc. and becomes positive later, but tends to remain positive longer.

Ornathine carbamyl transferase (OCT) is found mainly in liver and, to a much lesser extent, within intestinal mucosa. Since it takes rather extensive intestinal infarction to provoke significant OCT elevation, this enzyme is nearly specific for liver cell disease. It is even more sensitive than SGOT to hepatocellular injury, and reportedly may be elevated in some cases without histologic cell changes.

Isocitric dehydrogenase (ICD) behaves like the SGOT in liver disease. Although ICD is found in cardiac muscle and several tissues besides liver, it is not elevated in myocardial infarction, and usually is abnormal only in liver disease.

Alkaline phosphatase isoenzymes: Alkaline phosphatase can be separated into single enzymes which are relatively specific for bone, liver, placenta, and intestine. The easiest method is heat fractionation; bone isoenzyme is heat-inactivated, while liver is heat-stable. Placenta has the greatest heat stability. More than 30% heat-stable suggests liver origin; less than 30% heat-stable suggests bone. Normals are 15-35% heat-stable, creating overlap

with bone.  This method has not been reliable in my laboratory.
Chemical fractionation is too cumbersome.  Electrophoresis is just
becoming available, and promises to be the best separation method.
An interesting isoenzyme, called "Regan," migrates in the placenta
area and is found in some patients with cancer.

5-nucleotidase:  This is a member of the alkaline phosphatase
group, but is thought to be more specific (and possibly more sensitive) than alkaline phosphatase for hepatobiliary tract disease.  However, one study suggests elevation in some patients with bone lesions.

Gamma-glutamyl transpeptidase (GGTP):  This enzyme is found
primarily in liver and kidney, with a smaller amount in heart muscle.  Some reports have indicated an increased sensitivity over other
enzymes for hepatic metastases; at least one report, however, found
little difference from alkaline phosphatase.  GGTP may be elevated
in a wide variety of hepatic diseases but in no case with 100% sensitivity.  Elevations also occur with some frequency in diabetes, various neurologic and brain disorders, and alcoholism.  In general,
the majority of reports claim somewhat increased sensitivity in
acute hepatocellular damage and in obstruction, over standard liver
function enzymes.  Nonspecificity limits the attractiveness of GGPT
as a replacement for standard function tests.

Guanase is indicative of acute hepatocellular damage; sensitivity is somewhat greater than SGOT.  Guanase is also located in
brain, kidney, and intestine.

Aldolase has tissue specificity and sensitivity similar to that
of SGOT.

Alcohol dehydrogenase is said to be relatively (not completely)
specific for acute hepatocellular damage, although elevation may occur in fatty liver and metastatic tumor.  Infectious mononucleosis,
uncomplicated early extrahepatic obstruction, and inactive portal
cirrhosis are said to have normal levels.

Sorbital dehydrogenase is relatively specific for acute hepatocellular damage and is similar in this respect to SGPT.  Occasional
elevation is noted during infection.

Immunoglobulin levels:  Marked IgM increase has been reported
in 80% of biliary cirrhosis, but elevated levels may occur in extrahepatic obstruction and other diseases.  Reports of increased IgA in
alcoholic cirrhosis are even less  specific and frequent.  Immunoglobulins have not, therefore, been very helpful.

Cell component antibodies:  Antibodies have been described
which react against specific structures in cells, as demonstrated by
immunofluorescent technique.  Antimitochondrial antibodies are
found in 80-100% of biliary cirrhosis patients and may aid in the diagnosis of this uncommon disease.  False positive results have been
reported in some patients with drug-induced cholestasis and chronic
active hepatitis as well as in a relatively small number of patients
with extrahepatic obstruction, acute infectious hepatitis, rheumatoid
arthritis, and other conditions.  Anti-smooth-muscle antibodies

were reported in 45-70% of patients with chronic active ("lupoid") hepatitis and have been found in biliary cirrhosis and, less frequently, in other liver diseases (except alcoholic cirrhosis). An immunofluorescence expert is needed to set up and interpret these procedures. Liver biopsy is still needed.

Cholesterol and cholesterol esters: Cholesterol is synthesized in several tissues, but the liver is the chief organ in its manufacture, alteration, and degradation. Normally about 70% is esterified and about 30% in the free form. Esterification is affected much more than total cholesterol by liver damage. In moderate degrees of acute or chronic liver damage, cholesterol esters may decrease to the 40-50% range. They usually do not fall below 20% without severe liver parenchymal destruction. The total cholesterol is reduced below normal ranges (150-250 mg./100 ml.) only in severe damage, most often chronic. However, the usefulness of cholesterol as an index of liver function is severely handicapped by the technical difficulties of the test itself. Laboratories have considerable variation in accuracy even from day to day, so it is difficult to know if a slightly or moderately reduced value is genuine or not. Also the normal range is so wide that a patient could have his usual normal value decreased by one-third or more and still be within population normal ranges. Furthermore, other diseases such as hyperthyroidism, severe infections, and malnutrition will lower serum cholesterol. On the other hand, certain types of liver diseases are associated with increased cholesterol; these include biliary obstruction, especially biliary cirrhosis, and many cases of cholangitis. Nonhepatic diseases which cause elevated values are hypothyroidism, nephrotic syndrome, idiopathic hypercholesterolemia, and often diabetes.

References:

Breen, K. J., and Schenker, S.: Liver function tests, CRC Crit. Rev. Clin. Lab. Sc. 2:573, 1971.

Fitzgerald, M. X. M., et al.: Value of differential alkaline phosphatase thermostability in clinical diagnosis, Am. J. Clin. Path. 51:194, 1969.

Hanger, F. M.: The meaning of liver function tests, Am. J. Med. 16:565, 1954.

Sherlock, S.: Chronic active hepatitis, Postgrad. Med. 50:206, 1971.

Walker, G., and Doniach, D.: Antibodies and immunoglobulins in liver disease, Gut 9:266, 1968.

West, M., and Zimmerman, H. J.: Serum enzymes in hepatic disease, M. Clin. North America 43:1, 1959.

Zimmerman, H. J., and West, M.: Serum enzymes in gastrointestinal diseases, M. Clin. North America 48:189, 1964.

## CHAPTER 20. CARDIAC, PULMONARY, AND MISCELLANEOUS DIAGNOSTIC PROCEDURES

The ratio of total LDH to fast-moving (LDH-1) isoenzyme has been proposed as a test for myocardial infarct, to improve specificity of total LDH and to demonstrate increase in LDH-1 which is significant but does not exceed normal population range. There have been conflicting reports on the usefulness of this technique.

Arterial oxygen saturation has been proposed as an ancillary test for pulmonary embolization, giving support to the diagnosis if the arterial $pO_2$ is below 80 mm Hg. However, exceptions occur, and it is not yet clear whether the number of exceptions is great enough to seriously impair the usefulness of the test.

The protamine sulfate test (p. 81) may be positive in embolization. Sensitivity depends on which test modification is used; thus far, results have been variable with all techniques. My personal experience disclosed many false positives and negatives in embolization.

Radioisotope pulmonary function tests: Radioactive xenon is a gas which can either be inhaled or injected intravenously. Inhalation fills the alveoli for a few moments before the gas is exhaled. If injected intravenously, xenon quickly diffuses into the alveoli and then is exhaled. In either case a stationary rapid imaging device such as the Anger scintillation camera can photograph alveolar distribution of the gas. Conditions which alter ventilatory distribution, such as emphysema or space-occupying lesions, produce corresponding deficits in the distribution of xenon. In pulmonary embolization the xenon scan is typically normal in the presence of defects on perfusion scans using isotope-labeled particles which outline pulmonary blood distribution. However, if emphysema is present, both the ventilation and the perfusion scan will be abnormal, and this causes difficulty if embolization is suspected. Xenon tests are available at present only in large hospitals. The gas is very expensive and necessitates special apparatus to avoid contamination of the room.

Isotope-labeled particles can be inhaled via aerosol; this allows visualization of the pattern of the major bronchi. It is claimed that this method can distinguish pure emphysema from that secondary to bronchitis. The technique is still experimental.

C-reactive protein is produced during conditions which cause acute tissue destruction or inflammation. The protein gets its name from its ability to precipitate with pneumococcus somatic C-polysaccharide. The test is performed with antiserum against C-protein and is reported in a semiquantitative 0-4+ fashion. This technique has roughly the same usefulness as the ESR, but has never attained the same degree of popularity.

Digitalis toxicity screening: It has been reported that increased concentration of potassium and calcium in saliva is suggestive of digitalis toxicity. So far, there are conflicting data on the usefulness of this procedure.

The Gastrografin test for intestinal perforation: Several reports indicate that if Gastrografin (meglumine diatrizoate) is placed
into the stomach via nasogastric tube, it will be absorbed and excreted into the urine if GI tract perforation exists. The test is
simple and is said to be reasonably sensitive.

References:

Behringer, B. R., and Stephenson, H. E., Jr.: The diatrizoate precipitation test for intestinal perforation, Surg. Gynec.
& Obst. 129:475, 1969.

Blahd, W. H. (ed.): Nuclear Medicine (2d ed.; New York:
McGraw-Hill Book Company, Inc., 1971).

Dalen, J. E., et al.: Pulmonary angiography in acute pulmonary embolism: Indications, techniques, and results in 367
patients, Am. Heart J. 81:175, 1971.

Mills, J., and Drew, D.: Pulmonary embolism without arterial hypoxemia, Ann. Int. Med. 75:972, 1971.

Nutter, D. O.: The isoenzymes of lactic dehydrogenase. I.
Myocardial infarction and coronary insufficiency, Am.
Heart J. 72:315, 1966.

Wotman, S., et al.: Salivary electrolytes in the detection of
digitalis toxicity, New England J. Med. 285:871, 1971.

## CHAPTER 21.   SERUM PROTEINS

Several screening tests have been devised for the detection of
hyperlipoproteinemia. Two (K-agar and TEKIT precipitest) are
based on precipitation by a sulfated polysaccharide, the other (Beta-
L) involves precipitation of beta lipoprotein by specific antiserum.
Very little has been published regarding sensitivity and accuracy of
these procedures; however, each seems about 85-90% sensitive in
detecting hyperlipoproteinemia. More independent evaluation is
needed.

References:

Boyle, E., Jr., et al.: Evaluation of rapid screening methods
for the detection of abnormal lipid states related to atherosclerosis, Ann. Clin. Lab. Sc. 2:393, 1972.

Searcy, R., et al.: A screening procedure for detecting and
characterizing hyperlipoproteinemia, Clin. chim. acta
38:291, 1972.

## CHAPTER 22.   RHEUMATOID-COLLAGEN DISEASES

Serum complement: Total complement (C') can be measured
by hemolytic techniques, or C'-3 component alone can be assayed by
using specific antiserum. C' is said to decrease in approximately
75% of systemic lupus patients and to correlate best with renal in-

volvement. Other collagen diseases usually have normal values, although exceptions occur. Acute glomerulonephritis, some cases of nephrotic syndrome, and a few cases of severe rheumatoid arthritis may also have depressed levels.

Antinuclear antibodies (ANA) test morphology: A peripheral (nuclear border) antinuclear staining reaction (in contrast to a solid or a "speckled" nuclear staining pattern) is said to be fairly specific for systemic lupus. Most of these patients have active disease; the incidence is much less in treated or inactive cases. Treated or inactive lupus is more apt to have solid or speckled (broken) nuclear fluorescent patterns, and these may also be found in significant numbers of persons with other collagen diseases or in some persons with rheumatoid arthritis.

References:

Gewurz, H.: The immunologic role of complement, Hosp. Practice 2:45, 1967.

Rothfield, N. F.: Serologic tests in rheumatic diseases, Postgrad. Med. 45:116, 1969.

## CHAPTER 24. SERUM ELECTROLYTES

Magnesium deficiency may occasionally produce symptoms much like hypocalcemia, including tetany. The most common etiologies are steatorrhea, nasogastric suction accompanied by large quantities of magnesium-free intravenous fluids, diabetes, and alcoholism or alcoholic cirrhosis. Diagnosis is made by serum assay for magnesium; this generally requires atomic absorption equipment. Since this is relatively expensive and is not applicable to many other laboratory tests, most small hospitals do not have this equipment and therefore do not have magnesium determination readily available.

Serum water can be estimated by a refractometer (total solids meter), which measures the effects of serum proteins on the refractive index. Serum proteins constitute the major determinant of serum colloid osmotic pressure which regulates plasma and extracellular water equilibrium. Therefore, serum water estimates intravascular colloid osmotic pressure in contrast to serum osmolality, which measures intravascular osmotic pressure, an entity responding to electrolyte changes but not influenced significantly by colloid (protein). Serum water is influenced by changes in either protein or water. Elevated serum water suggests excess water; decreased serum water indicates water deficit. Unfortunately, decreased serum protein also leads to increased water values; and since decreased albumin is common in seriously ill patients, this fact plus the rather high cost of the instrument has limited the use of the test. Nevertheless, even protein abnormality does not totally destroy the usefulness of serum water determination, because a relative dilution

caused by hypoproteinemia may be treated by administration of albumin. Normal serum water values are 93-94 Gm./100 ml.

References:

> Mansberger, A. R., et al.: Refractometry and osmometry in
> clinical surgery, Ann. Surg. 169:672, 1969.
> Wacker, W. E. C., and Paresi, A. F.: Magnesium metabolism,
> New England J. Med. 278:658, 712, 772, 1968.

## CHAPTER 27.  TESTS FOR DIABETES AND HYPOGLYCEMIA

### Skin Tests for Hyperglycemia

A simple skin test utilizing glucose oxidase test paper has been
proposed for the detection of diabetes mellitus. Evaluation has disclosed such erratic results that, in its present form, this procedure
seems to have little value.

### Tolbutamide Tolerance Test

Tolbutamide (Orinase) is a sulfonylurea drug which apparently
has the ability to stimulate insulin production from pancreatic beta
cells. This drug has been used for treatment of mild diabetics who
produce insulin, but of insufficient quantity. In 1956, tolbutamide
was first proposed as a test for diabetes. A special water-soluble
form of tolbutamide is given intravenously. There is normally a
prompt and considerable fall in blood glucose levels with a maximum at 30-45 minutes, followed by a return to normal values between 1 1/2 and 3 hours. The counteracting forces responsible are
thought to be primarily liver production of glucose from glycogen
induced by epinephrine release in answer to the hypoglycemia. In
diabetics, there is both diminished and delayed response to intravenous tolbutamide. There is little correlation between the degree
of test abnormality and the likelihood that a patient would respond to
actual tolbutamide therapy. The test must be preceded by adequate
carbohydrate diet, as described in the GTT.

The tolbutamide test is regarded by some as the most specific
laboratory test for diabetes now available. However, this does not
mean that it is actually specific for diabetes. Some investigators
did find significant numbers of false positives, although reduced in
frequency, when abnormal GTTs from a variety of nonpancreatic
etiologies were retested with tolbutamide. Nevertheless, the nonpancreatic causes of abnormal GTT (oral or IV), mentioned earlier,
may give a normal tolbutamide curve. When they do produce abnormality, they may remain below tolbutamide levels diagnostic for
diabetes. The sensitivity of the tolbutamide test is apparently somewhat less than that of the oral GTT and definitely less than the C-
GTT. Many mild diabetics have abnormal response to tolbutamide,
but there is a definite overlap of results in the borderline area. A

considerable number of the very mild diabetics have close to normal tests.  The over-all sensitivity of the tolbutamide test seems to be about that of the intravenous GTT.

The tolbutamide test is not used in the last trimester of pregnancy,  due to a combination of increased insulin requirement and increased adrenal steroid levels.  The tolbutamide test has been used with the same schedule of steroid pretreatment as the C-GTT.  Results are too meager as yet, but there seems to be somewhat increased sensitivity at the expense of decreased specificity (some abnormal responses found in obesity and old age).  The tolbutamide test at present has not been widely accepted in clinical medicine for the diagnosis of diabetes, although it has proved one of the most reliable tests for insulin-producing tumors.  It is agreed that further evaluation is needed.

Hyperosmolar nonketotic coma is uncommon but is being reported with increased frequency.  The criterion for diagnosis is very high blood sugar (usually well over 500 mg./100 ml.) without ketones in either plasma or urine.  The patients usually become severely dehydrated.  Plasma osmolality is high due to dehydration and hyperglycemia.  Most patients are maturity-onset mild diabetics, but nondiabetics may be affected.  Associated precipitating factors include infections, severe burns, high-dose corticosteroid therapy, and renal dialysis.  Occasional cases have been reported due to Dilantin and to glucose administration during hypothermia.

Lactic acidosis syndrome is rare and may occur from several etiologies.  It is most frequently reported with phenformin (DBI) therapy of diabetes or as a nonketotic form of diabetic acidosis.  The most common cause of elevated blood lactate is tissue hypoxia from shock.  Arterial blood is said to be more reliable than venous for lactic acid determination.  Tourniquet blood stagnation must be avoided, and the specimen must be kept in ice until analyzed.

References:

Danowski, T. S. : Non-ketotic coma and diabetes mellitus, M. Clin. North America 55:913, 1971.

McCurdy, D. K. : Hyperosmolar hyperglycemic nonketotic diabetic coma, M. Clin. North America 54:683, 1970.

Oliva, P. B.: Lactic acidosis, Am. J. Med. 48:209, 1970.

Unger, R. H. , and Madison, L. L. : A new diagnostic procedure for mild diabetes mellitus, Diabetes 7:455, 1958.

CHAPTER 28.   THYROID AND PARATHYROID FUNCTION TESTS

I.  Thyroid Tests

TBG quantitative assay: Methods are now available for measuring actual TBG levels by means of electrophoresis-isotope combination techniques.  This was useful when thyroid tests abnormalities due to TBG alterations were suspected. With development of the "Corrected" T4 by isotope, TBG assay should rarely be needed.

Free thyroxine assay: Theoretically, free thyroxine levels should closely reflect thyroid function and not be affected by agents which alter TBG. Free thyroxine can be measured by performing a T4-by-isotope procedure, isolating the radioactive hormone which fails to bind to TBG (usually done by dialysis) and then calculating what percentage of radioactivity this fraction represents. This fraction has the same relationship to the radioactivity binding to TBG as free thyroxine has to thyroxine bound to TBG. If one then quantitates serum thyroxine via the PBI or some other method, the free thyroxine radioactive fraction multiplied by total thyroxine quantity yields the quantity of free thyroxine. The main drawback of this procedure is technical difficulty plus the unexpected finding that serum free thyroxine may be elevated in persons seriously ill from a variety of diseases. With development of the "Corrected" T4 by isotope, this test should rarely be needed.

Long-acting thyroid stimulator (LATS) assay: LATS is an IgG-type antibody whose origin is still debated but whose action results in stimulation of thyroid hormone production. There is especially good correlation with exophthalmos and pretibial myxedema. LATS is found only in Graves' disease, not in toxic nodular goiter. Elevated values have been reported in a small percentage of other thyroid diseases, but usually in low titer. At present, an average of 40-60% of patients with Graves' disease have significantly elevated LATS levels, although possibly current bioassay methods are not sensitive enough. Current methods are difficult and expensive, and the T3 suppression test gives similar information in borderline Graves' disease; so the necessity for LATS assay is rare. Nevertheless, there are reports of a few patients with exophthalmos, normal thyroid function tests, normal T3 suppression, and positive LATS assay.

"Dynamic" thyroid blood flow study (carotid-thyroid transit time): A technique has been described whereby a radioisotope compound is injected intravenously and the number of seconds' difference between the time when isotope appears in the common carotids and when it appears in the thyroid is measured. This test is said to be more accurate than the RAI, especially in hypothyroidism. It also has the advantage that less radiation is given to the patient. Both the study and a thyroid scan can be completed together in 1 day rather than the 2 days needed for the RAI. Disadvantages include the necessity for a stationary rapid imaging device such as the Anger camera and the fact that most conditions which affect the RAI likewise affect the "dynamic" flow study.

References:

Anderson, B. G.: Free thyroxine in serum in relation to thyroid function, J.A.M.A. 203:577, 1968.

Ashkar, F. S., and Smith, E. M.: The dynamic thyroid study—
A rapid evaluation of thyroid function and anatomy using
99m-Tc as pertechnetate, J. A. M. A. 217:441, 1971.
Gharib, H., and Mayberry, W. E.: Diagnosis of Graves' oph-
thalmopathy without hyperthyroidism: Long-acting thyroid
stimulator (LATS) determination as laboratory adjunct,
Mayo Clin. Proc. 45:444, 1970.
Kriss, J. P.: The Long-Acting Stimulator and Thyroid Disease, in Stollerman, G. H., et al. (eds.): Advances in Internal Medicine (Chicago: Year Book Medical Publishers,
Inc., 1970), Vol. 16, p. 135.

II.  Parathyroid Tests

Parathyroid hormone (Para-t-hormone; PTH) assay is theoretically the best way to diagnose hyperparathyroidism.  Both radioimmunoassay and bioassay techniques exist.  Unfortunately, such
procedures have achieved only mixed success and are available only
in reference or research laboratories.  Undoubtedly, radioimmunoassay reagents will improve in the next few years to the point of
routine clinical use.  Certain maneuvers, such as calcium or EDTA
infusion or combinations of PTH and serum calcium levels, have
been used to enhance specificity of PTH assay, but more extensive
evaluation is needed.  PTH specimens must be drawn fasting in the
morning without anticoagulants, processed at cold temperatures,
frozen immediately, and transported in dry ice.
Selenomethionine isotope scanning has been used to localize
hyperactive parathyroid glands.  Results have been rather disappointing for a majority of those who have tried this technique.
A modified calcium infusion procedure has been recently reported to improve specificity of the old Ellsworth-Howard infusion
test.  Independent evaluation is needed.

Reference:

Pak, C. Y. C., et al.: Simple and reliable test for diagnosis
of hyperparathyroidism, Arch. Int. Med. 129:48, 1972.


CHAPTER 29.  ADRENAL FUNCTION

Plasma aldosterone assay is just becoming available in a few
laboratories.  It is hoped that plasma measurement will avoid the
problems of 24-hour urine collection.  However, there are still major technical problems; furthermore, it will take time to discover
the drawbacks associated with this (as with any) new procedure.  Apparently there is a diurnal variation in plasma levels: afternoon
levels are half or less those of the morning.  Glucose ingestion
lowers plasma aldosterone temporarily.  Assuming an upright position increases levels over twice the recumbent values.  These fac-

tors require specimen collection in the morning before the patient is allowed to sit or stand.

## Tests in Primary Aldosteronism

The technical difficulty of aldosterone and renin determinations has led to various screening tests for Conn's syndrome and, in some instances, to procedures which might replace renin for diagnosis. Now that more reliable renin determination is becoming available through radioisotope immunoassay and while simplification of aldosterone technique continues, the need for replacement of aldosterone and renin determinations has greatly decreased. However, original good results from most of the screening procedures have not yet been sufficiently evaluated by others. The new procedures include the following:

1. Desoxycorticosterone (DOCA) suppression test: DOCA is reported to suppress aldosterone secretion in secondary aldosteronism but not in Conn's syndrome. DOCA is a precursor of aldosterone.

2. Alpha-fluorohydrocortisone (fludrocortisone) suppression test: This is similar to DOCA suppression. Fludrocortisone is a hydrocortisone analog with marked salt-retaining action.

3. Spironolactone test: Potassium clearance is measured before and after 3 days of oral spironolactone (with the patient on a high-salt diet). More than 50% reduction in clearance suggests aldosteronism (either primary or secondary).

4. Furosemide (Lasix) test: The patient remains upright for 4 hours following an oral dose of the diuretic furosemide. Plasma renin is then drawn. The original report states 80% agreement with low-salt diet renin response in hypertensive patients, with the 20% disagreement containing both false positives and false negatives.

5. Saline infusion: Large quantities of saline given intravenously over a 2-day period are said to suppress aldosterone to less than 50% of baseline values in conditions other than primary aldosteronism.

6. Twenty-four-hour urine potassium: In patients with hypokalemia, those with primary aldosteronism usually have normal potassium excretion (over 40 mEq./day), while most others have low excretion as the body attempts to conserve potassium.

7. Plasma aldosterone with saline infusion: Plasma aldosterone is reported to be suppressed to less than 50% of baseline (recumbent for 8 hours) values by infusion of 2 L. of saline over a 2-hour period, whereas levels in primary aldosteronism remain greater than 50%. Saline infusion causes more marked suppression than does a high-salt diet.

The 17-ketosteroids can be fractionated into alpha (androsterone and etiocholanolone) and beta (dehydroepiandrosterone). Increase of 17-KS in adrenal carcinoma is most often due to beta fraction increase. The normal ratio of beta to alpha is less than 0.2.

Alternatively, the "Allen Blue" test is a reasonable estimate of DHA. Not all carcinomas are positive with either of these procedures, and neither is indicated if urine 17-KS are normal; therefore the use of these tests is decreasing.

Tests for Cushing's Disease

1. Urinary free cortisol: Cortisol, like thyroxine, is predominantly bound to plasma proteins for storage, but a small amount (5%) exists in the free, metabolically active state. Twenty-four-hour free cortisol excretion is considered by some to be one of the best screening tests for Cushing's disease. Pregnancy causes "false positive" elevation. Analytical techniques are very difficult, and the test is not widely available.

2. Plasma ACTH assay is now becoming available in reference laboratories. ACTH is increased in Cushing's disease due to pituitary overactivity; is normal or increased in nonadrenal ACTH-secreting tumors ("ectopic ACTH" syndrome); and is decreased in Cushing's due to adrenal tumor.

References:

Biglieri, E. G., et al.: A preliminary evaluation for primary aldosteronism, Arch. Int. Med. 126:1004, 1970.

Birchall, R., and Batson, H. M., Jr.: Test for pathologic secretion of aldosterone, J.A.M.A. 206:2114, 1968.

Espiner, E. A., et al.: Effect of saline infusions on aldosterone secretions and electrolyte excretion in primary aldosteronism, New England J. Med. 277:1, 1967.

Frawley, T. F.: Cushing's Syndrome, in Clinician (Chicago: G. D. Searle & Co., 1971), Vol. 1, p. 37.

Leutscher, J. A., et al.: Effects of sodium loading, sodium depletion and posture on plasma aldosterone concentration and renin activity in hypertensive patients, J. Clin. Endocrinol. 29:1310, 1969.

MacDonald, W. G., and Todoroff, T. G.: Negative results: The urinary sodium-ACTH test for adrenal competence, Am. J. M. Sc. 252:446, 1966.

Smilo, R. P., and Forsham, P. H.: Diagnostic approach to hypofunction and hyperfunction of the adrenal cortex, Postgrad. Med. 46:146, 1969.

CHAPTER 30.  PITUITARY FUNCTION TESTS, MISCELLANEOUS HORMONE TESTS, AND TESTS IN OBSTETRICS

Metyrapone test measuring compound S: Recent reports suggest that the metyrapone test for pituitary function may be shortened and improved by obtaining a single plasma specimen for 11-deoxycortisol (compound S) plus cortisol measurement rather than standard multiple 24-hour urine specimens for 17-OH-CS or 17-KG steroids.

Plasma cortisol acts as a check on the validity of compound S data; unless cortisol decreases to less than 8 mg./100 ml. and comprises less than half of combined compound S and cortisol values, metyrapone is probably not functioning properly and abnormal compound S results are not reliable.

Growth Hormone (GH) levels are highest 1-2 hours after beginning sleep. A screening test for pituitary hypofunction has been suggested utilizing one GH specimen taken 90 minutes after beginning sleep.

Reference:

Doughaday, W. H.: Postgrad. Med. 45:84, 1969.
Spark, R. F.: Ann. Int. Med. 75:717, 1971.


## CHAPTER 31.  TESTS FOR SYPHILIS

A hemagglutination test has been developed which is said to have the same specificity as the FTA-ABS as well as equal sensitivity in all stages except primary syphilis. Since the test is considerably easier to perform in small numbers than the FTA-ABS, the technique may be more extensively used in the next few years. However, few evaluations have yet been published.

Reference:

Logan, L. C., and Cox, P. M.: Am. J. Clin. Path. 53:163, 1970.


## CHAPTER 32.  LABORATORY ASPECTS OF CANCER

Carcinoembryonic antigen (CEA): GI tract epithelium in early fetal life contains antigen which has recently been found in extracts from carcinomas of the adult GI tract. An immunologic test based on antibodies against this antigen was originally said to be specific for GI tract primary carcinoma. It was said to be highly sensitive for colonic and rectal adenocarcinoma but less so for other GI tract areas, and negative in benign GI tract diseases. Others have subsequently reported some positive results in tumor from organs other than the GI tract and in some persons with alcoholic liver disease, chronic renal disease, and benign GI tract conditions. In colonic carcinoma, different investigators have published widely divergent results, with percentages of tumors detected ranging from 59 to 97%. Reports indicate that smaller and earlier tumors are less likely to be positive. Much more extensive work must be done before the potential of this test can be assessed.

Urine lactic dehydrogenase (LDH) has been proposed as a screening test for urinary tract carcinoma. This procedure is not the same technique used for serum LDH, because urine contains an inhibitor which must be dialyzed out before assay is performed. Despite several enthusiastic reports, it has been found that other conditions such as urinary tract infection can also elevate urine LDH; this test has, to date, not been widely used.

Urine hydroxyproline: Hydroxyproline is a collagen component whose urinary excretion is increased in various disorders of increased osteoblastic activity as well as some diseases involving osteolysis and collagen metabolism. Significantly increased 24-hour excretion is reported in about half of patients with tumors having bone metastases, and normal results were obtained in most patients with tumors without bone involvement. Some of those with skeletal metastases and elevated urine hydroxyproline had normal alkaline phosphatase. Some investigators use hydroxyproline/creatinine ratios. The test may be useful in some cancer patients by suggesting occult bone metastasis, although a bone scan is probably more sensitive.

Calcitonin assay: Medullary carcinoma of the thyroid is frequently associated with pheochromocytoma and apparently produces a parathyroid-stimulating hormone called calcitonin. Although not currently available, calcitonin assay probably will appear in the next few years.

References:

Block, M. A.: Medullary thyroid carcinoma: A component of an interesting endocrine syndrome, CA 19:74, 1969.

Dhar, P., et al.: Carcinoembryonic antigen (CEA) in colonic cancer, J.A.M.A. 221:31, 1972.

Hosley, H. F., et al.: Hydroxyproline excretion in malignant neoplastic disease, Arch. Int. Med. 118:565, 1966.

Moore, T. L., et al.: Carcinoembryonic antigen assay in cancer of the colon and pancreas and other digestive tract disorders, Am. J. Digest. Dis. 16:1, 1971.

Schmidt, J. D.: Significance of total urinary lactic dehydrogenase activity in urinary tract disease, J. Urol. 96:950, 1966.

Stillman, A., and Zamcheck, N.: Recent advances in immunologic diagnosis of digestive tract cancer, Am. J. Digest. Dis. 15:1003, 1970.

## CHAPTER 33.  CONGENITAL DISEASES

Two reports indicate that x-ray techniques are very helpful in diagnosis and differentiation of various types of disaccharide malabsorption. This would probably have to be limited to adults. Confirmation by others is needed.

References:

Laws, J. W., and Neale, G.: Radiological diagnosis of disaccharidase deficiency, Lancet 2:139, 1966.

Preger, L., and Amberg, J. R.: Sweet diarrhea. Roentgen diagnosis of disaccharidase deficiency, Am. J. Roentgenol. 101:287, 1967.

# Appendix

A Compendium of Useful Data and Information

## EFFECTS OF AGE ON LABORATORY TESTS

Apparent age-related increase in abnormal results has been reported in a wide variety of tests in patients over the age of 50.

1. Antinuclear antibodies; rheumatoid factor; VDRL; serum globulin (Brit. J. Ven. Dis. 42:40, 1966; Ann. Rheumat. Dis. 28:431, 1969)
2. Cholesterol; triglyceride (p. 257)
3. BUN (J. Lab. & Clin. Med. 73:825, 1969)
4. Oral GTT values (p. 319)
5. ESR (p. 238)
6. Schilling test (p. 300)
7. D-xylose test (p. 301)
8. Serum calcium (New England J. Med. 281:367, 1969—however, most investigators do not find any significant difference)
9. Gastric acidity (p. 305)

## SUBSTANCES WHICH INTERFERE WITH CERTAIN LABORATORY TESTS
### (Compiled from various sources)

I. Pheochromocytoma tests
  A. Catecholamines
     Methyldopa (Aldomet)
     Certain "broad-spectrum" antibiotics (tetracyclines, Declomycin)
     Isuprel or epinephrine (inhalation)
     Formaldehyde-forming drugs (Mandelamine, Uritone)
     Quinine or quinidine
     Salicylates
     Large doses of B-complex vitamins
     Poor preservation during collection
     Bananas
     Hydralazine (Apresoline)
  B. Vanilmandelic acid (VMA)
    1. Screening tests (Gitlow method, etc.)
      Tea
      Coffee
      Citrus fruits
      Vanilla
      Bananas
      Chocolate
      Aspirin
      5-hydroxyindolacetic acid (5-HIAA)
    2. Fluorescent techniques
      Broad-spectrum antibiotics (e.g., tetracycline)
      Methyldopa

Quinine or quinidine
Mandelamine
C.  Metanephrines
1.  IVP x-ray media (Pisano method)
2.  Very few specific reports to date; presumably most
compounds which increase catecholamines would in-
crease metanephrines
II.  5-hydroxyindolacetic acid (5-HIAA)
A.  Substances which contain large amounts of serotonin (af-
fects any method)
Tomatoes
Red plums
Avocado
Eggplant
Bananas
B.  Method of Udenfriend
Methocarbamol (Robaxin)
Mephenesin carbamate (several proprietary muscle-
relaxant compounds)
Glyceryl guaiacolate (many proprietary cough medicines)
Phenothiazines (Thorazine, etc.)
P-hydroxyacetanalid
III.  17-hydroxycorticosteroids (17-OH-CS)
Acetone (in urine)                    Monase
Atarax                                Oleandomycin
Chloral hydrate                       Paraldehyde
Colchicine                            Quinine
Fructose (in urine)                   Reserpine
Glucose (in urine)                    Spironolactone
Librium                               Thorazine
Mandelamine
Meprobamate
Estrogens or contraceptive drugs
IV.  17-ketosteroids (17-KS)
Acetone (in urine)                    Oleandomycin
Amphetamine                           Pyridium
Atarax (Vistaril)                     Quinine
Diamox                                Reserpine
Digitoxin                             Seconal
Diuril                                Spironolactone
Doriden                               Thorazine
Librium                               Valmid
Meprobamate
Metabolites of progesterone (in urine)
Nalidixic acid (NegGram)

V. Anticoagulants
  A. Drugs which potentiate Coumadin (increase PT time)

Aldomet (methyldopa)
Anabolic steroids
Analexin (phenyramidol)
Antabuse (disulfiram)
Atromid-S (clofibrate)
Benemid
Butazolidin and Tandearil
Chloral hydrate
Choloxin and cholestyramine
Dilantin
Edecrin (ethacrynic acid)
Estrogens
Glucagon
Indocin
Isoniazid (INH)
MAO inhibitors

Orinase (tolbutamide)
PAS
Ponstel (mefenamic acid)
Quinidine and quinine
Reserpine
Ritalin (methylphenindate)
Salicylates (over 1 Gm./day)
Sulfas
Tempra, Tylenol (acet-
  aminophen)
Thiouracil drugs
Thyroid hormone
Vitamin B complex

Various antibiotics (chloromycetin, Kantrex, tetracycline, penicillin)

  B. Drugs which decrease response to Coumadin (decrease PT time)

Antacids
Barbiturates
Digitalis
Diuretics (except edecrin)
Doriden (glutethimide)
Estrogens
Griseofulvin

Haldol (haloperidol)
Meprobamate
Paraldehyde
Placidyl (ethchlorvynol)
Rimactane (rifampin)
Steroids

  C. Drugs which antagonize action of heparin

Antihistamine (large doses)
Digitalis
Penicillin

Phenothiazines (Thorazine,
  etc.)
Polymyxin-B (Coly-Mycin)
Tetracycline

VI. Drugs which interfere with absorption
  Dilantin: blocks folic acid; decreases $B_{12}$ and D-xylose
  Colchicine: decreases $B_{12}$, carotene, D-xylose
  Neomycin: blocks folic acid; decreases $B_{12}$ and D-xylose

VII. Effects of estrogens (birth control pills)
  Decreases albumin, glucose tolerance, $T_3$ test; may decrease
    folic acid
  Increases transferrin, TBG, and various thyroxine tests, tri-
    glycerides, total lipids, serum iron, iron-binding capacity,
    plasma cortisol, urine aldosterone, serum alpha-2 globulins,
    growth hormone, alpha-1 antitrypsin, neutrophil alkaline
    phosphatase
  Potentiates Coumadin (increases PT time); invalidates
    metyrapone test

VIII.  Technicon Autoanalyzer drug effects
       SGOT increased by diabetic acidosis, PAS, Vistaril, barbitu-
          rates
       Glucose increased by reducing substances (15 mg./100 ml.
          creatinine plus 10 mg./100 ml. uric acid raises glucose
          20 mg./100 ml.)
       Lipemia decreases cholesterol, bilirubin, albumin, LDH,
          alkaline phosphatase
  IX.  Miscellaneous
       Alkaline phosphatase: increased by many brands of human
          serum albumin (derived from placental tissue)
       SGOT: erythromycin increases colorimetric method, but not
          UV methods
       Heparin: antagonized by ascorbic acid; increases thyroxine
          temporarily
       Plasma cortisol: spironolactone produces increase by fluoro-
          metric method
       Urine estriol: false positive from glucosuria, urinary tract
          infection, Mandelamine
       Porphobilinogen: false positive from phenothiazines
   X.  Digitalis
       A.  Conditions which decrease digitalis requirements
           Renal failure (BUN over 50 mg./100 ml.; decreased
              digitalis excretion)
           Hemodialysis
           Hypothyroidism
           Liver disease (hypokalemia and thiamine deficiency)
           Hypokalemia (diuretic therapy, cirrhosis, diabetic acidosis,
              etc.)
       B.  Drugs which potentiate digitalis effects
           Adrenergic drugs (ephedrin,      Propranolol
              Isuprel, etc.).               Quinidine
           Calcium intravenous              Serpasil (reserpine)
              therapy                        Thyroid hormone
           Dilantin
           Diuretics
           Insulin
           Ismelin (guanethidine)
           Laxatives (prolonged use)
  XI.  Drugs which affect kidney function
       Amphotericin B
       Cephaloridine
       Diuretics
       Guanethidine (Ismelin)
       Indomethacin (Indocin)
       Kanamycin
       Methacillin
       Methyldopa (Aldomet)

Neomycin
Polymyxin B or colistin
Tetracyclines (intravenous)
XII. Serum cholinesterase (decrease)
Atropine
Barbiturates
Chloroquin
Epinephrine
Opiates
Phenothiazines
Prostigmine
Quinidine
XIII. Effects of ascorbic acid (vitamin C)
Increases tests which depend on reducing-substance reactions
  such as:
Creatinine
Glucose by Folin-Wu, ferricyanide or neocuproine methods
Uric acid
Urine glucose by Benedict's or Clinitest methods
Interferes with blood volume determination using RBC tagging.
XIV. Drugs which may affect liver function
  A. Exclusively cholestatic (androgenic/anabolic steroids,
      estrogens)
     Dianabol (methandrostenolone)
     Enovid (norethynodrel)
     Halotestin (methyltestosterone)
     Nilevar (norethandrolone)
     Norlutin (norethindrone)
  B. Cholestatic plus hepatocellular toxic component
     Butazolidine                 Nicotinic acid
     Dilantin                     Nilevar (nortestosterone)
     Ilosone                      Phenothiazines (Thorazine)
     Librium                      Tapazole (methimazole)
     Marsalid (iproniazid)        Tetracycline (intravenous)
     Meprobamate
  C. Cytotoxic
     Diabinase (chlorpropamide)   Nitrogen mustards
     Dialose (laxative)           Novobiocin
     Gold salts                   Oxacillin
     Halothane                    Oxyphenisatin acetate (stool
     Imuran (azathioprine)          softener ingredient)
     Indocin                      PAS
     Isoniazide (INH)             Probenecid
     Methotrexate                 Phenurone (phenacetylurea)
     Methyldopa                   Zoxazolamine (Flexin)
     Monamine oxidase inhibitor
       (Marsalid, Nardil)

D.  Reported but not in detail

Allopurinol                  Papaverine
Carbenicillin                Procainamide
Clofibrate                   Rifampin
Florantyrone                 Thiothixene
Lincomycin                   Tolazamide
Metaxalone                   Troleandomycin

XV.  Digitalis assay

Current reports indicate that when oral digoxin is given, serum digoxin levels used to monitor therapy should be obtained just prior to the daily dose and not sooner than 6 hours after a previous dose.

References:

Martin, E. W. , et al. : Hazards of Medication (Philadelphia: J. B. Lippincott Co. , 1971).

Sode, J. , and Walsh, F. M. : CAP-ASCP Annual Meeting, October 1972.

Sunderman, F. W. , Jr. : Drug interference in clinical biochemistry, CRC Crit. Rev. in Clin. Lab. Sc. 1:427, 1970.

Young, D. S. , et al. : Effects of drugs on clinical laboratory tests, Clin. Chem. 18:1041, 1972.

NORMAL (AVERAGE) BLOOD VALUES AT VARIOUS AGES
(Compiled from various sources)

|  | Birth | 5 days | 2 weeks | 3 months | 6 months | 2 years | 8 years |
|---|---|---|---|---|---|---|---|
| Red blood cells (millions/cu.mm.) | 5.5 | 5.5 | 5.0 | 4.1 | 4.5 | 4.8 | 5.0 |
| Hemoglobin (Gm. /100 ml.) | 18.0 | 18.0 | 17.0 | 11.0 | 11.5 | 13.0 | 14.0 |
| White blood cells (thousands/cu.mm.) | 16.0 | 20.0 | 12.0 | 10.0 | 9.5 | 9.0 | 8.0 |
| Platelets (thousands/cu.mm.) | 350.0 | 400.0 | 300.0 | 260.0 | 250.0 | 250.0 | 250.0 |
| Differential on peripheral blood |  |  |  |  |  |  |  |
| % Neutrophils | 45 | 55 | 35 | 35 | 40 | 40 | 60 |
| % Lymphocytes | 25 | 20 | 55 | 55 | 53 | 50 | 30 |
| Nucleated RBC (per 100 WBC) | 5 | 3 | 0 | 0 | 0 | 0 | 0 |

LABORATORY DIFFERENCES IN PROTHROMBIN TIME (PT TIME)
DUE TO REAGENTS FROM DIFFERENT MANUFACTURERS
Suggested "Therapeutic Ranges" for
Various Thromboplastins*

| Thromboplastin | Suggested Therapeutic Range (Seconds) |
|---|---|
| 1. Thrombotime (Pfizer) | 23 -29.5 |
| 2. Manchester (Poller) | 25 -41.0 |
| 3. Dried (Hyland) | 20 -27.0 |
| 4. Fibroplastin (BioQuest) | 19 -28.0 |
| 5. Simplastin (Warner-Lambert) | 20 -29.0 |
| 6. Brain (Ortho) | 18 -24.5 |
| 7. Dried (Dade) | 16.5-21.5 |
| 8. Activated (Dade) | 13.5-18.0 |
| 9. Simplastin-A (Warner-Lambert) | 20.0-29.0 |

*Each is equivalent to a range of 10 to 20% reduction in the coagulation factors affected by oral anticoagulants.
(From Miale, J. B., and Kent, J. W.: Standardization of the therapeutic range for oral anticoagulants based on standard reference plasmas, Am. J. Clin. Path. 57:80, 1972 [Table 8]).

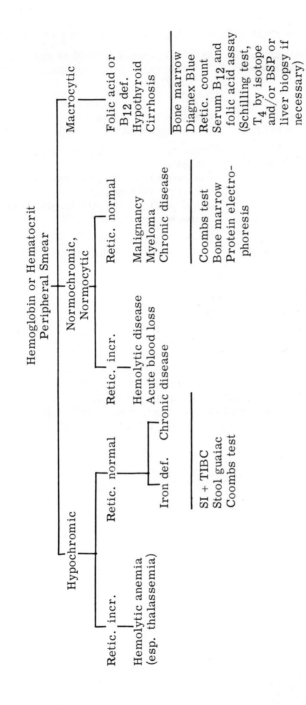

SIMPLIFIED GUIDE TO ANEMIA DIAGNOSIS USING A MINIMUM OF
TESTS—AIMED AT MOST IMPORTANT DISEASE CATEGORIES

Hemoglobin or Hematocrit
Peripheral Smear

Hypochromic

Retic. incr.

Hemolytic anemia
(esp. thalassemia)

Retic. normal

Iron def.    Chronic disease

SI + TIBC
Stool guaiac
Coombs test

Normochromic,
Normocytic

Retic. incr.

Hemolytic disease
Acute blood loss
Chronic disease

Retic. normal

Malignancy
Myeloma
Chronic disease

Coombs test
Bone marrow
Protein electro-
phoresis

Macrocytic

Folic acid or
B$_{12}$ def.
Hypothyroid
Cirrhosis

Bone marrow
Diagnex Blue
Retic. count
Serum B$_{12}$ and
folic acid assay
(Schilling test,
T$_4$ by isotope
and/or BSP or
liver biopsy if
necessary)

## SERUM IRON (SI) AND TOTAL IRON-BINDING CAPACITY (TIBC)

| | |
|---|---|
| SI decreased;<br>TIBC decreased | Chronic diseases (including chronic infections, cirrhosis, rheumatoid-collagen, nonbleeding cancer)<br>Uremia |
| SI decreased;<br>TIBC increased | Iron deficiency anemia<br>Pregnancy in third trimester |
| SI increased;<br>TIBC decreased | Hemachromatosis (a minority say that the TIBC is increased)<br>Iron therapy overload (TIBC may be normal)<br>Hemolysis (if severe)<br>*Hemolysis (mild); thalassemia; lead poisoning; sideroachrestic anemia |
| SI increased;<br>TIBC increased | Estrogen medication<br>Acute hepatitis (some report TIBC low normal) |

*SI may be normal or (more often) increased; TIBC may be normal or increased

Notes:
1. There is considerable (rather inexplicable) difference of opinion in the literature, sometimes quite contradictory, on findings in a variety of conditions
2. SI has diurnal variation, highest values in A. M. ; some report considerable day-to-day variation
3. Combination of disease may exist; e. g. , chronic blood loss anemia (which increases TIBC) superimposed on some other chronic disease (which depresses TIBC)

## NEPHRITOGENIC STRAINS OF
## LANCEFIELD GROUP A STREPTOCOCCI

4
12 (most frequent)
18
25
Red Lake

## ENTEROPATHOGENIC STRAINS OF E. COLI
## (SEROTYPES REPORTED TO CAUSE INFANT DIARRHEA)

O26:B6
O55:B5
O86:B7
O111:B4
O119:B11
O119:B17
O125:B15
O126:B16
O127:B8
O127:B12

Note:  O refers to somatic antigen; B refers to one of the
       "capsule" antigens

## THE WIDAL TEST—SEROLOGIC GROUPS (O ANTIGENS)
## OF THE PATHOGENIC SALMONELLAE

| Group | Organism |
|---|---|
| A | Paratyphi A |
| B | Paratyphi B<br>Typhimurium |
| C | Paratyphi C<br>Choleraesuis<br>Newport |
| D | Typhi (Typhosa)<br>Enteritidis<br>Sendai |
| E | Anatum |

## CLASSIFICATION OF ENTEROBACTERIACEAE

| TRIBE | GENERA |
|---|---|
| Escherichieae | Escherichia (incl. E. coli and<br>    Alkalescens-Dispar)<br>Shigella |
| Edwardsielleae | Edwardsiella |
| Salmonelleae | Salmonella<br>Arizona<br>Citrobacter (incl. E. freundii) |
| Klebsielleae | Klebsiella<br>Enterobacter (formerly Aerobacter)<br>Serratia |
| Proteeae | Proteus<br>Providencia (Proteus inconstans) |

Reference:

Douglas, G. W., and Washington, J. A.: Identification of
    Enterobacteriaceae in the Clinical Laboratory (Atlanta:
    Microbiology Branch, National Communicable Disease
    Center, 1969)

## DISTRIBUTION OF MONOCLONAL GAMMOPATHIES

| Disease | % of Total |
|---|---|
| Multiple Myeloma ...................... | 65% |
|    IgG = 60% | |
|    IgA = 25% | |
|    Bence-Jones | |
|     only = 14% | |
| Waldenström's ........................ | 10 |
| Franklin's disease.................... | 1 |
|   (Heavy chain disease) | |
| Lymphomas and leukemias .............. | 6 |
| Cancer ............................... | 8 |
| Not associated with neoplasia ........... | 10 |

References:

Osserman, E., and Takatsuki, K.: Plasma
cell myeloma: Gamma globulin synthesis
and structure, Medicine 42:357, 1963.

Mattioli, C., and Tomasi, T. B., Jr.: Human Serum Immunoglobulins, in Disease-
a-Month (Chicago: Year Book Medical
Publishers, Inc., April 1970).

### RHEUMATOID FACTOR TESTS
(Average % positive and reports from various publications)

|  | Rose-Waaler Sensitized Sheep Cell | Plotz-Singer Latex | Hyland RA Test | Eosin Slide |
|---|---|---|---|---|
| Adult RA | 64% (58-78)* | 76% (53-94) | 82% (78-98) | 90% (88-92) |
| Normal | 5.6 (0.3-13) | 1.0 (0.2-3) | 8 (0.7-15) | 5 (0.2-8.6) |
| Collagen disease | 15-39 | 17-20 | 14-67 | 10-50 |
| Procedure | Tube | Tube | Slide | Slide |

*Numbers in parentheses refer to the range of values found in different reports.

## TESTS FOR SYSTEMIC LUPUS ERYTHEMATOSIS (S. L. E.)
### (Approximate % positive)

| | SLE | Scleroderma | Other Collagen Diseases | Rheumatoid Arthritis | Other |
|---|---|---|---|---|---|
| L. E. cell | 60-80 | 0-20 | <5 | 5-25 | Lupoid hepatitis drugs (hydralazine, procainamide) |
| Antinuclear antibody | 95-100 | 75-80 | 10 | 10-50 | Chronic liver disease Thyroid disease Acquired hemolytic anemia Old age |
| Serum complement (C') | Low in 60% with active disease | Normal (rarely low) | Normal or high | Normal or high | Normal |

## USEFUL FLUID AND ELECTROLYTE INFORMATION
### (Compiled from various sources)

Normal Daily Output

Insensible loss (skin and lungs)—600-1000 ml./day
Urine—500-1500 ml./day

Average Composition of Certain Body Fluids ($\pm$ 20%)

|  | Na | K | Cl (mEq. /L.) |
|---|---|---|---|
| Gastric | 50 | 10 | 100 |
| Bile | 150 | 5 | 100 |
| Small intestine | 100 | 5 | 100 |
| Perspiration (visible sweating) | 30 | 0 | 30 |

Normal Production of Certain Body Fluids

| Saliva | 500-1500 ml./day |
|---|---|
| Gastric | 1000-3000 ml./day |
| Bile | 300-1000 ml./day |
| Pancreas | 1000-1500 ml./day |
| Small intestine | 1000-2000 ml./day |
| Visible sweating (at bed rest and/or high fever) | 1000-2000 ml./day |

Note: Normally, most GI secretions (fluid and electrolytes) are re-absorbed before they reach the rectum.

Daily Nutritional Requirements:

A. Caloric requirements
1st 10 kg. body weight: 100 calories/kg.
10-20 kg. body weight: 100 calories plus 50 calories for
every kg. over 10
Over 20 kg. body weight: 1500 calories plus 20 calories for
every kg. over 20

B. Fluid requirements
1 ml. fluid for every calorie needed

C. Electrolyte requirements
Na: 3 mEq. /100 cal.
K:  2 mEq. /100 cal.
Cl: 2 mEq. /100 cal.

## DATA FOR DIABETES TOLERANCE TESTS

I.  Oral Glucose Tolerance Test

The ideal body weight dosage which may be used for adults is
1.75 Gm./kg.  For infants and children, 2.5 Gm./kg. up to
age 1 1/2; then 2.0 Gm./kg. up to age 3 years has been recommended.

II. Intravenous Glucose Tolerance Test

Most investigators use a standard dose of glucose (in a 50%
solution) amounting to 1/3 Gm./kg. of ideal body weight.
Some use a standard dose of 25 Gm., regardless of weight.
For children, the recommended dose is 0.5 Gm./kg.

III. Cortisone-Glucose Tolerance Test

After a standard 3-day carbohydrate diet, oral cortisone acetate is given 8 1/2 hours and again at 2 hours before the test
glucose dose.  A person over 160 lb. gets 62.5 mg. cortisone
and under 160 lb. 50 mg. (at each time period).  Afterward,
the standard oral GTT is performed.  Normal values are less
than 160 mg./100 ml. at 1 hour, 150 mg./100 ml. at 1 1/2
hours, and less than 140 mg./100 ml. at 2 hours (whole blood).

IV. Tolbutamide Tolerance Test for Diabetes

Inject 20 ml. of sterile "Orinase Diagnostic" (1 Gm. of water-
soluble sodium tolbutamide) intravenously over 2-3 minutes'
time.  Blood samples are taken fasting and at 20 and 30 minutes after tolbutamide.  At 20 minutes, normal values are
less than 75% of FBS.  Between 75 and 85% (of FBS) is considered borderline, between 85 and 89% highly suspicious
(90% of patients in this group have diabetes), and over 89%
are thought to show definite diabetes.  At 30 minutes, over
76% of FBS is said to be virtually (99%) diagnostic.  Either
the 20 or 30 minute value is diagnostic when within the diabetic zone, even if the other is not.

Note:  These are not the normal values to be used when
investigating hypoglycemia.

COMPOUNDS THAT INTERFERE WITH RESULTS OF THYROID TESTS

| | PBI | | RAI | | T₃ |
|---|---|---|---|---|---|
| | Effect | Duration | Effect | Duration | Effect |
| **Inorganic Iodides** | | | | | |
| Lugol's, KI, SSKI, etc. | Incr. | 1-4 wk. | Decr. | 1-3 wk. | None |
| Ornade | | | | | |
| **Organic Iodine** | | | | | |
| 1) X-ray contrast media | | | | | |
| Teridax (gallbladder) | Incr. | 30 yr. | None | | None |
| Cholografin (gallbladder) | Incr. | 3-4 mo. | Decr. | 3 mo. | None |
| Telepaque (gallbladder) | Incr. | 6-12 wk. | Decr. | 2 mo. | None |
| Diodrast | Incr. | 2 wk. | Decr. | 1-3 mo. | None |
| Dionosil (bronchogram) | Incr. | 1-5 mo. | Decr. | 2-5 mo. | None |
| Lipiodol (bronchogram) | Incr. | 1-2 yr. | Decr. | 1-3 yr. | None |
| Pantopaque (myelogram) | Incr. | 3-12 mo. | Decr. | 3-12 mo. | None |
| Hypaque (IVP) | Incr. | 4-7 days | Decr. | 1-2 wk. | None |
| Renografin (IVP) | Incr. | 1-4 wk. (?) | Decr. | 1-2 wk. | None |
| Salpix (uterosalpingogram) | Incr. | 2 wk. | Decr. | 1 mo. | None |
| 2) Iodinated vaginal suppositories | | | | | |
| Floraquin, Vioform, etc. | Incr. | 4 wk. | Decr. | 4 wk. | None |
| **Other Medications** | | | | | |
| Thyroxine | Incr. | 2-4 wk. | Decr. | 1-2 wk. | Incr. |
| Thyroid extract | Incr. | 4-6 wk. | Decr. | 1-2 wk. | Incr. |
| Iodothiouracil | Incr. | sev. wk. | Decr. | 2-8 days | Decr. |
| Estrogens | Incr. | 2-4 wk. | Occ. Incr. | | Decr./Nl. |
| Triiodothyronine (T₃) | Decr. | 2-4 wk. | Decr. | ? | Incr. |
| Propylthiouracil or Tapazole | Decr. | 5-7 days | Decr. | 2-8 days | Decr. |
| Thiocyanate | Decr. | 2-3 wk. | Decr. | 2-8 days | Decr. |
| Dilantin | Decr. | 7-10 days | None | | Incr. |
| Androgens | Decr. | 3 wk. | None | | Incr. |
| Adrenal corticoids or ACTH | Decr. | 1-2 wk. | Decr. | 1 wk. | Incr. |
| Salicylates (large doses) | Decr. | ? | Decr. | ? | Incr. |
| Phenylbutazone | Decr. | 2 wk. | Decr. | ? | Incr. |
| Perphenazine (Trilafon) after 6-10 weeks' treatment | Occ. Incr. | | ? | | Occ. Decr. |
| Chlorpromazine (Thorazine) | None | | Decr. | ? | None (?) |
| Mercurial diuretics | Decr.* | 1-3 days | ? | | None |
| Thiazide diuretics | Decr.# | ? | None | | None |
| Antihistamines (without iodine) | None | | Decr. | 2-7 days | None |
| Orinase | None | | Decr. | 2-7 days | None |
| Dicumarol or heparin | None | | None | | Incr. |
| Sulfonamides | Decr. (?) | ? | Decr. | 1 wk. | ? |
| PAS or isoniazid (prolonged Rx) | Occ. Decr. | | Decr. | 1-2 wk. | ? |
| Pentothal | ? | | Decr. | 1 wk. | ? |
| Penicillin (large doses only) | None | | None | | Incr. |
| Gold salts | Decr. | sev. wk. | None | | None |
| Metrecal | Incr.## | ? | ? | | ? |
| Lithium carbonate | Decr. | ? | Incr. | ? | ? |

*The alkaline (dry) ash PBI method is not affected.
#Not affected by 2-3 days therapy.
##BEI is also increased.

There is disagreement as to whether or not the PBI or RAI is affected by the minute amounts of inorganic iodide in the barium sulfate used for x-rays. Because of this uncertainty, and the possibility of excessive iodine contamination of individual supply lots of barium sulfate, it may be advisable, in the interest of accuracy, to withhold a PBI or RAI for a week after performance of a GI series or a barium enema. Blood contaminated with bromsulphalein (BSP) dye should not be submitted for a PBI study. Interference by BSP is related to the percentage retained in the serum, and also to occasional organic iodine contamination of individual supply lots.

(From Ravel, R.: Bulletin of Pathology 8:172, 1967.)

## PLASMA RENIN

Plasma renin determination may be very helpful in the diagnosis (or exclusion) of primary aldosteronism. However, in order to interpret results, it is necessary to keep in mind certain technical aspects of current methods. Renin is an enzyme. Most enzymes cannot be measured directly, but are estimated indirectly by observing their effect on a known quantity of substrate. In the case of renin, the situation is even more complex, since the substrate (which results in production of angiotensin) cannot be directly measured and must be estimated indirectly by observing its effect on an indicator system and comparing the results with a known amount of angiotensin. In addition, renin is a very unstable enzyme and must be kept at freezing temperature as much as possible to preserve its activity. Collection methods are very important; if the specimen is not collected and processed correctly, a false low value may result.

One possible collection protocol is outlined below. It incorporates a provocative test-low sodium diet plus upright posture—to help differentiate primary from secondary aldosteronism. Urinary aldosterone determinations should not be collected during a low-salt diet because sodium deficiency stimulates aldosterone secretion. In fact, urine sodium should be obtained on all aldosterone specimens as a check on possible sodium deficiency. The protocol, therefore, incorporates a section with a high salt diet to insure proper collection of aldosterone. If desired, a plasma renin specimen may be obtained during this time to help rule out unilateral renal disease. If unilateral renal disease is not a possibility, step 2 may be omitted. If aldosterone collection is not desired, steps 1-3 may be omitted.

### Protocol for Plasma Renin and Urine Aldosterone

1. Patient off medications, placed on 9 Gm. (180 mEq.) high sodium (normal potassium) diet for 4 days. (Note: can use normal diet plus 6 Gm. salt tablets extra per day).
2. Fasting plasma renin specimen drawn the morning of the fourth day before patient stands or sits up (specimen #1). (Note: this can be omitted if unilateral renal disease screening is not desired).
3. Twenty-four-hour urine for aldosterone and sodium collected during the fourth day. (Note: can also get metanephrine determination on the same specimen to rule out pheochromocytoma).
4. Patient then placed on a 0.5 Gm. (10 mEq.) low sodium (normal potassium) diet for 3 days.
5. After awakening the morning of the fourth day, the fasting patient is placed upright (standing or leaning; not allowed to sit or lie down) for 2 hours. Lab notified when the 2-hour period will end; patient kept upright until lab draws blood specimen.

6.  Plasma renin specimen drawn while patient is still upright (specimen #2); test ends.

Note:  Heparinized collection tube is placed in ice water before obtaining the specimen and kept in ice bath as long as possible before actually drawing the blood.  The tourniquet should be released for a few seconds before blood is drawn, since it has been reported that venous stasis may decrease blood renin.  The tube is returned to the ice bath immediately after the specimen is drawn and kept in ice water.  The tube is centrifuged still packed in ice; the plasma withdrawn, frozen immediately, and sent to the reference laboratory packed in dry ice (do not send specimen on week end).

A high sodium diet decreases aldosterone secretion in normal persons.  In patients with hypertension due to primary aldosteronism or unilateral renal disease, aldosterone is elevated.  Plasma renin should be decreased in normal persons and those with primary aldosteronism, and increased in hypertension due to unilateral renal disease.  A low sodium diet should confirm results.  Renin levels should be high in normal persons, whereas the previous elevation of renin seen in unilateral renal disease remains elevated and the decrease seen in primary aldosteronism remains decreased.

References:

Bath, N. M., et al.:  Plasma renin activity in renovascular hypertension, Am. J. Med. 45:381, 1968.

Conn, J. W.:  Aldosteronism in hypertensive disease, M. Times 98:116, 1970.

Conn, J. W., et al.:  Preoperative diagnosis of primary aldosteronism, Arch. Int. Med. 123:113, 1969.

SURVEY OF PREGNANCY TESTS

| Test | Type | Time | Sensitivity (% Pregnant Women Detected) | | Accuracy (% Negative in Nonpregnant Women) | | Sensitivity (Nonconc. Urine IU/L.) | Protein | Affected by: Phenothiazines | Other |
|---|---|---|---|---|---|---|---|---|---|---|
| | | | Average | Range | Average | Range | | | | |
| Gravindex | Slide | 2 min. | 92.5% | 70-99% | 98% | 92-100% | 3000 | Yes | No++ | |
| Hyland HCG | Slide | 2 min. | 83 | 50-94 | 94 | 93-100 | 2000 | Yes | Yes | |
| Natatel | Slide | 2 min. | - | 95 | - | 100 (?) | ? | No | No | |
| Pregslide | Slide | 2 min. | - | 91-96 | - | 95.3-98.7 | 3000 | Yes | Yes | |
| DAP | Slide | 2 min. | - | 97 | - | 97 | 2000 | No++ | No++ | ## |
| Prequest | Slide | 2 min. | - | 96 | - | 96 | 5000 | ? | ? | |
| Prognosis | Slide | 2 min. | 96.5 | 96.2-97.1 | 99 | 98.9-100 | 2000 | No | No** | |
| Planotest (Pregnosticon slide) | Slide | 2 min. | 98.5 | 98-99 | 98.5 | 96.0-99.5 | 2500 | No | No | |
| Pregnosticon Dri-Dot | Slide | 2 min. | - | 100 | - | 94 | 1000-2000 | ? | ? | |
| Pregnosticon | Tube | 2 hr. | 98.5 | 86-100 | 99 | 97-100 | 1000 | No | Occ. | |
| Pregnosticon-Accusphere | Tube | 2 hr. | - | 98 | - | 90 | 750-1000 | No | ? | |
| UCG | Tube | 2 hr. | 93.5 | 69-97 | 96 | 90-100 | 2000 | No | No | |
| Prepurin | Tube | 2 hr. | 98.5 | 96-99 | 97 | 94-100 | 4000 | ? | No | |
| Twentisec | Chemical-color | 20 sec. | - | 89.5 | - | 94 | ? | ? | ? | * |
| LPT | Chemical-color | 5 min. | - | 93** | - | 93** | ? | ? | Yes | *# |
| A-Z | Mouse | 96 hr. | 98 | 83-100 | 98 | 90-100 | 600-700 | ? | ? | |
| Friedman | Rabbit | 48 hr. | 98 | 86-100 | 99 | 95-100 | 1000-5000 | ? | ? | |
| Frog, male | Frog | 2 hr. | 94-97 | 62-100 | 98 | 93-100 | 1000-5000+ | ? | Yes | |
| Frog, female | Toad | 2 hr. | 90-97 | 80-99 | 99 | 78-100 | 1000-5000+ | ? | Yes | |

No average % accuracy given if fewer than 3 evaluations.
+Concentrated; 3-5 times less sensitive unconcentrated (Postgrad. Med. 42:A-48, 1967).
*False positive results with oral contraceptives.
++One report differs from others.
**Manufacturer's data only available.
#False positive results in some persons with hepatitis or with salicylate or chloramphenicol therapy.
##One report indicates high incidence of false positive reactions in postmenopausal women.

## LIPID STORAGE DISEASES

| Disease | Lipid | WBC | Diagnosis by: Fibroblast Culture | Liver Biopsy |
|---|---|---|---|---|
| **A. Glycolipid Storage Diseases** | | | | |
|   1. Ganglioside storage | | | | |
|     Tay-Sachs | $G_{m-2}$ | No | Yes | No |
|     Tay-Sachs variant | Globoside and | ? | Yes | Yes |
|     (hexosamidase A+B deficiency) | $G_{m-2}$ | | | |
|     Metachromatic | Sulfatide | Yes | ? | Yes |
|     leukodystrophy | | | | |
|     Generalized gangliosidosis | $G_{m-1}$ | Yes | ? | Yes |
|   2. Ceramide storage | | | | |
|     Gaucher's | Glucosyl | Yes | Yes | Yes |
|     Krabbe's | Galactosyl | Yes | ? | Yes |
|     (globoid leukodystrophy) | | | | |
|     Fabrey's | Trihexoside | Yes | ? | Yes |
|     Lactosyl ceramidosis | Lactosyl | No | Yes | Yes |
|     Niemann-Pick | Sphingomyelin | Yes | ? | Yes |
| **B. Other Lipid Storage Diseases** | | | | |
|   Wolman's* | Triglyceride (neutral lipid) and cholesterol esters | No | ? | Yes |
|   Refsum's+ | Phytanic acid | No | Yes | Yes |

*Calcification in adrenals on x-ray is typical.
+Plasma fatty acids can be analyzed for phytanic acid.

References:
Brady, R. O.: The genetic mismanagement of complex lipid metabolism, Bull. New York Acad. Med. 47:173, 1971.
Danes, B. S.: The use of WBC cultures in the study of genetic metabolic disease, Hosp. Practice 5:52, 1970.

## DISORDERS OF CONNECTIVE TISSUE
(Mucopolysaccharidoses)

| Name | Physical Anomalies | Mental Deficiency | Urinary Mucopolysaccharides |
|------|--------------------|--------------------|------------------------------|
| Hurler | Marked | Moderate | Dermatan sulfate (chondroitin sulfate B) Heparan (heparitin) sulfate (approx. 2:1) |
| Hunter | Moderate | Variable or none | Dermatan sulfate Heparan sulfate (approx. 1:1) |
| Sanfillipo A and B | Mild | Marked | Heparan sulfate |
| Morquio | Marked | None | Keratan sulfate |
| Scheie | Mild | None | Dermatan sulfate Heparan sulfate (approx. 2:1) |
| Maroteaux-Lamy | Moderate | None | Dermatan sulfate |
| "Atypical" | Moderate | None | ? |

Note: All are transmitted as autosomal recessive except for Hunter, which is sex-linked.

References:

Neufield, E. F.: Mucopolysaccharidoses: The biochemical approach, Hosp. Practice 7:107, 1972.
McKusick, V. A., et al.: The genetic mucopolysaccharidoses, Medicine 44:1, 1965.

## SELECTED SKIN TESTS

| Disease | Test | Antigen | Time | Positive |
|---|---|---|---|---|
| Brucellosis | Brucella | Brucellergen (killed bacteria) | 24-48 hr. | Over 5 mm. reaction |
| Tularemia | Foshay | Killed bacteria | 48 hr. | Over 5 mm. reaction |
| Lymphogranuloma venereum | Frei | Killed virus | 48 hr. | (P. 195) |
| Echinococcosis | Casoni | Fluid from hydatid cyst | 15-30 min. | "Immediate" reaction |
| Scarlet fever | Schultz-Charlton | Antitoxin | 24 hr. | Blanched area |
| Diphtheria susceptibility | Schick | Diphtheria toxin | 3-6 days | Reaction over 10 mm. |
| Scarlet fever susceptibility | Dick | Erythrogenic toxin | 24 hr. | Reaction over 10 mm. |
| Sarcoidosis | Kveim | Sarcoid tissue | 6 weeks | (P. 237) |
| Tuberculosis | Mantoux | PPD or OT | 24-48 hr. | (Pp. 167-168) |
| Systemic fungal infection | Histoplasmin, etc. | Killed fungi | 48 hr. | (Pp. 178-180) |
| Trichinosis | Trichinella | Killed larvae | 15 min. | (P. 201) |

## CURRENT AVAILABILITY OF SPECIAL
## LABORATORY PROCEDURES

It is difficult to obtain certain tests, either because of unusual technical complexity or because the test is currently new and not yet widely accepted. Therefore, it may be useful to have the names and addresses of several United States laboratories which advertise facilities to provide these tests.

The following points must be emphasized:

1. This listing is not an endorsement. The author does not guarantee results from any of these laboratories, and has not checked any of them for accuracy.
2. More laboratories than the ones listed may provide identical services. These are only the ones presently known to the author.

Bio Science Laboratories
7600 Tyrone Avenue
Van Nuys, Calif. 91405

Bio-Assay Laboratory
P. O. Box 6113
Dallas, Texas 75222

Biochemical Procedures
12020 Chandler Boulevard
North Hollywood, Calif. 91607

Reference Laboratory
12926 Saticoy
North Hollywood, Calif. 91609

Inter Science Institute
2000 Cotner Avenue
Los Angeles, Calif. 90025

Linden Laboratories, Inc.
731 West Peachtree Street N. E.
Atlanta, Ga. 30308

Leary Laboratory, Inc.
43 Bay State Road
Boston, Mass. 02215

Clin-Chem Laboratories
1106 Commonwealth Avenue
Boston, Mass. 02215

Laboratory Medicine Data
P. O. Box 22282
Houston, Texas 77027

New England Nuclear Corp.
Biomedical Assay Laboratories Div.
15 Harvard Street
Worchester, Mass. 01608

Bioanalysis
1701 Berkeley Street
Santa Monica, Calif. 90404

Center for Laboratory Medicine
16 Pearl Street
Metuchen, N. J. 08840

United Medical Laboratories
Portland, Oregon

## SPECIMEN COLLECTION

To a pathologist, nothing is quite as upsetting as listening to an outraged complaint about laboratory results and tracing the difficulty to improper specimen collection. Sometimes this is the correct specimen but not collected at the proper time or in the proper way. Even when these criteria are met, the specimen may appear in the laboratory with inadequate identification or instructions, or be delayed in transit enough to cause damage. Finally, at times the test or specimen ordered is not what would be best in the particular situation. It is surprising, although understandable, how one can order the most complicated series of diagnostic manipulations and not realize that the specimens on which all results depend are being collected by personnel who may not have the slightest idea how to perform their task. Even when collection routine is optimum, the patient may be confused, incontinent, or otherwise fail to provide the specimen in its entirety without close supervision. This is especially important for 24-hour collections. In some cases, such as PSP, BSP, or clearance tests, exact timing to the minute is essential to calculate results.

24-Hour Urine Specimens: The patient should void; the collection period begins when this is completed. At the end of the time period, the patient voids, and this specimen is added to the others collected during the time period. Most 24-hour urine specimens should be refrigerated or kept in an ice water bath during the collection, to control bacterial growth. In some cases, a preservative may be added instead.

It is usually advisable to have a creatinine excretion determination done in order to provide an additional check on completeness of collection. A 24-hour creatinine value below normal range suggests incomplete collection. Although there is moderate fluctuation in daily excretion, 24-hour cretainine values should vary less than 10-15% from day to day.

Fresh specimens are needed in some cases, such as culture, cytology, or enzyme tests.

A partial list of special collection situations discussed in the book are noted below.

ALA, p. 241.
Aldosterone (urine), p. 452.
Bacterial culture, routine, p. 170.
Bacterial meningitis, p. 207.
Blood culture, pp. 170; 173-174.
Blood sugar, pp. 315-318.
Cryptococcus, p. 207.
Cytomegalic inclusion disease, p. 190.
Entameba histolytica, p. 199.
Fungus culture, p. 180.
Gastric contents for cytology, p. 384.

Growth hormone, p. 366.
Hemolysis effects on blood specimens (on LDH, p. 232).
Lactic acid, p. 423.
Lipoproteins, p. 260.
Renin, p. 452.
Sputum for cytology, p. 386.
Trichomonas, p. 201.
Tuberculosis culture (urine, p. 131; sputum and gastric, p. 167).
Urine culture, p. 170-172.
Urine urobilinogen, p. 124.
Venous blood pH specimens, p. 275.
Virus culture, pp. 185-187.

## TABLE OF REPRESENTATIVE NORMAL VALUES

This section appears reluctantly, because there are usually several methods for assaying any substance, and each method has different normal values; for example, enzyme procedures have different values depending on the temperature and conditions of assay. In addition, modifications of every basic technique inevitably appear (sometimes modifications of modifications), each with its own normal range. Nevertheless, there seems to be sufficient demand for a normal-value table to justify providing one here. The figures listed represent "classic" procedures. The values are in some cases rounded off in order to be representative, rather than exact transcription of a single method. In some cases the reader is referred to passages in the text. Each laboratory must provide normal values for the particular techniques that it uses.

A.   Blood
   1.   Chemistry

| | |
|---|---|
| A/G ratio | 1.5-2.5 |
| Albumin | 4.0-5.5 Gm./100 ml. (Biuret) |
| | 3.5-5.0 Gm./100 ml. (electrophoresis) |
| Ammonia | 30-70 $\mu$g./100 ml. |
| Bilirubin: total | 0.2-1.5 mg./100 ml. |
|         direct | 0.1-0.5 mg./100 ml. |
| BSP (45 min.) | 0-5% |
| BUN | 10-20 mg./100 ml. |
| Calcium | 8.5-10.5 mg./100 ml. |
| Ceph. floc. (24 hr.) | 0-1+ |
| Chloride | 96-106 mEq./L. |
| Cholesterol: total | 150-300 mg./100 ml. (p. 257) |
|         esters | 65-75% |
| $CO_2$ (comb. power) | 20-30 mEq./L. |
| Cortisol, plasma | 5-20 g./100 ml. |
| Creatinine, serum | 0.8-2.0 mg./100 ml. |

| | |
|---|---|
| Globulin | 1.2-3.0 Gm./100 ml. |
| Glucose tolerance test, oral | (p. 319) |
| Iron, serum | 60-150 mg./100 ml. |
| Iron-binding capacity | 250-350 mg./100 ml. |
| Lipids: total | 400-1000 mg./100 ml. |
|       phospholipids | 200-300 mg./100 ml. |
|       triglycerides | 30-190 mg./100 ml. (p. 257) |
| Magnesium | 1.5-2.5 mEq./L. |
| Osmolality, serum | 285-300 mOsm./L. |
| Phosphorus (inorg.) | 2.5-4.5 mg./100 ml. |
| Potassium | 4.1-5.6 mEq./L. |
| Sodium (serum) | 136-145 mEq./L. |
| Sugar (fasting) | 70-110 mg./100 ml. (p. 316) |
| Sugar (2-hr. postprandial) | Less than 140 mg./100 ml. (p. 319) |
| Thymol turbidity | 0-5.5 SH units |
| Total protein | 6-8 Gm./100 ml. |
| Triglyceride | 190 mg./100 ml. (p. 257) |
| Uric acid | 2.5-8 mg./100 ml. |

2. Thyroid Tests

| | |
|---|---|
| BEI or $T_4$ by column | 3-7 µg./100 ml. |
| PBI | 4-8 µg./100 ml. |
| RAI uptake | 10-40% |
| $T_3$ | Below 0.87, hyper; above 1.13, hypo (Res-O-Mat) |
| | 25-35% (Triosorb) |
| | 39-64% (Trilute) |
| | 90-110% (Thyopac) |
| $T_4$ by isotope | 4-11 µg./100 ml. (Murphy-Pattee) |
| | 5.5-14.5 µg./100 ml. (Tetrasorb) |
| | 5.3-12.2 µg./100 ml. (Tetralute and Res-O-Mat) |

3. Serologies

| | |
|---|---|
| Antistreptolysin-O | 0-200 units |
| Febrile agglutinins (Weil-Felix) | 0-1:40 (p. 195) |

4. Enzymes

| | |
|---|---|
| Amylase | 60-180 units/100 ml. (Somogyi) |
| Acid phosphatase | 0.5-2 units/100 ml. (Bodansky) |
| | 0.1-5 units/100 ml. (King-Armstrong) |
| | 0.1-0.8 units/100 ml. (Bessey-Lowry) |
| | 0.1-2 IU/L. (Babson) |
| | 0.1-2 units/100 ml. (Gutman) |

| | |
|---|---|
| Alkaline phosphatase | 1-4 units/100 ml. (Bodansky) |
| | 4-13 units/100 ml. (King-Armstrong) |
| | 0.8-2.5 units/100 ml. (Bessey-Lowry) |
| | 30-85 mU/ml. (SMA 12/60) |
| CPK: | 1-12 IU/L. (Okinaka-activated) |
| males | 5-50 mU/ml. (Oliver-Rosalki) |
| females | 5-30 mU/ml. (Oliver-Rosalki) |
| | 0-12 units (Sigma) |
| | 0-1.5 IU/L. (Tanzer-Gilvarg - nonactivated) |
| | 1-12 IU/L. (Tanzer-Gilvarg - activated) |
| males | 5-70 IU/L. (Hughes - activated) |
| females | 5-45 IU/L. (Hughes - activated) |
| | 25-145 mU/ml. SMA 12/60 |
| HBD | 150-300 units/100 ml. (Rosalki-Wilkerson) |
| | 95-210 mU/ml. (Rosalki-Wilderson) |
| | 55-125 units (Sigma) |
| LAP: males | 75-230 units (Goldberg-Rutenberg) |
| females | 80-210 units (Goldberg-Rutenberg) |
| | 70-200 units (Sigma) |
| LDH, total | 200-500 units/ml. (Wroblew-sky-LaDue) |
| | 200-600 O.D. units (Teller) |
| | 25-80 IU/L. (Babson) |
| | 5-50 IU/L. (Wacker U.V.) |
| | 30-110 mU/ml. (Wacker U.V.) |
| | 100-225 mU/ml. (SMA 12/60) |
| LDH, heat stable | 20-40% of total |
| Lipase | 0-1.0 Sigma units |
| SGOT | 8-40 units/100 ml. (Reitman-Frankel) |
| | 1-12 IU/L. (Reitman-Frankel) |
| | 15-36 units/ml. (Henry) |
| | 9-36 IU/L. (Babson) |
| | 5-40 units/100 ml. (Karmen U.V.) |
| | 5-20 mU/ml. (Karmen U.V.) |
| | 10-40 mU/ml. (SMA 12/60) |

SGPT                                  5-35 units/ml. (Reitman-
                                           Frankel)
                                        1-12 IU/L. (Reitman-Frankel)
                                        12-55 units/ml. (Henry)
                                        5-25 mU/ml. (Wroblewski)

5. Blood gases (arterial)
   pH                                   7.38-7.42
   $pCO_2$                              35-45 mm. Hg.
   $pO_2$                               80-90 mm. Hg. (under age 65)
                                        75-85 mm. Hg. (over age 65)
   $O_2$ sat.                           96-97% (room air)
   B. E.                                $0 \pm 2$
6. Clearances
   Urea: standard                       40-65 ml./min.
         maximal                        60-100 ml./min.
   Creatinine                           90-120 ml./min.
   Phosphate reabsorption               Over 80%
      (TRP, PRI)
7. Hematology and coagulation
   Hgb: males                           12-17 Gm./100 ml.
        females                         11-15 Gm./100 ml.
   Hematocrit: males                    40-54%
               females                  37-47%
   RBC: males                           4.5-6.0 million
        females                         4.0-5.5 million
   MCH                                  26-34 (p. 13)
   MCHC                                 31-37% (p. 13)
   MCV                                  80-100 cu. $\mu$ (p. 12)
   Platelets                            150-300 thousand
   WBC                                  4500-11,000/cu. mm.
   Dif.: lymphs                         20-40%
         seg.                           50-70%
         bands                          0-7
         eos.                           0-5%
         monos.                         0-7%
   Sed. rate: male                      0-15 mm. /hr.
              female                    0-20 mm. /hr.
   Fibrinogen (quant.)                  200-400 mg./100 ml.
   Coagulation time (Lee-               5-15 min.
      White)
   PT control                           $\pm$ 2 sec. (p. 440)
   PT                                   40-100 sec.(nonactivated)
   PRT                                  90-130 sec.
8. Protein electrophoresis (cellulose acetate)
   Albumin                              3.5-5.0 Gm. (50-65%)
   Alpha-1                              0.2-0.4 Gm. (2.5-5.5%)
   Alpha-2                              0.6-1.0 Gm. (7-12%)
   Beta                                 0.6-1.0 Gm. (7-15%)
   Gamma                                0.7-1.3 Gm. (11-21%)

B.    Spinal Fluid (CSF)

      Sugar                       40-70 mg./100 ml.

      Protein                     20-40 mg./100 ml.

      WBC                       0-5 mononuclears

      RBC                       Zero

      Colloidal gold          No number more than 1

      Chloride                  20 mEq./L. higher than
                                  serum

C.    Urine

   1.  Adrenal chemistry

       Aldosterone         2-26 μg./24 hr. (Kliman and
                                 Peterson)

       Catecholamines     5-150 μg./24 hr.
                                   5-100 μg./25 hr. (Lund)

       Metanephrines      0.3-0.9 mg./24 hr. (Pisano)

       VMA                     0.5-12 mg./24 hr.
                                   0.5-7 mg./24 hr. (Pisano)

       17-KS:  male         10-25 mg./24 hr.

             female under 50    5-15 mg./24 hr.

             female over 50     4-8 mg./24 hr.

       17-OH-CS:  male    3-12 mg./24 hr.

                female        3-10 mg./24 hr.

       17-KG:  male        8-25 mg./24 hr.

                female        5-18 mg./24 hr.

   2.  Miscellaneous chemistry

       Amylase             Up to 300 units/hr. (p. 310)

       Calcium             Less than 250 mg./24 hr.
                                   (reg. diet)

       Creatinine          1.0-1.8 Gm./24 hr.

       Glucose             0-0.3 Gm./24 hr.

       Potassium          26-123 mEq./24 hr.

       Protein             0-0.1 Gm./24 hr.

       Sodium             40-100 mEq./L./24 hr. (p. 153)

       Uric acid           250-750 mg./24 hr.

       5-HIAA            1-7 mg./24 hr. (Goldenberg)

   3.  Urinalysis

       Protein             0-30 mg./100 (random)
                                   0-0.1 Gm./24 hr.

       WBC                   0-5/HPF

       RBC                   0-1/HPF

       Urobilinogen        0-1 Ehrlich unit
                                   0-1:20

       Sugar                 Neg.

       Acetone             Neg.

# Index